Property of

Winifred N. Iglsic M.D

1374 S. Pleasant Valley

Westminster Md. 21157

816-1651

ADVANCES IN SURGERY

VOLUME 12

ADVANCES IN SURGERY

ADVANCES *in* SURGERY

EDITOR

CHARLES ROB
Greenville, North Carolina

ASSOCIATE EDITORS

JAMES D. HARDY
Jackson, Mississippi

GEORGE L. JORDAN, JR.
Houston, Texas

WILLIAM P. LONGMIRE, JR.
Los Angeles, California

LLOYD D. MACLEAN
Montreal, Canada

G. THOMAS SHIRES
New York, New York

CLAUDE E. WELCH
Boston, Massachusetts

VOLUME 12 • 1978

YEAR BOOK MEDICAL PUBLISHERS • INC.
CHICAGO • LONDON

Library of Congress Catalog Card Number: 65-29931

International Standard Serial Number: 0065-3411

International Standard Book Number 0-8151-7366-0

Editor's Preface

An international panel of authors has contributed to this volume of ADVANCES IN SURGERY, which has been designed for both the practicing and academic surgeon. Chapters range in content from the practical aspects of common problems to new research material.

Doctor Boijsen and his colleagues from Sweden have written an interesting and provocative chapter on the relatively new field of therapeutic techniques in diagnostic radiology. The final value and place of these techniques in the clinical management of patients awaits a longer follow-up period, but in many instances early results have been encouraging. Frank Cockett of London, a well-known expert in his field, describes clearly the current management of ulcers of the lower limb. And from Canada, Dr. Hinchey and his associates have contributed an authoritative chapter on the current status of the treatment of perforated diverticular disease of the colon.

Eight chapters covering a wide field of surgery come from the United States. The group headed by Frank Spencer at New York University gives us its views on the present status of the coronary bypass operation. The controversy surrounding this procedure appears to be resolving to a position that most patients should have the operation. However, there is still a need for clarification of some of the indications for it. In my opinion this operation has proved itself and is here to stay.

From Denver comes a much needed chapter on the current status of the vascular laboratory. Although the literature contains many papers on the functions of such a laboratory, many of the authors are individuals who have helped in the development of laboratory equipment. The advantage of the chapter in this volume is that the authors have not developed any special piece of equipment. Doctors Kempczinski and Rutherford have considerable experience in the field and present an expert but unbiased assessment of the place of the vascular laboratory in clinical medicine today.

Two chapters cover surgery of the alimentary tract. Dr. Thompson of Galveston discusses the important subject of hormonal influences on gastric secretion. And Dr. Ferguson and his colleagues describe in a clear and practical way the hospital and office management of patients with hemorrhoids, fistulae and fissures.

Dr. Beahrs and associates from the Mayo Clinic have written a fine chapter based on their vast experience with the management of parotid gland tumors. Dr. Wylie's group from San Francisco discuss the problem of renovascular hypertension, also based on considerable personal experience. An outstanding chapter on metabolism during the hypermetabolic phase of thermal injury has been contributed by Douglas Wilmore, Howard Aulick and Basil Pruitt. Dr. Penn from the University of Colorado, a pioneer in his field, discusses the problem of the development of cancer in transplantation patients.

We thank our contributors and believe that the 12th volume of ADVANCES IN SURGERY is a fine book that will be useful to all surgeons, from those in training to those long established in practice.

CHARLES ROB
EDITOR

Table of Contents

Current Status of the Vascular Diagnostic Laboratory

RICHARD F. KEMPCZINSKI, M.D. AND ROBERT B. RUTHERFORD, M.D.

University of Colorado School of Medicine; Denver Veterans Administration Hospital; and Colorado General Hospital, Denver, Colorado

During the past 10–15 years, rapid developments in medical instrumentation have made it possible to accurately and noninvasively measure the physiologic alterations produced by peripheral vascular disease. Although much of the developmental work and initial clinical experience was accumulated in a few large centers, this technology has now become available in most hospitals and even in some physicians' offices.

Patients with symptoms suggestive of peripheral vascular disease often pose challenging questions for the physician:

1. Is there objective evidence of arterial occlusion?
2. Is it responsible for the patient's symptoms?
3. In patients with combined arterial occlusive disease and neuropathy, which condition is more likely responsible for the pain or ulceration?
4. Will an ulcer or amputation heal at a specific level?
5. Is a patient's impotence hormonal, psychogenic, neurogenic or arterial?
6. Which of multiple in-series arterial occlusions is hemodynamically most significant?
7. Is an asymptomatic patient with a carotid bruit at high risk to suffer a stroke?

8. Is leg swelling due to deep venous thrombosis or some other cause?

Since the traditional diagnostic tools of clinical history and physical examination often are inadequate in answering such questions, and since angiography is painful and provides no physiologic information, increasing attention has been focused on the vascular diagnostic laboratory. Planning a vascular reconstruction without obtaining hemodynamic data seems as unreasonable as contemplating cardiac valve replacement without preoperative catheterization. To quote Lord Kelvin: "When you can measure what you are speaking about and express it in numbers, you know something about it, but when you cannot measure it, when you cannot express it in numbers, your knowledge is of a meager kind."

This chapter will review the instrumentation that currently is of proven value in the evaluation of patients with peripheral vascular disease. Emphasis will be on those instruments and studies with which the authors have personal experience; and the application of these procedures to commonly encountered clinical situations will be discussed. Those techniques that presently are research tools or that more appropriately belong in nuclear medicine or radiology, such as isotope clearance studies and computerized tomographic scanning, will not be discussed.

Instrumentation

The Subcommittee of Peripheral Vascular Disease of the American Heart Association[1] has suggested that instruments for the clinical vascular laboratory be: (1) simple, reliable and reproducible; (2) capable of intrinsic standardization; (3) easily used by paramedical personnel; (4) suitable for measurements during and/or after exercise; and (5) adaptable to current recording devices.

ULTRASOUND

The use of low intensity ultrasound in the range of 1 – 10 mHz for medical diagnosis has become widespread since its introduction 17 years ago.[2] Current instruments either use the Doppler effect to detect flow velocity or rely on tissue reflectance of transmitted sound waves (B-mode scans) to produce acoustic images of internal organs and vessels.

The Doppler effect can be stated

$$\overline{V} = \frac{C \, \Delta f}{2 \, fo \, \cos\theta}$$

where $\overline{V}$ = average flow velocity; C = velocity of sound in tissue; Δf = Doppler frequency shift; fo = transmitting frequency of ultrasound beam; and θ = angle of incident sound beam to blood vessel being examined. Since transmitting frequency, angle of incidence and sound velocity in tissue can be kept constant, frequency shift (Δf) becomes proportional to the velocity of blood flow.

In practice, a hand-held Doppler probe is coupled with the skin with an acoustic gel. When the transmitted sound waves strike moving erythrocytes, they are shifted in frequency in direct proportion to the velocity of the blood flow. This back-scattered sound is detected by a receiving crystal mounted in the probe adjacent to the transmitting crystal and is passed through a differential amplifier which, in effect, "filters" out sound not shifted in frequency by more than 50 – 60 cycles/second. The filtered sound can be then amplified to provide an audible signal, which is perfectly adequate for most clinical purposes. The same Doppler-shift flow signal may also be processed by two additional methods to provide a visible display for graphic analysis of velocity waveforms: (1) the zero-crossing, frequency-to-voltage converter,[3] and (2) audio-frequency analysis or sonography.[4] Two types of Doppler instruments are produced: continuous-wave and pulsed.

CONTINUOUS-WAVE DOPPLER INSTRUMENTS. — Only continuous-wave Dopplers currently are available for clinical use. The ultrasound beam is generated by electrically exciting a ceramic piezoelectric crystal. Depending on the probe selected, the transmitting frequency will be 2, 5, 8 or 10 megacycles/second. The 2 – 5 mHz instruments provide better penetration of tissue and are more suitable for examination of intra-abdominal structures such as the iliac veins or inferior vena cava. The 8 – 10 mHz instruments, on the other hand, give shallower penetration but can be focused sharply, thus making them more useful for precise examination of extremity vessels. Although most continuous-wave Dopplers are nondirectional, they are portable, simple, inexpensive and perfectly adequate for survey of extremity vessels or measurement of segmental limb systolic pressures.

By introducing a phase-shift network prior to flow detection, positive and negative Doppler shifts can be identified and separated, thus permitting the direction as well as the velocity of blood flow to be determined.[5] Although directional Dopplers are more expensive, the added versatility is especially useful in studying patients with extracranial arterial disease[6] and venous valvular insufficiency of the lower extremity.[7]

By coupling the directional Doppler with a position-sensing arm and a storage oscilloscope, luminal imaging of superficially placed vessels or "ultrasonic angiography"[8] is possible. This application of ultrasound, which has been explored more thoroughly using the pulsed Doppler, holds great promise, especially in the study of extracranial carotid disease.

PULSED DOPPLER INSTRUMENTS. — Pulsed Dopplers, unlike continuous-wave instruments, use the same piezoelectric crystal to alternately transmit and receive the back-scattered signal. By sampling the reflected signals at discrete time intervals after transmission, they are capable of analyzing individual points along the course of the sound beam with a resolution of 1.0 – 1.5 mm. As the probe is moved across the vessel, two-dimensional velocity data can be collected for small intraluminal volumes rather than mean cross-sectional areas as with continuous-wave instruments.

When such an instrument is coupled with a position sensing arm and a storage oscilloscope, a precise "velocity image" of the moving blood can be obtained in either the vertical or horizontal plane.[9] This technique has been applied extensively to the carotid bifurcation,[10, 11] but its widespread clinical application is limited by calcification within the arterial wall, which inhibits the transmission of ultrasound and produces acoustic shadows, by a lack of resolution adequate to demonstrate nonstenosing, ulcerated plaques which may be the source of cerebral emboli, and by artifacts as a result of patient motion.

The pulsed ultrasound Doppler velocity meter (PUDVM) can also be adapted for the transcutaneous measurement of velocity profiles and blood flow.[12]

ULTRASONIC SCANNING. — Ultrasonic scanning, a second common application of diagnostic ultrasound, also uses a pulsed beam. Unlike the PUDVM, however, its application is not based on Doppler effect. Rather, the image it produces represents spatial differences in ultrasound reflectance from tissue interfaces of differing acoustic impedance. Combining such a device with a position-sensing arm and a storage oscilloscope permits acoustic imaging of organs and blood vessels within many parts of the body. Modern B-mode scanners utilize brightness modulation and scan converter memory systems to permit display of a wide range of tissue densities in grey scale images. This refinement allows accurate definition of the luminal thrombus contained within aortic or peripheral aneurysms, thus permitting measurement of their diameter with a resolution of 2–5 mm.

The B-mode scanner has been further modified by using multiple rotating transducers to produce real time vessel images.[13] When combined with a PUDVM, the resulting "duplex scanner" is capable of not only imaging the vessel under study, but also exploring the velocity of blood flow at multiple points within its lumen. Although such sophisticated and expensive instruments are beyond the resources of most vascular diagnostic laboratories, their further development and clinical application should be observed with interest.

PLETHYSMOGRAPHY

Plethysmography, the measurement of the volume change of an organ or region of tissue, was one of the earliest methods used for the measurement of extremity blood flow. Various applications of this principle are available for use in the vascular laboratory. They include volume displacement (air or water), strain gauge (mercury-in-Silastic), impedance, mechanical, photoelectric and ocular plethysmographs.

Only the volume (air or water) plethysmographs, which enclose completely the part being studied, measure volume change directly. However, they are too cumbersome for routine clinical use. A more practical form of volume (air) plethysmography[14] utilizes pneumatic cuffs placed at multiple levels around the extremity. By standardizing the injected volume of air and the pressure within the cuff, momentary volume changes of the limb result in pulsatile pressure changes within the air-filled bladder.

These changes can be displayed as segmental pressure pulse contours which correspond closely to a direct intra-arterial recording at that level.

By adding venous occlusion to plethysmography, indirect measurements of arterial flow are possible. A pneumatic cuff placed on the proximal extremity is inflated to a pressure that temporarily arrests venous outflow without impeding arterial inflow. Under these circumstances, the initial rate of volume change in the distal extremity, as measured by any of the plethysmographic techniques, is equal to the rate of arterial inflow. It usually is expressed as cc flow/100 ml tissue/minute. Since resting arterial flow is not reduced until an advanced degree of ischemia is present,[14] this technique has not found wide clinical application.

Strain-gauge plethysmographs encircle the part being studied with a thin Silastic tube filled with mercury. Volume change is then measured indirectly by the changing electric resistance of the mercury loop as a function of its changing length. This technique is less cumbersome than standard volume plethysmography and has become the accepted method for measuring limb blood flow.[15] It also can be used to obtain pulse volume waveforms, which are of proven value in the diagnosis of arterial occlusive disease (see below).

Impedance plethysmography is based on the principle that blood is an excellent conductor of electricity and therefore changes in limb blood volume should result in measureable alterations in electric resistance (impedance) of the extremity. In theory, the more blood present, the less the resistance to the passage of a current. Unfortunately, the change in impedance produced by volume changes of the limb is such a small proportion of its total resistance that calibration becomes difficult. In addition, movement of the electrodes or loss of skin contact result in frequent artifacts. As a result, the technique has not been adopted widely for arterial disease but is still useful in the detection of deep venous thrombosis.[16]

The term mechanical plethysmography or phleborheography has been applied to a device* developed by Cranley et al.[17] for the detection of deep venous thrombosis of the lower extremities. It is, in fact, a modified form of segmental air plethys-

---

*Grass Instrument Co.; Quincy, Mass.

mography. It relies on the detection of transmitted, spontaneous respiratory waves from above and those generated by intermittent mechanical compression of the distal extremity to diagnose and localize venous occlusions.

Photoplethysmography (PPG) uses an infrared light-emitting diode and a phototransistor to detect the back-scattered light. In much the same indirect manner that impedance plethysmography records volume change through its effect on electric resistance, so PPG measures pulsatile flow through the ability of the cutaneous microcirculation to alter the back-scattering of an infrared light beam transmitted through the skin. When such a device is applied to the periorbital region, it has been found useful in the diagnosis of hemodynamically significant carotid occlusive disease.[18] It has also been used to monitor the pulse rate of patients in intensive care units or to obtain an end point when measuring segmental limb pressures.

Ocular plethysmography (OPG) detects phasic changes in eye volume caused by pulsatile flow in the ophthalmic artery. Since this vessel is a branch of the internal carotid artery, alterations in ocular pulse volume can result from hemodynamically significant corotid arterial occlusive disease. Two general types of OPG currently are available.

The first type,* developed by Kartchner, McRae and Morrison[19] utilizes saline-filled plastic cups placed on the anesthetized cornea of both eyes and held in place by a negative pressure of 40 – 45 mmHg. Pulse waveforms are simultaneously recorded from both eyes while light opacity ear lobe sensors (PPG) provide concomitant timing of external carotid pulses. Pulse volume contour and arrival time (pulse wave velocity) in the two eyes are then compared relative to each other and to the ear. To facilitate detection of minor differences, an electronically generated differential tracing is also displayed. Under normal circumstances, there is no delay between the two eyes and the differential tracing appears as a relatively straight line.

Recently a second instrument† based on this approach has been introduced. It differs inasmuch as it uses air-filled corneal cups which allow the patient to lie comfortably supine during the study. Furthermore, it has been automated so that delays in

*Medical Electronic Devices, Inc.; Tucson, Ariz.
†Zira International; Tucson, Ariz.

pulse arrival time between the two eyes, between both ears and between the "earliest" eye and ear are digitally displayed for each cardiac cycle and automatically are averaged every eight cycles. These refinements reduce the time required for technician training and analysis of the results. Although comparative studies with this instrument are not yet available, preliminary experience in one of our laboratories (R.B.R.) indicates that it has an accuracy comparable to that of the Kartchner/McCrae OPG.

The second type, ocular pneumoplethysmograph,[*20] uses air-filled cups applied to the anesthetized sclera of both eyes, lateral to the cornea. A vacuum (>300 mmHg) is then applied to both cups. As the sclera is drawn into the cup by the suction, the globe is distorted and intraocular pressure (IOP) rises. A reproducible relationship exists between the vacuum applied and the corresponding increase in IOP, with a vacuum of 300 mmHg equivalent to an IOP of 110 mmHg. If this induced IOP exceeds systolic pressure, the in-line transducer displays an absence of eye pulsation. As the vacuum is reduced, pulsations return when IOP falls below systolic pressure. Thus, the systolic pressure for each eye and, by implication, each internal carotid artery, can be determined. An ocular pneumoplethysmograph attachment is also available for the pulse volume recorder.† It differs primarily in that each eye must be studied separately. In our laboratory (R.F.K.), accuracy with this instrument has been comparable to that reported by Gee, Smith and Hinson.[20]

PHONOANGIOGRAPHY

Diagnostically useful information regarding the presence or absence of extracranial carotid arterial occlusive disease is contained in the precise localization and characterization of cervical bruits.[21] The phonoangiograph‡ was developed to facilitate the collection of this information. A sensitive, high-fidelity microphone is used to detect bruits along the course of the carotid artery. The hand-held microphone is placed over the carotid artery at three different levels: (1) immediately above the clavicle; (2) in the mid-carotid, near its bifurcation; and (3) high in the

---

*Electro-diagnostic Instruments; Burbank, Calif.
†Life Sciences, Inc.; Greenwich, Conn.
‡Medical Electronic Devices, Inc.; Tucson, Ariz.

neck, behind the angle of the mandible. The audio signals are displayed simultaneously on paired oscilloscopes, permitting a Polaroid photograph to be made from one screen while the examiner continues to monitor the signal on the second screen. By making three separate exposures and by shifting the camera angle slightly between them, the tracing from all three levels of each carotid can be recorded on a single photograph.

MISCELLANEOUS

Oscillometry, ophthalmodynamometry and thermography have, at one time, all enjoyed some popularity in the noninvasive evaluation of vascular disease. However, because of a lack of specificity and sensitivity, they largely have been abandoned. Electromagnetic flowmeters require surgical exposure of the vessel to be studied and therefore are not applicable to the vascular diagnostic laboratory.

Clinical Applications

The application of the aforementioned instruments to clinical situations will be discussed under three separate headings: (1) peripheral arterial disease; (2) extracranial cerebrovascular insufficiency; and (3) extremity venous disease. In each of these areas, experience has shown that no single test or instrument is sufficiently accurate to be recommended to the exclusion of the others. Invariably, greater diagnostic accuracy has been achieved by a combination of tests with each, in effect, serving as a check or balance on the other. Several instruments capable of providing similar information often are available. Selection of a particular one usually is based on such factors as cost, ease of operation, compatability with available equipment or, simply, individual preference.

PERIPHERAL ARTERIAL DISEASE

Doppler Arterial Survey

The Doppler can be used to study all major peripheral arteries. A normal arterial velocity signal (Fig 1) contains two, often three, component sounds. The first sound, corresponding to rap-

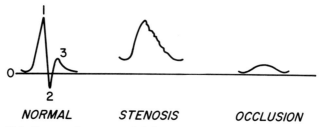

Fig 1.—Velocity waveforms recorded from normal, stenotic and occluded arteries. The three major deflections that correspond to audible sounds are indicated for the normal artery.

id inflow of blood during systole, is high pitched. It is followed by a brief second sound which probably represents flow reversal in early diastole. Finally, there is a low-pitched third sound as forward flow returns. If peripheral resistance is markedly reduced, e. g., in reactive hyperemia, flow reversal may be abolished and velocity signals will be higher pitched but monophonic. When a high-pitched multiphasic signal is audible over a peripheral vessel, significant proximal stenosis is unlikely.

Immediately distal to a stenosis, the peak frequency of the first sound is increased, reflecting the increased velocity of blood flow; and the second sound is muffled by turbulence. In the presence of a complete proximal arterial occlusion, the Doppler can assess patency of distal vessels, despite the absence of palpable pulses. The flow signal in such vessels is low-pitched and monophonic with absence of the second sound. However, such information is qualitative and of limited practical value.

Segmental Limb Pressures

Winsor[22] introduced the concept of measuring segmental limb systolic pressures (SLP) to assess the level and significance of arterial occlusions. The test requires: (1) appropriately sized pneumatic cuffs; (2) a manometer to measure cuff pressure; and (3) a means of detecting distal arterial flow.

The pneumatic cuff must be of a size appropriate to the limb segment under study. The American Heart Association[23] has recommended that the inflatable bladder should be 20% wider than the segmental limb diameter. Standard adult-sized cuffs, as used in most hospitals to record brachial blood pressures, have a pneumatic bladder 12 cm wide and are suitable for measuring SLP at the calf and ankle in average-sized adults. The measurement of thigh pressure, however, requires a larger cuff with a bladder 18–20 cm in width. In small adults or children, or for transmetatarsal measurements in normal adults, a "child-size" cuff with a 9-cm bladder is recommended.

When an appropriate thigh cuff is used, it is impractical to place a second cuff lower on the thigh. Accordingly, we place a single, large cuff (18×36 cm) as high as possible on the thigh, a calf cuff (12×23 cm) immediately below the knee and an ankle cuff (12×23 cm) just above the malleolus. A standard mercury-gravity or aneroid manometer is used to measure cuff inflation pressure.

The return of flow distal to the deflating cuff can be determined using a stethoscope (which is difficult in the lower extremity), one of the plethysmographic devices or the Doppler

Fig 2.—Placement of the pneumatic cuffs for measurement of segmental limb pressures and pulse volume recordings in the lower extremity.

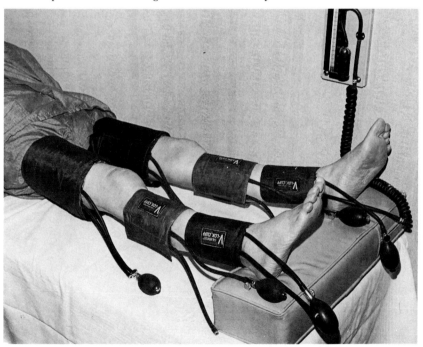

velocity detector, which is, by far, the simplest and most sensitive method.

After cuff placement, the heel is elevated slightly on a cushion (Fig 2). Using the Doppler, the posterior tibial and dorsalis pedis arteries are both surveyed and the one giving the loudest signal is chosen. The thigh cuff is then inflated until detectable blood flow ceases. Cuff pressure is gradually reduced until flow is detected again. The pressure in the cuff at that point is recorded as the thigh systolic pressure. The thigh cuff is then completely deflated and the procedure is repeated for the remaining cuffs on both lower extremities. If a baseline Doppler flow signal cannot be detected, a mercury strain gauge or segmental air plethysmograph on the foot may be used as an alternative means of detecting the return of blood flow.

Although resting diastolic pressure in a limb segment does not fall until a severe degree of proximal arterial stenosis is present, peak or systolic pressure decreases with lesser degrees of narrowing. It has been found to be reduced, even at rest, in all limbs with complete arterial occlusion and in the majority with symptomatic proximal stenosis.[24] For this reason, only systolic pressures need be determined.

Subtracting the SLP at any given level from the one immediately proximal to it will determine the "vertical gradient" or pressure differential between the two. If SLP is instead compared to one measured at the same level in the opposite extremity, a "horizontal gradient" can be determined.

Since many laboratories still prefer to use four cuffs in measuring SLP in the lower extremities, we have listed our normal standards for both methods (Table 1). Gradients >20 mmHg are strongly suggestive of a hemodynamically significant lesion in the intervening artery. Results will vary significantly, depending on the size of the pneumatic cuffs used; and each laboratory should develop its own standards.

Since SLP varies with systemic systolic pressure, it is common

TABLE 1.—SEGMENTAL PRESSURE GRADIENTS (mmHg) IN NORMAL
SUBJECTS (MEAN ± SD)

	ARM-UPPER THIGH	UPPER THIGH-LOWER THIGH	THIGH-CALF	CALF-ANKLE
4-cuff technique	25 ± 11	−4 ± 10	−7 ± 8	−7
3-cuff technique	7 ± 11		4 ± 13	−8 ± 6

practice to divide each SLP by the higher brachial systolic pressure and obtain a segmental pressure index. The ankle pressure index has been especially valuable in the diagnosis of lower extremity arterial insufficiency. In the absence of occlusive disease, it should be 1.0 or greater. It correlates more closely with patients' symptoms and provides a better index of the severity and extent of arterial occlusive disease than resting calf muscle blood flow, as measured by venous occlusion plethysmography.[15] In a large series of patients,[24] it was always below normal in limbs with complete arterial occlusion. With unisegmental occlusions, it was 0.5–0.8 but was invariably lower (<0.5) in limbs with multiple, in-series occlusions.

However, the ankle pressure index does not localize proximal occlusions nor can it determine the relative significance of multiple, in-series stenoses. To obtain such information, we measure SLP at multiple levels and look for gradients between them. Typical SLPs, as seen with representative unisegmental occlusions, are depicted in Figure 3. Significant (>20 mmHg) gradients clearly localize the isolated iliac artery occlusion, the distal superficial femoral artery (SFA) occlusion and distal tibial artery disease. Unfortunately, SLPs alone may be misleading

Fig 3. – **A,** typical segmental limb pressures (SLP) in a normal right extremity and one with isolated iliac artery occlusion *(left).* **B,** SLPs seen in distal, segmental occlusion of the right superficial femoral artery (SFA) compared to proximal occlusion of the left SFA. **C,** SLPs in distal *(right)* tibial artery occlusions and tibial disease extending into the proximal left popliteal artery.

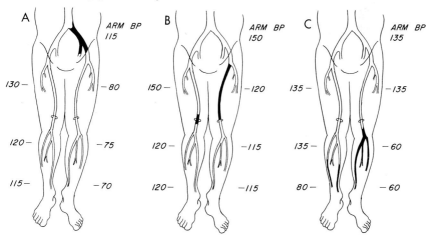

TABLE 2.–ACCURACY OF SLP
USING 3-CUFF TECHNIQUE AT
VARIOUS ΔPs

	ΔP mmHg	>25	>20	>15
AI	false +	33%	39%	41%
	false –	14%	11%	8%
SFA	false +	3%	9.7%	23%
	false –	47%	28%	23%

under the following circumstances: (1) clinically significant
stenoses may be so well collateralized that resting pressures are
normal[25]; (2) occlusion of the entire SFA may result in an arm-
thigh gradient indistinguishable from that seen with iliac artery occlusion; similarly, tibial artery occlusive disease that
extends into the proximal popliteal artery can mimic SFA occlusion; and (3) the arteries of patients with calcific medial sclerosis
can be so rigid that pneumatic compression is difficult or impossible, resulting in falsely elevated SLPs. For these reasons, we
have found that reliance on SLP alone is associated with significant inaccuracy in distinguishing aortoiliac (AI) and SFA occlusion, especially when they are present in combination (Table 2).
Therefore, we have incorporated two additional techniques into
our evaluation of patients with extremity arterial insufficiency:
the response of SLPs to reactive hyperemia (exercise testing)
and waveform analysis.

Exercise Testing

After exercise, there is a significant increase in total limb
blood flow in the normal lower extremity, with little or no decrease in ankle systolic pressure. However, when there is a major arterial occlusion or stenosis, blood flow is diverted around it
into high-resistance collateral vessels. Although flow through
such collaterals may be adequate in the resting extremity, during and immediately after exercise, the increased pressure drop
across the high-resistance, collateral bed in response to the increased blood flow and the redistribution of limb blood flow into
vasodilated proximal muscles, both combine to result in a pronounced and prolonged decrease in ankle pressure.

Although a similar degree of reactive hyperemia can be induced by occluding arterial flow into the extremity with a pneumatic cuff placed around the upper thigh and inflated to 50 mmHg above brachial systolic pressure for 5 minutes,[26] we prefer treadmill exercise for the following reasons: (1) it duplicates the clinical setting in which the patient normally becomes symptomatic and allows measurement of his impairment under standardized conditions; and (2) it permits assessment of the individual's total response to exercise in addition to his extremity circulation, thus facilitating identification of patients more limited by musculoskeletal or cardiopulmonary disease than by claudication.

After SLPs have been determined for both resting extremities with the patient supine on the examining table, the thigh and the calf cuffs are removed and the patient is exercised on the treadmill at a rate of 2 mph with a 10% incline. Five minutes, under these conditions, is considered standard walking time (SWT). However, if symptoms force the patient to stop sooner, that time is recorded as the maximum walking time (MWT). Following completion of exercise, the patient immediately resumes the supine position and a single postexercise determination of brachial and ankle SLP is made. In those persons who cannot use the treadmill because of foot lesions, amputations or recent extremity surgery, we induce reactive hyperemia with a pneumatic cuff on the thigh as previously described and then follow the above procedure.

Sumner and Strandness[27] have demonstrated that, after exercise, the increase in calf blood flow, the fall in ankle SLP and the rate of return of these parameters to baseline levels permitted patients with lower extremity arterial occlusive disease to be divided into three groups: (1) those with unisegmental occlusions; (2) patients with multisegmental occlusions; and (3) those with severe rest pain and claudication. However, since ankle systolic pressures must often be followed for 20–30 minutes after exercise before returning to baseline levels, it is impractical, in a busy vascular laboratory, to make such determination routinely. We have found that the combination of SLPs and segmental pulse volume waveforms, before and after exercise, can localize and grade occlusive lesions with greater speed and accuracy.

Exercise testing, therefore, is used preoperatively to reveal those arterial stenoses that may be fully compensated at rest and to quantitate the extent of a patient's disability under standardized conditions. It is unnecessary in patients with rest pain or gangrene.

Waveform Analysis

Two types of waveform analysis are presently in use: velocity and pulse volume. Velocity waveforms (VWFs) are commonly obtained with a directional Doppler which utilizes a zero-crossing, frequency-to-voltage convertor to produce an electric signal which is then transcribed on a standard strip chart recorder.[3] By adjusting the angle of the probe to the vessel until a "maximized" tracing is obtained, reproducible waveforms can be recorded from any peripheral artery. The dimensions of these waveforms are then analyzed in a quantitative manner. Johnston[28] has criticized the use of instruments featuring the zero-crossing device on the grounds that it introduces artifacts in the velocity profile, may be distorted by movement and radiofrequency interference, and can reflect velocity information emanating from adjacent veins. Although it is true that data obtained with such instruments do not permit precise, quantitative analysis of the entire spectrum of blood flow velocities in a vessel or the accurate conversion of this data to flow using the Doppler equation, it does not preclude the dimensional analysis of the VWF from having empiric diagnostic value. Indeed , Fronek et al.[29] and others[3, 30] have shown that analysis of the VWFs of extremity arteries can accurately diagnose the presence of occlusive lesions. However, for more precise quantitation, the velocity signal should be processed through a frequency analyzer. By this approach, Johnson and Taraschuk[31] have produced a "pulsatility index" which is a sensitive measure of arterial occlusive disease. However, this technique is too complicated, expensive and time-consuming for routine clinical application.

Regardless of the method used to process the velocity signal, VWF analysis has several other drawbacks that limit its clinical application in the diagnosis of arterial occlusion: (1) obtaining reproducible VWFs demands considerable technical skill; (2) dimensional analysis often requires a computer program; (3) excess fat, hematoma, scar and calcification all interfere with ultrasound transmission; (4) VWFs analyze single vessel flow rather than total segmental flow; and (5) VWFs may not be obtainable distal to multiple, in-series occlusions.

Despite these serious limitations in the diagnosis of extremity arterial occlusive disease, carotid VWFs significantly complement the other noninvasive techniques in the diagnosis of extracranial carotid artery occlusive disease (see below).

For these reasons, we rely on pulse volume waveforms to sup-

Fig 4.—Normal arterial supply to the right lower extremity (*CIA* = common iliac artery; *CFA* = common femoral artery; *PFA* = profunda femoris artery; and *SFA* = superficial femoral artery). The segmental limb pressures and the pulse volume recordings (PVRs) from the thigh and calf levels are displayed opposite the appropriate limb segment. The contour for each segment is normal and the characteristic augmentation in the amplitude of the calf PVR is evident.

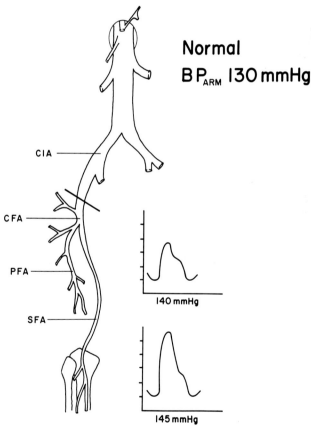

Normal
BP$_{ARM}$ 130 mmHg

CIA

CFA

PFA

140 mmHg

SFA

145 mmHg

plement SLP in the diagnosis of extremity arterial occlusive disease. Using the same cuff placement as previously described and a segmental air plethysmograph,* pulse volume recordings (PVRs) are obtained at three levels on each resting extremity.

The normal waveform (Fig 4) is characterized by a rapid upstroke (anacrotic limb), a sharp peak, a brisk decline (catacrotic limb) and a clearly visible reflected diastolic wave. These characteristics are generally evident in the tracing at each level.

A second important feature of the normal lower extremity study is a consistent augmentation in the amplitude of the pulse volume waveform from thigh to calf. The thigh cuff contains 400–500 cc of air when inflated to the standard pressure of 65 mmHg, whereas the calf cuff contains only 75 cc. Thus the segmental, limb volume changes with each cardiac cycle result in a smaller pressure increase in the thigh cuff relative to the calf cuff. Although this augmentation is an artifact due to differences in cuff volume, it is a reliable and reproducible finding in the presence of a patent superficial femoral artery (SFA).

With increasing degrees of arterial narrowing, the contour of the PVR distal to the lesion demonstrates characteristic alterations (Fig 5). First, there is loss of the reflected diastolic wave and prolongation of the slope of the catacrotic limb. This is followed by rounding of the peak and decrease in the slope of the anacrotic limb. Lastly, the amplitude of the entire tracing is decreased and flattened.

Comparing these features of the PVR with the findings in 200 femoral arteriograms,[32] we found overall accuracy of 97% in diagnosing SFA occlusion. The 1.5% false positives were associated with such severe inflow disease that the thigh tracing was

Fig 5. – Pulse volume recordings indicating the changes seen in waveform contour with progressive arterial narrowing (see text).

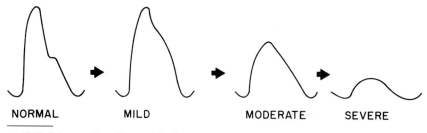

NORMAL   MILD   MODERATE   SEVERE

*Life Sciences, Inc.; Greenwich, Conn.

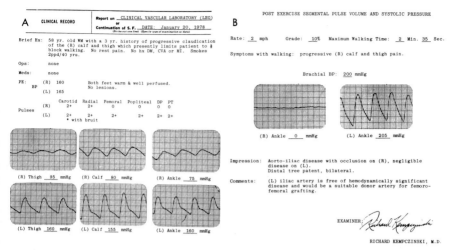

Fig 6. – **A,** typical vascular laboratory study on a patient with claudication of the right leg. **B,** exercise testing in the same patient.

virtually flat making it impossible to assess augmentation. The 1.5% false negatives occurred in patients with large profunda femoris collaterals that had effectively bypassed short segmental occlusions of the SFA.

Thus, our standard evaluation for lower extremity arterial insufficiency presently includes: (1) Doppler survey of all major extremity vessels in which a pulse cannot be palpated; (2) resting SLP and PVRs at thigh, calf and ankle levels in both extremities; (3) standardized, treadmill exercise; and (4) immediate postexercise determination of ankle pressures and PVRs (Fig 6).

Specific Clinical Situations

CLAUDICATION. — Extremity pain following exercise may be due to arterial insufficiency, musculoskeletal disease or neurospinal compression. Occasionally, two or more of these problems may coexist. It can be extremely difficult to distinguish between these conditions by history and physical examination alone. Furthermore, even when true claudication is present, it is important to determine the degree of the patient's objective disability, not only as a baseline against which the results of medical or surgical therapy can be judged, but also to provide objective information upon which to base a decision for arterial reconstruction. A patient whose postexercise ankle pressure is >50 mmHg with a good PVR is unlikely to be having disabling claudication[33] and other explanation for his symptoms should be sought.

REST PAIN. — Extremity pain at rest also may have diverse causes. It is important to differentiate between arterial insufficiency and neuropathy, especially in diabetic patients in whom these two conditions frequently coexist.

Raines et al,[33] studied 71 patients with ischemic rest pain and found ankle pressures <35 mmHg in nondiabetics and <55 mmHg in diabetics with severely attenuated ankle PVRs. Others[34] have not distinguished between diabetics and nondiabetics and have suggested that ischemic rest pain should not occur unless ankle pressures are <50 mmHg.

OCCULT AORTOILIAC STENOSIS. — The inadequacy of aortography, especially in a single plane, to recognize aortoiliac (AI) stenosis has been long known.[35] The diagnosis is even more difficult when concomitant SFA occlusion is present. In our laboratory,[32] one-third of patients with proximal SFA occlusion and no iliac disease had a significant gradient between the SLPs of arm and thigh, thus making it difficult to distinguish them from patients with isolated AI stenosis.

To overcome this problem, others[35, 36] have proposed inserting a needle in the common femoral artery and measuring direct arterial systolic pressure before and after induced reactive hyperemia. Although accurate, this approach is invasive. The value of velocity waveforms in making similar distinctions has already been discussed.[3]

We have found that segmental PVRs have enabled us to accurately distinguish the various combinations of AI and SFA disease (Fig 7). Patients with AI occlusion alone have an abnormal contour in the thigh waveform but the amplitude of the PVR augments from thigh to calf. If isolated SFA occlusion is present, the contour of the thigh tracing shows only minor abnormality limited to the catacrotic or "runoff" portion of the curve, but there is moderate to severe alteration in the calf PVR and the characteristic augmentation in its amplitude is absent. With combined AI and SFA disease, the thigh PVR is moderately to severely abnormal while the calf tracing shows further alteration in contour and lack of augmentation. Comparing these fea-

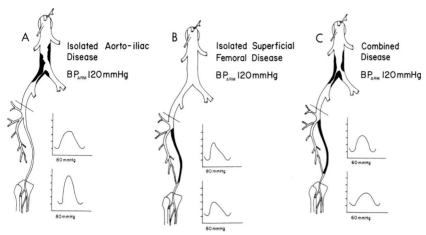

Fig 7.—Segmental limb pressures (SLPs) and pulse volume recordings (PVRs) in limbs with aortoiliac (AI) and superficial femoral artery (SFA) occlusion. **A,** isolated AI stenosis is characterized by a vertical pressure gradient, arm-thigh, on SLPs and a moderately abnormal thigh waveform with normal augmentation in the amplitude of the calf PVR. **B,** isolated SFA occlusion causes only mild abnormality of the thigh waveform, but augmentation in the amplitude of the calf tracing is absent. When SFA occlusion involves the entire artery to its origin from the common femoral artery, SLPs often show a vertical gradient, arm-thigh, indistinguishable for AI stenosis. **C,** Combined AI and SFA occlusion demonstrates a moderately abnormal contour of the thigh waveform with further abnormality and lack of augmentation of the calf PVR.

tures with biplanar arteriography in the lower extremities of more than 200 patients,[32] the overall accuracy of the PVR in diagnosing AI disease was 95%. Five percent false positives were due to high-grade stenosis of the profunda femoris artery (PFA) in the presence of coexisting SFA occlusion. There were no false negative results.

IMPOTENCE.—The etiology of impotence may be hormonal, psychogenic, neurogenic or arterial. In the past, the inability to separate and distinguish between these various causes has made therapy difficult. Measurement of testosterone levels may identify hormonal insufficiency, while the documentation of nocturnal erections points to a psychogenic etiology.

However, the differentiation between neurogenic and vascular impotence remains difficult. This is especially true in the diabetic since both elements may coexist. With the development of epigastricocavernous anastomosis[37] to treat impotence due to arterial insufficiency, the distinction becomes even more important.

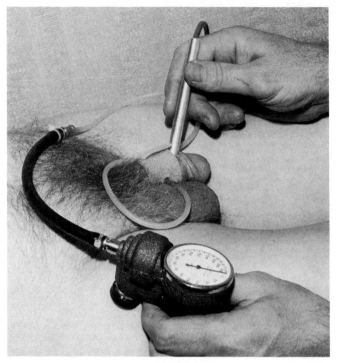

Fig 8.—Position of the pneumatic cuff and Doppler probe for measurement of penile systolic pressure and pulse volume recording.

Impotence may result from arterial occlusion of the penile blood supply even in the absence of demonstrable lower extremity arterial insufficiency. To identify this group of patients, several authors[38, 39] have emphasized the diagnostic value of measuring penile systolic pressure (PSP), as shown in Figure 8.

We have obtained PSPs and penile PVRs in a group of 50 patients.[40] Analysis of these data (Table 3) supports several preliminary conclusions. (1) The difference between PSP and brachial systolic pressure in potent males was small (10 mmHg mean).

TABLE 3.—RELATIONSHIP OF PENILE AND
BRACHIAL SYSTOLIC PRESSURES

	NO. PATIENTS	MEAN AGE (YRS)	MEAN ΔPMMHG (RANGE)
Potent	23	42	-10 ($+5$ to -45)
Impotent	27	53	-45 (-15 to -90)

As also reported by Gaskell,[39] PSP was always greater than mean brachial pressure in potent males. Therefore, if PSP is equal to or greater than brachial pressure in an impotent male, penile arterial insufficiency is extremely unlikely. (2) Although the mean penile-brachial systolic pressure gradient was four times greater in impotent patients, there was enough overlap with the potent males that documentation of a moderate (30–40 mmHg) penile-brachial gradient alone is insufficient evidence for vascular impotence. (3) Although normal penile waveforms (PVRs) were generally seen in young, potent males and appeared to become more abnormal in contour with increasing age, even in the face of continued potency, there were enough exceptions to preclude meaningful conclusions at this time. (4) Sufficient vascular laboratory criteria do not yet exist to select those impotent patients who would clearly benefit from penile revascularization. We are continuing our studies in this area in the hope of developing more discriminate criteria.

ARTERIAL ENTRAPMENT SYNDROMES. — Patients with symptoms of thoracic outlet compression are frequently referred to the vascular laboratory for evaluation. However, since the pain associated with this entity is almost entirely due to compression of the lowest trunk of the brachial plexus rather than to the subclavian artery, and since arterial compression can be documented, in certain positions, in 40–60% of asymptomatic patients, we have not found the laboratory very useful in diagnosing thoracic outlet compression.

In young athletes with symptoms of intermittent claudication despite palpable pulses, SLP and PVR at the ankle should be obtained both at rest and during sustained, active plantar flexion. Decrease in ankle SLP or dimunition of the PVR during this maneuver strongly suggests the diagnosis of popliteal artery entrapment syndrome.[41]

HEALING OF LEG ULCERS OR FOOT LESIONS. — Ulcerating lesions of the lower extremity may be due to arterial insufficiency, venous insufficiency, neuropathy, infection or a variety of systemic diseases. The vascular laboratory is useful not only in distinguishing between these diverse etiologies, but also in predicting whether arterial inflow is adequate to permit healing with conservative therapy, regardless of etiology.

Raines et al.[33] suggest that foot lesions are unlikely to heal, without arterial reconstruction, if ankle pressure is <55 mmHg in nondiabetics and <80 mmHg in diabetics, and if ankle PVRs are severely attenuated. This requirement for higher perfusion pressures in diabetics may reflect the more extensive small vessel involvement or may suggest that SLP in diabetics are falsely elevated because of calcific medial sclerosis. These criteria are in good agreement with those suggested by Carter.[42]

HEALING OF AMPUTATIONS. — Selection of the proper level for amputation is important not only to preserve the maximal amount of viable tissue, but also to minimize morbidity from futile attempts to obtain healing of amputations performed through ischemic tissue.

Ankle pressures have shown little or no correlation with the healing of below-knee amputations (BKA).[43] However, several authors[43, 44] have found that a calf or distal thigh pressure of 50 – 70 mmHg was associated with a high (88 – 100%) likelihood of primary healing. As in previous examples, diabetics appear to require a higher calf pressure (>80 mmHg) to achieve the same degree of successful healing.

This situation is complicated, however, by the fact that patients have been seen who achieved primary healing of BKA despite calf pressures <50 mmHg. Accordingly, we feel that an attempt at BKA is justified in all patients with measureable pressure and/or a pulsatile waveform at the calf. Although one should be very cautious in recommending above-knee amputations (AKA), in otherwise favorable situations based solely on vascular laboratory data, in a borderline clinical situation, the absence of measureable calf pressure and pulsatile flow would strongly support proceeding directly with AKA.

Prediction of successful healing of transmetatarsal or toe amputations is even more difficult. Verta et al.[45] reported that in the absence of invasive infection, ankle pressure >35 mmHg was associated with eventual healing of single toe amputations in 83% of their 39 patients. This is surprising, as most patients with ankle pressure <50 mmHg usually have ischemic rest pain and would not be expected to heal a toe amputation. By contrast, Baker and Barnes[46] noted that none of 4 patients with ankle pressures <60 mmHg were able to heal forefoot amputations, and that even with ankle pressures >70 mmHg, only 86% healed. Diabetics who failed to heal their amputations had higher (mean, 79 mmHg) ankle pressures than nondiabetics (mean, 48 mmHg).

The apparent discrepancy between these two reports may be explained by the failure of ankle pressure alone to accurately assess the plantar arch and digital circulation. We agree with Raines et al.[33] that the best index of successful healing of forefoot amputations appears to be the presence of a pulsatile PVR at the transmetatarsal level. Lacking this, even ankle pressures >60 mmHg provide no assurance of healing.

RESPONSE TO SYMPATHECTOMY. — Because of the variable response to sympathectomy of patients with arterial insufficiency in whom reconstructive surgery is not feasible, there is need for a predictive vascular laboratory test. To this end, a number of techniques have been developed, including: measurement of galvanic skin resistance and its response to various stimuli;[47] digital plethysmography before and after lumbar sympathetic or peripheral nerve block; and measurement of skin temperature change after reflex heating.[48] These methods are all time-consuming and of questionable reliability.

Yao and Bergan[49] found that although measurement of skin blood flow before and after administration of an intravenous α-blocking agent (moxisylyte) correctly predicted the result of subsequent sympathectomy in only 40% of patients, all patients with an ankle pressure index >0.35 responded to sympathectomy. Only 4% of those whose index was <0.20 benefited.

Using a mercury-in-Silastic strain gauge, Strandness[50] measured preoperative digital blood flow. Subsequent lumbar sympathectomy was found to be most successful in patients who were able to increase the amplitude of their digital pulse volume >50% following reactive hyperemia, which was induced by occluding arterial inflow with pneumatic compression at the ankle for five minutes.

These studies emphasize the importance of preoperative documentation both of adequate perfusion pressure into the ischemic segment and of a collateral bed capable of further dilation. Although, in our experience, neither of these techniques has proven completely accurate, they have been helpful in selecting those patients most likely to benefit from sympathectomy.

PREDICTING THE RESULTS OF ARTERIAL RECONSTRUCTION. — In patients with combined aortoiliac and distal arterial occlusive lesions, it may be difficult to assess their relative hemodynamic significance and to predict the outcome of correcting only the aortoiliac occlusion. Bone et al.[51] demonstrated that one could anticipate a successful result following aortofemoral bypass in all patients with a thigh pressure index of 0.85 or less. He also observed that an increase in ankle pressure index of 0.1 or more during the first 12 hours after aortofemoral bypass was an excellent predictor of subsequent symptomatic improvement.

Similarly, Dean et al.[52] reported that 91% of patients with ankle pressure index <0.20, who subsequently underwent femoropopliteal reconstructions experienced early graft thrombosis. On the other hand, arteriographic evaluation of the runoff vessels in these same patients failed to predict subsequent graft failure.

Although such prognostic information cannot supersede surgical judgment in selecting patients for revascularization, particularly in limb salvage situations, it can be useful to the surgeon in formulating a more realistic appraisal of the likelihood of success or, conversely, the need for an alternative form of treatment. Furthermore, in the appropriate clinical setting, it might be used to advise against futile attempts at revascularization.

PERIOPERATIVE MONITORING. — Recognition and correction of technical misadventure in the operating room is facilitated by measurement of SLPs or PVRs. Garrett et al.[53] reported the use of ankle pressure measurements immediately following aortofemoral grafting in assessing the need for concomitant distal bypass. He suggests this approach should be considered in patients who fail to show an intraoperative increase in ankle pressure index of 0.1 or more. However, in addition to the difficulty of obtaining accurate ankle pressures in these vasoconstricted patients with uncorrected distal occlusive lesions, we have often seen progressive increases in the ankle pressure index over the first 24 hours postoperatively. Therefore, we are unwilling to recommend an additional distal reconstruction based solely on this single intraoperative determination.

The pulse volume recorder can easily serve as an intraoperative monitor with much less risk of contaminating the operative field. Appropriately sized cuffs are placed on the limb segment immediately beyond the anticipated distal anastomosis. A baseline tracing is obtained after induction of anesthesia. The patient is prepped and draped in the conventional manner with the connecting tubing lead out to the foot of the operating table. After completion of the anastomoses and restoration of flow, a postoperative PVR is easily obtained by the circulating nurse while the wounds are still open. In our experience, absence of a pulsatile tracing, albeit dampened, invariably has been associated with some technical complication.

O'Donnell, Raines and Darling[54] assessed the physiologic capability of the runoff bed in the operating room during femoropopliteal grafting by obtaining an ankle PVR while pulsing an injection of heparinized saline — first, through the opened popliteal artery and then, through the vein graft following completion of the distal anastomosis. This technique permitted rapid assessment of the technical adequacy of the distal anastomosis without need for time-consuming operative arteriography.

In the recovery room, serial determinations of ankle SLPs or PVRs can provide objective evidence of continued graft function. This is especially valuable in following those patients in whom uncorrected distal disease precludes the return of palpable pulses. Not only is the surgeon reassured of a successful reconstruction in the cool, vasoconstricted patient, nursing personnel are provided with objective parameters to follow. Early detection or prediction of graft failure thus can allow the surgeon to take prompt corrective action and salvage the reconstruction. Simply documenting distal arterial flow or graft flow with the Doppler in such patients provides no functional information and will not warn of impending graft thrombosis.

POSTOPERATIVE FOLLOW-UP. — All patients with arterial reconstructions are restudied routinely in our laboratory immediately before discharge or as soon as wound healing permits; at 3, 6 and 12 months postoperatively, and then annually thereafter unless new symptoms develop. Each study includes SLPs and PVRs before and after exercise. Exercise testing has proven especially sensitive in revealing early functional deterioration or impending graft failure even in the absence of obvious symptomatic progression.

Such routine follow-up permits objective documentation of the continued hemodynamic improvement coincident with collateral development, disease progression distal to a functioning reconstruction, or impending graft failure. These data are of value not only in understanding the changing hemodynamics of individual patients but also in intelligently planning their postoperative management.

UPPER EXTREMITY ARTERIAL OCCLUSIVE DISEASE. — Although

chronic arterial occlusion in the upper extremity is relatively infrequent, digital vasospasm, emboli and trauma may cause arterial insufficiency and prompt vascular laboratory evaluation.

After placing a pneumatic cuff (12×23 cm) on the upper arm, on the forearm below the elbow, and at the wrist (9×18 cm), Doppler survey of the radial or ulnar artery or digital plethysmography is used to detect distal flow. SLPs and PVRs are then obtained as in the lower extremity. In our laboratory, vertical gradients in normal upper extremities are 0–1 ± 10 mmHg; therefore, a 15–20 mmHg gradient definitely would be abnormal.

Since it is more difficult to develop a standardized exercise test for the upper extremity, we use five minutes of pneumatic compression of the upper arm to induce reactive hyperemia. Specially designed digital cuffs* (9×3 cm and 7×2 cm) or mercury strain gauges are needed to measure digital systolic pressures and to obtain digital PVRs.

The Doppler alone can accurately assess patency of the palmar arch as a modified Allen test.[55] Such a study should be considered in all patients suspected of intrinsic small vessel disease of the hand or prior to cannulation of either the radial or ulnar arteries. Similarly, Doppler survey of the digital arteries can document the presence of organic occlusion.

Sumner and Strandness[56] have described a characteristic "peaked pulse" seen in the digit volume pulse contours of patients with cold sensitivity as a result of collagen vascular disease or other forms of intrinsic digital artery disease. This is in contrast to patients with pure vasospasm where the contour is normal in configuration but of decreased amplitude. At room temperature, digital perfusion may be normal in early vasospastic disease. In such cases, baseline PVRs of all digits are obtained in a warm room. The hands are then immersed in ice water for three minutes. Serial digital PVRs are measured as rewarming occurs. If they fail to return to baseline levels within five minutes, a pathologic degree of vasospasm is likely.[57]

The response to dorsal sympathectomy in such patients can be predicted by comparing digital PVRs before and after either dorsal sympathetic block or intra-arterial vasodilators. If no

---

*Life Sciences, Inc.; Greenwich, Conn.

increase in amplitude of the tracing is seen following these maneuvers, it is most unlikely that dorsal sympathectomy would be of benefit and intrinsic small vessel occlusive disease should be suspected. This test also can be used to objectively follow the response to vasodilating drugs.

ARTERIOVENOUS FISTULAS. — Little consideration generally has been given to the noninvasive diagnosis of extremity arteriovenous (AV) fistulas. However, three of the studies already described can serve as an effective diagnostic screen: SLPs, plethysmography (PVRs) and velocity waveform analysis (VWF).[58]

The reduced peripheral resistance associated with AV fistulas decreases mean arterial pressure proximally, but increases pulse pressure. Therefore, proximal to a fistula, systolic pressures are usually increased compared to the contralateral, normal extremity. Beyond the fistula they are normal, except in the case of "stealing" from distal arterial flow, under which circumstance they may be decreased.

An AV fistula will increase the segmental limb volume changes normally produced by pulsatile arterial flow. This increase can be detected plethysmographically. We have found that PVRs proximal to the fistula are uniformly of greater amplitude. In addition, the anacrotic slope and peak are sharper with loss of the dicrotic "notch." Distal to the fistula, PVRs often are normal down to the digital level.

As previously noted, the VWF of a resting extremity normally is multiphasic with major systolic and minor diastolic forward components. Flow in late diastole generally is negligible so that the VWF ordinarily rests on the zero velocity baseline. Decreased peripheral resistance eliminates reversed flow and increases forward flow, particularly during diastole.[59] Consequently, the end-diastolic VWF is elevated above the zero baseline in direct proportion to the decrease in peripheral resistance. This pattern can be seen with reactive hyperemia, vasodilator drugs, artificial warming of the extremity, inflammation and sympathectomy. However, in the absence of these conditions, it is diagnostic of an AV fistula.

These tests are particularly valuable in evaluating patients with premature or atypical varicose veins, unequal limb growth or hemangiomas of the extremity. Since such conditions commonly occur in children or young adults, avoidance of unnecessary diagnostic arteriography is especially important.

Finally, by using the PUDVM to estimate mean velocity, vessel diameter and the angle of incidence of the ultrasound beam, velocity data can be converted to actual flow with the Doppler equation. This approach has been used not only to measure normal arterial flow transcutaneously,[60, 61] but also in evaluating AV fistulas.[58]

In practice, the difference between flow measured in the major artery proximal to the fistula and the same vessel in the contralateral extremity provides a good estimate of fistula flow. Such information is particularly useful in managing fistulas created for angioaccess. It allows one to determine whether fistula flow is sufficient to support dialysis, whether it is progressively decreasing, indicating imminent thrombosis, or whether it is too high, resulting in high output cardiac failure.

Extracranial Cerebrovascular Insufficiency

Stroke remains a leading cause of death and morbidity in our population. The recognition that a large percentage of such strokes result from potentially correctable lesions in the extracranial carotid artery has stimulated widespread interest in their early detection. Since cerebral angiography is accompanied by a small but definite morbidity and mortality, attention has turned to noninvasive diagnostic methods. Several different but complementary studies currently enjoy widespread popularity: (1) periorbital Doppler study; (2) carotid velocity waveform analysis (VWF); (3) carotid phonoangiography (CPA); and (4) ocular plethysmography (OPG).

Periorbital Doppler Study

Because the ophthalmic artery is a branch of the internal carotid artery (ICA), its potential value as a monitor of ICA flow has long been recognized. As shown (Fig 9), the supraorbital artery (SOA), a branch of the ophthalmic and thus, in turn, of the ICA, courses upward through its notch on the medial side of the supraorbital ridge to supply the medial forehead. The lateral portions of the supraorbital ridge and forehead are supplied primarily by branches of the superficial temporal artery (STA) which, in turn, are the terminal branch of the external carotid artery (ECA). Normal SOA flow is upward or antegrade. Since it

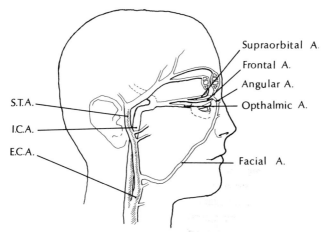

Fig 9. — Schematic representation of the normal periorbital blood supply (*STA* = superficial temporal artery; *ICA* = internal carotid artery; and *ECA* = external carotid artery). The important collateral communication between the supraorbital artery and STA; and between the frontal artery and the facial artery, are indicated.

anastomoses on the forehead with the terminal branches of the STA, compression of the latter results in augmentation of the antegrade SOA flow.

At the opposite extreme, with severe occlusive disease of the ICA, flow in the SOA is directed into the eye or retrograde. Since this flow originates in collateral branches of the STA, it will greatly diminish or cease when the latter is compressed. Thus, in the simplest clinical application of this test as introduced by Brockenbrough,[62] antegrade flow which augments with STA compression is normal and retrograde flow, which diminishes with SFA compression, is abnormal.

However, there are intermediate findings between these two extremes: in order of increasing ICA occlusive disease, SOA flow may be antegrade but reduced in magnitude, and may fail to augment in response to STA occlusion. Alternately, it may be retrograde but reverse, and may become weakly antegrade after STA compression.

The accuracy of this test in diagnosing carotid artery occlusive disease varies greatly in published reports. These variations are related not so much to differences in the skill of the examiner as to the degree of carotid occlusion which was present in the sample population. For example, Wise et al.[63] reported

94% accuracy in patients with >50% stenosis of the ICA. However, 13 of 19 cases of ">50% stenosis" were actually totally occluded.

Barnes et al.[64] also relate the high degree of inaccuracy reported in the literature to the fact that the study had been limited to only SOA flow and that only the STA was compressed. He points out that many extracranial and intracranial sources of collateral circulation may be recruited in the face of ICA occlusion and recommends additional compressive maneuvers. Furthermore, since it may be difficult to determine the direction of flow in the SOA because of improper probe angle or inadvertent monitoring of a palpebral branch of the STA, he recommends that the more medially placed frontal (FA) or supratrochlear artery, which is also a branch of the ophthalmic artery, be used. Moore et al.[65] found that this combination of both SOA and FA testing yielded a diagnostic accuracy, in patients with >50% ICA stenosis, of 93%. Supraorbital testing alone showed only an 86% specificity. The complete examination, therefore, consists of three basic steps: (1) determination of resting flow in the FA; (2) sequential compression of all branches of the ECA supplying this area (i. e., the STA, infraorbital and FA) bilaterally; and (3) brief compression of each common carotid artery (CCA) low in the neck.

If resting FA flow is antegrade, the study probably is normal, but this impression must be confirmed by sequential compression of the branches of the ECA, which usually results in either no change or augmentation of antegrade flow. If, instead, flow diminishes or ceases with compression of any of these branches, that branch represents an abnormal collateral source of FA flow. Reversed resting FA flow is always abnormal and sequential compression of the ECA branches will result in its cessation or diminution when the appropriate collateral is occluded.

Common carotid compression is indicated only if FA flow is not reversed by any of the other compressive maneuvers in order to identify the remaining alternative collateral pathways. Normally, ipsilateral CCA compression will diminish, obliterate or, occasionally, cause reversal of FA flow. In the presence of such a normal response, the contralateral CCA need not be compressed. If, however, FA flow is unchanged or actually augmented by ipsilateral CCA compression, significant obstruction of the ICA is present. When FA flow diminishes or ceases in response to contralateral CCA compression, the latter vessel, through its intracranial and facial communications, is the collateral source of FA flow. Finally, if FA flow is unaffected or actually is augmented by sequential compression of both CAAs, there must be occlusion of the ICA with intracranial collateralization via the vertebrobasilar arteries.

According to the results of Barnes et al.,[64] this type of comprehensive Doppler examination had a specificity of 98.7% in 152 ICAs with arteriographically proven stenosis or occlusion. With STA compression alone and a nondirectional Doppler, 36% of the abnormal studies would have been missed. However, if a directional Doppler had been used, reversal of FA flow would have identified 90% of the abnormals even without the additional compressive maneuvers.

In general, the examination begins to become positive at 50% ICA stenosis (by diameter) and should be 100% positive at >75% stenosis. The test is quick, simple, inexpensive, portable and highly specific. Its disadvantages are its low sensitivity and the necessity for CCA compression to achieve this accuracy. However, Barnes et al. have noted only one transient ischemic episode with this maneuver in almost 1,000 examinations; and Brockenbrough[62] reported only two in more than 4,000 examinations.

Velocity Waveform Analysis

Carotid VWF analysis is based on the fact that the ECA, which supplies skin, muscle and bone, has insignificant end-diastolic flow similar to extremity arteries, and, therefore, its VWF rests on the zero baseline. On the other hand, the ICA which is a high-flow, low-resistance conduit, even under basal conditions, normally has a velocity profile which is elevated well above the zero baseline during diastole. It has been reasoned[66] that since 80–90% of CCA flow goes through the ICA, its velocity pattern should largely reflect the ICA. Significant occlusive disease of that vessel then would result in a reduced diastolic velocity of the CCA with alteration of its ratio of systolic to diastolic flow. Thus, the concept of a carotid velocity index was introduced and the suggestion made that values above the normal range (>0.75) were diagnostic of CAOD.

In a series of 36 cases of arteriographically documented

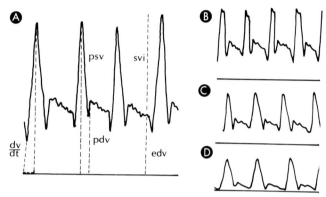

Fig 10. — Carotid velocity waveforms (CVWF) in various clinical situations. **A,** normal waveform illustrating five of the dimensions that have proven valuable in discriminant analysis (*psv* = peak systolic velocity; *svi* = systolic velocity increase; *pdv* = peak diastolic velocity; *edv* = end diastolic velocity; and dv/dt = systolic acceleration). **B,** actual CVWF in a patient with mild (30–40%) stenosis of internal carotid artery (ICA). **C,** CVWF with moderately severe (70–75%) stenosis of ICA. **D,** complete occlusion of ICA results in CVWF characteristic of the external carotid artery.

CAOD,[67] we found this ratio reliably elevated only with very high-grade stenosis or complete occlusion. However, in an experimental dog model, when the ICA diameter was progressively narrowed, every major dimension of the CCA waveform underwent stepwise reduction, suggesting the potential value of multidimensional analysis. Subsequent clinical studies[68] demonstrated the changes in the CCA velocity waveform that occurred with progressive degrees of ICA occlusion: the systolic peak became lower, broader and more notched while the diastolic velocity slope flattened and dropped towards the zero baseline (Fig 10). When divided into five clinical categories (young normal, old normal, <50% stenoses, >50% stenoses and occlusions), statistically significant differences between the values of adjacent groups were found for seven of nine dimensions measured. Discriminant analysis identified the five most sensitive of these and, by using weighted equations with discriminant function coefficients for each, a "score" was produced which retrospectively separated these five groups from each other with 91% accuracy. In a prospective study, 134 arteriographically documented cases were assigned to the correct clinical category with 85% accuracy. Of these cases, 59% had normal periorbital Doppler examinations.

With increasing experience, several sources of diagnostic error have been identified. First, any hemodynamic factor that affects the rate or strength of the systolic ejection can cause alterations in the dimensions of the carotid VWF. We now use the VWF from the patient's own normal brachial artery to standardize the waveform dimensions. Second, hemodynamically significant occlusive disease of the contralateral carotid may result in a compensatory increase in ipsilateral carotid flow, mask a stenosis or cause its severity to be underestimated. Finally, intracranial lesions such as subdural hematoma, cerebral edema, etc. may reduce CCA flow. Therefore, it should be appreciated that carotid VWF analysis detects changes in carotid blood flow, but does not identify or localize the cause.

Although this method can detect lesser degrees of CAOD than Doppler exam or OPG and although it does so with inexpensive, portable equipment, one must be careful to obtain a "maximized" tracing. Furthermore, separate standards must be established for each particular instrument and power source used. Approaches to eliminate these variables are actively being explored.

Phonoangiography

The technique of phonoangiography is the most sensitive, but least specific, of all the tests utilized to detect CAOD, and has been used primarily to supplement Doppler examination or OPG. It is capable of detecting lesser (40–60%) degrees of ICA stenosis which may not alter arterial hemodynamics sufficiently to be detected by any of the other tests.

A bruit transmitted up into the neck from the thorax appears at the clavicular level and either diminishes in intensity or remains unchanged at higher positions (Fig 11). A bruit originating at the carotid bifurcation is typically not audible at the clavicular position, but appears at the midcarotid level and gets louder above the bifurcation (Fig 12). As the degree of ICA stenosis increases, the resulting bruit occupies a progressively greater portion of systole. At 70–80% stenosis, it fills systole and extends into early diastole with loss of the second heart sound. When the stenosis is >95% of the lumen, flow through it may be so insignificant that the bruit disappears.

Stenosis of the ECA alone is infrequently (4–14%) responsi-

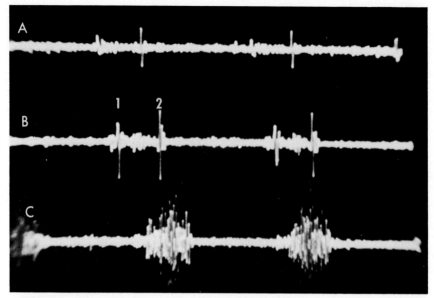

Fig 11.—Carotid phonoangiogram demonstrating a transmitted thoracic bruit that is visible immediately above the clavicle (**C**). At the midcarotid level (**B**) and at the angle of the jaw (**A**), both first and second heart sounds are evident and systolic turbulence is negligible.

ble for a midcervical bruit.[69] When present, it may mimic lesser degrees of ICA stenosis. However, it never completely fills systole or extends into diastole, since forward flow in the ECA, as in extremity arteries, ceases during late systole and the second heart sound is generally audible. These distinctions usually permit differentiation from bruits due to significant ICA stenosis.

This technique has been most carefully studied by Kartchner et al.[70] In his experience, it complemented the findings of OPG by permitting detection of 40% or greater stenosis of the ICA. Decrease in the intensity of a carotid bruit on serial determinations, if associated with a strongly positive OPG, indicated progression toward total ICA occlusion. Although we have not been as impressed with its ability to detect lesser degrees of carotid stenosis, it has indeed proven useful in identifying transmitted, cervical bruits and supporting the findings of OPG.

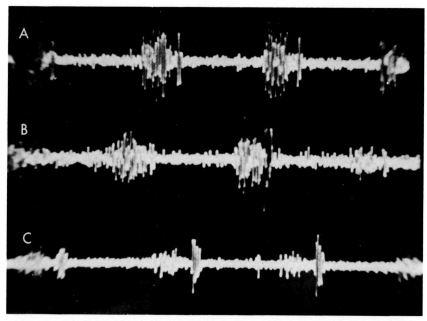

Fig 12. — Phonoangiogram of a bruit originating at the carotid bifurcation. The recording above the clavicle (C) shows no turbulence but a loud bruit, filling systole appears at the bifurcation (B) and is transmitted up to the angle of the jaw (C). However, it does not extend into diastole, suggesting that it is due either to a moderate stenosis of the internal carotid artery (ICA) or, as in this case, severe stenosis of the external carotid artery with ICA occlusion.

Ocular Plethysmography

The details of the two principal types of OPG have already been discussed. Both are able to detect hemodynamically significant (>50% by diameter) stenosis of the ICA with an accuracy of 85–95%.

Kartchner and McRae[71] reviewed the carotid arteriograms of 148 patients who had had positive OPG tests. A positive test was defined as a delay in pulse arrival comparing either one eye to the other or eye to ear. Small differences were accentuated by a phase shift of the differential tracing. The presence of bilateral, equal ICA stenosis was suggested by absence of delay in pulse arrival between the two eyes, with a significant delay between eye and ear. Of such patients, 89% had a significant stenosis of the ICA (11% false positive results). In a second group of 147 patients whose OPG had been negative, carotid arteriograms revealed that 11% had a >40% stenosis of the ICA (11% false negatives). However, only 4% had a >60% stenosis and were thus felt to be at high risk for major stroke. When the findings of CPA were added to these with OPG, accuracy in detecting >40% stenosis of the ICA, was increased to 97%, if both tests were positive. A second important finding from this study related to patients with "asymptomatic" bruits. When both CPA and OPG were positive, 12% of patients subsequently developed strokes, over a mean follow-up period of 24 months, as compared to only 2–3% of those in whom either of the two tests was negative.

The ocular pneumoplethysmograph is only capable of generating an IOP up to 110 mmHg. This limitation previously has restricted its use in patients with significant hypertension. To compensate for this problem, Gee et al.[72] have recently reported the following additional criteria for significant ICA stenosis:

(1) a >5 mmHg difference in IOP between the two eyes; (2) an OPG/brachial systolic ratio of 0.77 or less; and (3) a >2 mm difference in the ocular pulse amplitude between the two eyes. If one or more of these criteria was fulfilled, he reported an accuracy of 95% in detecting hemodynamically significant stenosis of the ICA. This contrasted sharply with the 31% accuracy of this technique previously reported by Gross et al.,[73] who had used the single criterion of a 15% or greater difference in IOP between the two eyes.

If the ipsilateral CCA is compressed during the measurement of IOP, a carotid "stump" pressure can be determined noninvasively. It has been used to predict whether patients with recurrent or extensive head and neck tumors are likely to tolerate elective carotid resection.[74]

We have used an OPG attachment, based on the Gee technique, for the pulse volume recorder* and have analyzed our results in 104 arteriographically studied carotid arteries.[75] Overall accuracy in detecting a >50% stenosis of the ICA was 94%. Since CPA was abnormal in both false negatives, the combined accuracy of these techniques was 100%.

In summary, it is apparent that all the various techniques of OPG have a comparable accuracy in detecting 50% or greater (diameter) stenosis of the ICA. However, no technique is yet

---

*Life Sciences, Inc.; Greenwich, Conn.

capable of detecting the nonstenosing, ulcerated carotid atheroma. Therefore, in a patient with appropriate lateralizing cerebral symptoms, carotid arteriography must be obtained regardless of the results of vascular laboratory tests.

The greatest value of the noninvasive tests presently available is in screening patients with asymptomatic cervical bruits or atypical, nonhemispheric symptoms. The demonstration of a hemodynamically significant ICA stenosis in such patients identified those persons whom Kartchner has shown are at high (12%) risk of subsequent major stroke. They are also useful in evaluating patients who develop a neurologic deficit in the immediate postoperative period following carotid endarterectomy, and for the long term follow-up of postendarterectomy patients.

Vertebral Artery Occlusive Disease

Relatively little has been done to apply the technology of the vascular diagnostic laboratory to vertebral artery occlusive disease. This is, in part, due to the difficulty of noninvasively studying vertebral artery flow. In addition, in a given situation, documented alterations in this flow may have little or no bearing on symptomatology.

Keller, Meier and Kumpe[76] studied vertebral artery flow using the directional Doppler in 90 patients, 40 of whom underwent subsequent arteriography. The probe was positioned in the dorsal oropharynx, after appropriate topical anesthesia, and the following four determinations were made: (1) flow direction in each vertebral artery; (2) relative amplitude of both signals; (3) the cessation of flow in either vertebral during any part of the cardiac cycle; and (4) the response of vertebral flow to ipsilateral CCA compression.

Under normal circumstances, vertebral flow was always craniad and of equal amplitude in both vessels. It never reached zero during any phase of diastole, and it did not change with CCA compression. Alterations in any of these normal observations were diagnostic of vertebral artery occlusive disease with a specificity of 82%. The test was most reliable in detecting vertebral artery occlusion or aplasia, subclavian steal and normalcy. It was less reliable in stenosis or hypoplasia. The technique has been simplified by avoiding the transoral route and, hence, the need for topical anesthesia. Using a probe positioned just below the mastoid process and directed toward the contralateral eye, Kaneda et al.[77] reported a diagnostic reliability of 92%.

However, Corson, Menzoian and LoGerfo[78] felt that the mastoid approach was unreliable since the spatial relationship between the probe and the vessel axis was less easily defined and more intervening structures were present. Instead, he positioned the probe in the region of the Chassaignac tubercle and was easily able to demonstrate reversal of vertebral flow in two patients with subclavian steal.

Although these early studies are interesting, it is worth reemphasizing that the demonstration of vertebral reversal in the presence of subclavian stenosis or occlusion does not imply a decrease in basilar artery blood flow and is not, of itself, an indication for surgery.

Extremity Venous Disease

Superficial thrombophlebitis usually is obvious on clinical examination. However, when there is considerable associated edema and inflammation, exploring the course of the vein with the Doppler, while using various compressive maneuvers to augment flow, can be helpful in distinguishing it from cellulitis or lymphangitis.

The diagnosis of deep venous thrombosis (DVT), on the other hand, is notoriously inaccurate. It has been shown by Haeger[79] and Cranley, Canos and Sull[80] that the "classic" clinical findings of DVT occur with approximately equal frequency in symptomatic patients whether their venograms were positive or negative. Such experiences have caused most physicians to rely heavily on contrast phlebography. However, the numerous disadvantages of venography for the routine diagnosis of DVT are well recognized.

Obviously, there is a need for an accurate, noninvasive bedside test for acute DVT which is both practical and inexpensive. Presently, the major alternatives to venography are radionuclide phlebography, I^{125} fibrinogen scanning, Doppler venous examination and venous plethysmography. Radionuclide phlebography[81] has a lower morbidity than contrast venography and, if labeled albumin microspheres are used, it can also provide a concomitant lung scan. However, it gives poor definition and is inaccurate for calf vein thromboses. Furthermore, it requires expensive, complicated, cumbersome equipment and is not suitable as a bedside screening test. I[125] fibrogen scanning[82] can detect calf vein thromboses with great accuracy and is suitable as a serial bedside screening test. However, because of numerous other drawbacks, its application is limited to investigating the relative efficacy of various regimens in the prophyllaxis of DVT. Only the Doppler venous examination and venous plethysmography have proven themselves of practical clinical value in the diagnosis of DVT.

Venous valvular insufficiency may be congenital, occurring primarily at the saphenofemoral or saphenopopliteal junctions, and may result in varicose veins. Less commonly isolated incompetence of communicating veins can occur on a congenital basis. However, the most common cause of deep venous and/or perforator valvular incompetency is DVT. Although subsequent recanalization of thrombosed veins restores patency, it destroys valvular integrity. Therefore, identifying the cause of varicose veins is important both in predicting the likelihood of success and in defining the indications for surgery. Both Doppler examination and plethysmography can objectively evaluate the valvular competency of extremity veins.

Doppler Venous Examination

When evaluating the deep venous system for obstruction or valvular incompetency,[83] the common femoral, popliteal and posterior tibial veins are examined with the Doppler for the presence and quality of spontaneous venous flow and its augmentation with both respiratory and manual compressive maneuvers. The examiner asks four questions at each level: (1) is spontaneous flow present or absent? (2) is it continuous or phasic with respiration? (3) is it augmented by compression? and (4) is there an ipsilateral increase in superficial venous flow? Considerable experience is required to achieve maximum accuracy, and subtle differences may often be detected only by comparing both extremities. All abnormal observations should be repeated to assess reproducibility.

The femoral vein is studied first. Its Doppler shift sounds should be loud and clearly synchronous with respiration, rising and falling like the sound of wind whistling through the trees.

Although one cannot perform proximal compressive maneuvers, both deep inspiration and a Valsalva maneuver should cause cessation of flow. This indicates that not only is the femoral vein patent, but so are the proximal iliac vein and inferior vena cava. If the femoral vein were thrombosed there would simply be no signal. If the iliac vein were occluded, the sounds would not be phasic with respiration but would be continuous, and there would be little augmentation of flow following respiratory maneuvers. Finally, manual compression of the thigh muscles normally results in augmentation of femoral venous flow. The absence of such augmentation should lead one to suspect femoral vein thrombosis distal to the monitoring probe, which can be confirmed by examining the popliteal vein.

Ileofemoral valvular incompetence results in flow reversal or reflux, rather than cessation, with a Valsalva maneuver. Some degree of incompetency has been observed with this maneuver in 16% of normal patients, in 32% of children of patients with varicose veins[84] and in 100% of patients with "primary" varicose veins.[85] This concurs with Ludbrook's and Beale's[86] pressure and Basmajian's[87] anatomic studies suggesting congenital absence of iliofemoral venous valves as the cause of primary varicose veins. Therefore, the demonstration of iliofemoral and saphenous incompetence in the presence of popliteal, posterior tibial and perforator competence, provides assurance that one is dealing with primary varicose veins and that high ligation and stripping should provide excellent long-term results.

Examination of the popliteal vein differs from the femoral vein only in that manual compression of the proximal thigh replaces the Valsalva maneuver and the patient is in a prone position with the knee slightly bent and the calf relaxed by supporting the foot on a small pillow or foam pad. The placement of the Doppler probe is more perpendicular to the skin than usual because the popliteal vein already lies in an oblique plane.

Study of the posterior tibial vein completes the examination. Although spontaneous respiratory sounds often can be heard at this level, their absence does not have the same diagnostic significance as in more proximal veins. At times, it is only possible to confirm posterior tibial patency by distal compression, i.e., squeezing the forefoot. Otherwise, the interpretation of spontaneous flow signals and their augmentation by proximal and distal compression maneuvers is identical to that described for the other deep veins.

The diagnostic accuracy of such a Doppler examination in detecting DVT varies with clinical reports but, in a review of nine major clinical evaluations,[83] mean diagnostic accuracy was 87% for proximal DVT, i. e., thrombi at or above the level of the popliteal vein. However, it was very inaccurate in distal or calf vein thrombosis, with an average of 73% false negatives.

Doppler survey utilizes inexpensive, portable equipment and can serve as an effective bedside screening exam for DVT. It also provides information regarding venous valvular competence not routinely obtained by impedance plethysmography. If a directional Doppler is available, one can also detect and localize incompetent communicating veins.[84] However, it does not supply objective, quantitative information; it requires considerable skill and experience to achieve maximum potential accuracy; and it is not reliable if excessive fat, scar tissue, edema or hematoma separate the monitoring probe from the underlying vein.

Venous Plethysmography

Since 80% of lower extremity blood volume resides in the veins, plethysmographic measurement of invoked changes in limb volume has been used to diagnose obstruction and valvular incompetency of the deep veins of the lower extremities. The techniques used include mercury strain gauge, volume displacement, mechanical and impedance plethysmography. All are similar in application and comparable in accuracy. The strain gauge method of Barnes provides quantitative estimates of either reflux[88] or the maximum rate of venous outflow,[89] while the pulse volume recorder (volume displacement) obtains similar data using an instrument which is equally suitable for diagnosing arterial occlusive disease. However, since the technique of impedance plethysmography (IPG) enjoys wide clinical application and has been evaluated thoroughly in venographically documented cases by Wheeler et al.[90] and Hull et al.,[91] it will be described in detail as the prototype of this method.

Originally the diagnosis of deep venous thrombosis by IPG was based only on the recognition of a significant dampening (i. e., >20%) in the phasic volume shifts associated with sponta-

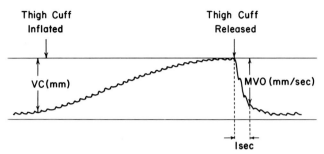

Fig 13.—A normal venous study, obtained by segmental plethysmography, demonstrating the gradual increase and plateau of the baseline, venous capacitance *(VC)* after temporary occlusion of venous return. Upon release of the thigh cuff it falls rapidly, maximum venous outflow *(MVO)*, back to its previous level. A tracing produced by impedance of strain-gauge plethysmography would be similar in appearance.

neous respiration. Subsequently, Wheeler et al.[92] introduced the practice of measuring the initial rate of venous outflow following its temporary interruption by a deeply held inspiration. Because of excessive variability in patients' performance of this maneuver, it was replaced by inflation of a thigh cuff for 45 seconds to 45 cm H_2O to provide temporary venous occlusion.

During such occlusion, the baseline rises as the volume of the calf increases in response to the venous obstruction. The plateau in calf volume after 45 seconds of thigh occlusion is considered the venous capacitance (VC). Following release of the thigh cuff, the initial slope of venous outflow, or, more precisely, the decrease in volume within the first second of cuff release, is called the maximum venous outflow (MVO) (Fig 13).

Hull et al.[91] have established that because of variability in the degree of venous pooling during thigh occlusion, it is more accurate to plot MVO against VC than to simply measure both parameters separately (Fig 14). Using discriminant analysis, they were able to determine a slope for this ratio which separated normal cases from those with proximal DVT with 98% accuracy. In a prospective series of limbs, all studied with venography, they report a specificity of 97% in 397 normal limbs and an overall sensitivity of 93% in the 133 limbs with proximal DVT. This decreased to 83% in asymptomatic limbs with proximal DVT and to 78% if the proximal thrombi were nonocclusive. Wheeler et al.[90] have reported comparable accuracy. Both groups have a high (83%) false negative rate in detecting documented distal or

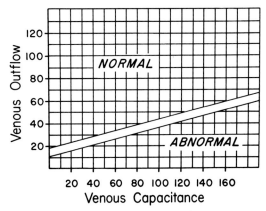

Fig 14. — Graphic representation of the relationship between venous capacitance and maximum venous outflow. The discriminant line separates limbs with normal deep veins from those with occluding proximal thrombi with >90% accuracy (modified after Hull et al.[91]).

calf vein thrombi. In addition, there is an increasing rate of false negative studies with the passage of time following DVT as collateral channels bypass the obstructing thrombus. False positive tests have been noted in patients with congestive heart failure, arterial insufficiency and the postphlebitic syndrome.

The study is easily performed at the bedside and, although the equipment is more costly than a Doppler, it provides more objective information. The importance of having the leg slightly elevated to eliminate differences in venous pooling, having the leg externally rotated to encourage muscle relaxation, and having it slightly flexed to avoid extrinsic popliteal vein compression should be stressed. The degree of accuracy reported in the literature can be achieved only by repeating the study until reproducible results are assured.

Even assuming that most vascular diagnostic laboratories will not achieve the high levels of accuracy reported by the developers of these methods, it is likely that the combined accuracy of both venous plethysmography and Doppler examination should still approach 90% for proximal DVT. Therefore, in practice, if both tests are negative, venography need only be performed if the clinical suspicion of DVT is extremely strong. If they are both positive, treatment for DVT may be begun without venographic confirmation. Venography is required only in those cases in which these two tests disagree with each other or a strong clinical impression.

Although the diagnosis of venous valvular insufficiency by plethysmography has been reported by Barnes,[88] we have found this technique cumbersome. Since the diagnosis of deep venous valvular insufficiency often is clinically obvious and since it can be readily confirmed by simple Doppler examination, we no longer use plethysmographic methods unless more quantitative data are required. Two useful methods for obtaining such inforation have been reported.[93, 94]

Practical Considerations

The Inter-Society Commission for Heart Disease Resources[95] has made several valuable recommendations — which we strongly endorse — pertaining to the organization and operation of the vascular diagnostic laboratory. They suggest that any hospital of 200 or more beds which is performing angiography, receiving trauma patients and doing arterial reconstructive surgery should establish a vascular diagnostic laboratory. The laboratory should be institutionally based but readily available to out-patients and should be able to provide diagnostic tests in cere-brovascular and extremity arterial and venous problems. Ideally, at least 200 square feet of space should be available for the laboratory equipment and furniture. However, at a time when in-hospital floor space is severely limited, we find this recommendation unnecessarily generous. Both the authors' laboratories average less than 150 square feet and are perfectly adequate for clinical purposes. The location of the laboratory must provide easy access to the operating rooms, recovery rooms and intensive care areas, and must have an adequate outpatient waiting area.

The vascular laboratory, a diagnostic service, administratively should be a part of the department of surgery or medicine. It should be directed by an independent, preferably full-time physician or Ph.D., and should not become the private domain of any single physician or group of clinicians. The director should have adequate personal experience in both the performance and interpretation of all tests available in the laboratory.

If the director is a physician, technical support can be provided by a medical technician after a 4 – 6 week training period in an established laboratory. We feel that this recommendation, while ideal, is impractically long. Adequate technical competence for most clinical purposes usually can be acquired with a week of intensive instruction and practical demonstration.

The laboratory should be capable of performing bedside, out-of-laboratory examinations, and a call schedule is suggested to ensure that its services are available on an emergency basis at all times. Its reports should contain all pertinent diagnostic information and should become part of the patient's permanent medical record. Referring physicians must maintain control over all therapeutic decisions. Re-examination is their prerogative and not that of the laboratory.

Initial equipment costs will naturally vary, but generally range between $10,000 and $20,000. The yearly operating budget of a typical vascular diagnostic laboratory is approximately $30,000, including the technician's salary.

The decision to establish a vascular diagnostic laboratory does not require that a specific amount of space, technical assistance or expensive instrumentation be made available. Rather, it can simply represent a commitment to study the hemodynamic alterations produced by vascular disease, to intelligently plan their correction and to document the results of therapy. Whether this goal is achieved with a simple pocket-model Doppler or with the most sophisticated instrumentation will depend on each individual physician's experience and clinical needs.

REFERENCES

1. Spittell, J. A., DeWolfe, V., Hume, M., Winsor, T., and Wylie, E. J.: Prevention and early detection of peripheral vascular disease, Circulation 42: A-42, 1970.
2. Satomura, S., and Kaneko, Z.: Ultrasonic blood rheograph, *Proceedings of the Third International Conference on Medical Electronics*, 1960, p. 254.
3. Nicolaides, A. N., Gordon-Smith, I. C., Dayandas, J., and Eastcott, H. H. G.: The value of Doppler blood velocity tracings in the detection of aortoiliac disease in patients with intermittent claudication, Surgery 80: 774, 1976.
4. Woodcock, J. P., Goslin, R. G., and Fitzgerald, D. E.: A new noninvasive technique for assessment of superficial femoral artery obstruction, Br. J. Surg. 59:226, 1972.
5. McLeod, R. D.: Directional Doppler demodulation, 20th Ann. Conf. Eng. Med. Biol. 27:1, 1967.
6. Brockenbrough, E. C.: *Screening for the prevention of stroke: Use of a Doppler flowmeter* (Seattle: Parks Electronics, 1970).

7. Folse, R., and Alexander, R.: Directional flow detection for localizing venous valvular incompetency, Surgery 67:114, 1970.
8. Spencer, M. P., Reid, J. M., Davis, D. L., and Paulson, P. S.: Cervical carotid imaging with a continuous-wave Doppler flowmeter, Stroke, 5:145, 1974.
9. Fish, P. J., Corrigan, T., Kakkar, V. V., and Nicolaides, A. N.: Arteriography using ultrasound, Lancet 1:1269, 1972.
10. Mozersky, D. J., Hokanson, D. E., Sumner, D. S., and Standness, D. E.: Ultrasonic visualization of the arterial lumen, Surgery 72:253, 1972.
11. Barnes, R. W., Bone, G. E., Reinertson, J., Slaymaker, E. E., Hokanson, D. E., and Strandness, D. E.: Noninvasive ultrasonic carotid angiography: Prospective validation by contrast arteriography, Surgery 80:328, 1976.
12. Histand, M. B., Miller, C. W., and McLeod, F. D.: Transcutaneous measurement of blood velocity profiles and flow, Cardiovasc. Res. 7:703, 1973.
13. Green, P. S.,and Marich, K. W.: Real-time orthographic ultrasonic imaging for cardiovascular diagnosis, in Harrison, D. E., Sandler, H., and Miller, H. A. (eds.): *Cardiovascular Imaging and Image Processing: Theory and Practice,* Vol. 72 (Palos Verdes Estates, Calif.; Society of Photo-Optical Instrumentation Engineers, 1975).
14. Darling, R. C., Raines, J. K., Brener, B. J., and Austen, W. G.: Quantitative segmental pulse volume recorder: A clinical tool, Surgery 72:873, 1972.
15. Yao, J. S. T., Needham, T. N., Gourmoos, C., and Irvine, W. T.: A comparative study of strain-gauge plethysmography and Doppler ultrasound in the assessment of occlusive arterial disease of the lower extremities, Surgery 71:4, 1972.
16. Wheeler, H. B., Pearson, D., O'Connell, D., and Mullick, S. C.: Impedance phlebography: Technique, interpretation and results, Arch. Surg. 104:164, 1972.
17. Cranley, J. J., Gay, A. Y., Grass, A. M., and Simeone, F. A.: A plethysmographic technique for the diagnosis of DVT of the lower extremities, Surg. Gynecol. Obstet. 136:385, 1973.
18. Barnes, R. W., Clayton, J. M., Bone, G. E., Slaymaker, E. E., and Reinertson, J.: Supraorbital photoplethysmography. Simple, accurate screening for carotid occlusive disease, J. Surg. Res. 22:319, 1977.
19. Kartchner, M. M., McRae, L. P., and Morrison, F. D.: Noninvasive detection and evaluation of carotid occlusive disease, Arch. Surg. 106:528, 1973.
20. Gee, W., Smith, C. A., and Hinson, C. E.: Ocular pneumoplethysmography in carotid artery disease, Med. Instrum. 8:244, 1974.
21. Kartchner, M. M., and McRae, L. P.: Auscultation for carotid bruits in cerebrovascular insufficiency, JAMA 210:494, 1969.
22. Winsor, T.: Influence of arterial disease on the systolic blood pressure gradients of the extremity, Am. J. Med. Sci. 220:117, 1950.
23. Kirkendall, W. M., Burton, A. C., Epstein, F. H., and Freis, E. D.: Recommendations for human blood pressure determination by sphygmomanometers, Circulation 36:980, 1967.
24. Carter, S. A.: Clinical measurement of systolic pressures in limbs with arterial occlusive disease, JAMA 207:1869, 1969.

25. Carter, S. A.: Response of ankle systolic pressure to leg exercise in mild or questionable arterial disease, N. Engl. J. Med. 287:578, 1972.
26. Johnson, W. C.: Doppler ankle pressure and reactive hyperemia in the diagnosis of arterial insufficiency, J. Surg. Res. 18:177, 1975.
27. Sumner, D. S., and Strandness, D. E.: The relationship between calf blood flow and ankle blood pressure in patients with intermittent claudication, Surgery 65:763, 1969.
28. Johnston, K. W.: In Discussion (section of reference 3).
29. Fronek, A., Johansen, K. H., Dilley, R. B., and Bernstein, E. F.: Noninvasive physiologic tests in the diagnosis and characterization of peripheral arterial occlusive disease, Am. J. Surg. 126:205, 1973.
30. Waters, K. J., Chamberlain, J., and McNeill, I. F.: The significance of aortoiliac atherosclerosis as assessed by Doppler ultrasound, Am. J. Surg. 134:388, 1977.
31. Johnston, K. W., and Taraschuk, I.: Validation of the role of pulsatility index in quantitation of the severity of peripheral arterial occlusive disease, Am. J. Surg., 131:295, 1976.
32. Kempczinski, R.: Use of the pulse volume recorder in the detection of aorto-iliac disease (manuscript in preparation).
33. Raines, J. K., Darling, R. C., Buth, J., Brewster, D. C., and Austen, W. G.: Vascular laboratory criteria for the management of peripheral vascular disease of the lower extremities, Surgery 79:21, 1976.
34. Lennihan, R., and Mackereth, M. A.: Ankle pressures in arterial occlusive disease involving the legs, Surg. Clin. North Am. 53:657, 1973.
35. Moore, W. S., and Hall, A. D.: Unrecognized aorto-iliac stenosis: A physiologic approach to the diagnosis, Arch. Surg. 103:633, 1971.
36. Brenner, B. J., Raines, J. K., Darling, R. C., and Austen, W. G.: Measurement of systolic femoral arterial pressure during reactive hyperemia: An estimate of aorto-iliac disease, Circulation 49/50:II-259, 1974.
37. Michal, V., Kramar, R., Pospichal, J., and Hejhal, L.: Arterial epigastricocavernous anastomosis for the treatment of sexual impotence, World J. Surg. 1:515, 1977.
38. Abelson, D.: Diagnostic value of the penile pulse and blood pressure: A Doppler study of impotence in diabetics, J. Urol. 113:636, 1975.
39. Gaskell, P.: The importance of penile blood pressure in cases of impotence, Can. Med. Assoc. J. 105:1047, 1971.
40. Kempczinski, R.: Role of the vascular diagnostic laboratory in the management of impotence (manuscript in preparation).
41. Darling, R. C., Buckley, C. J., Abbott, W. M., and Raines, J. K.: Intermittent claudication in young athletes: Popliteal artery entrapment syndrome, J. Trauma 14:543, 1974.
42. Carter, S. A.: The relationship of distal systolic pressures to healing of skin lesions in limbs with arterial occlusive disease, with special reference to diabetes mellitus, Scand. J. Clin. Lab. Invest. 31 (suppl 128):239, 1973.
43. Dean, R. H., Yao, J. S. T., Thompson, R. G., and Bergan, J. J.: Predictive value of ultrasonically derived arterial pressure in determination of amputation level, Am. Surg. 41:731, 1975.
44. Barnes, R. W., Shanik, G. D., and Slaymaker, E. E.: An index of healing in

below-knee amputation: Leg blood pressure by Doppler ultrasound, Surgery 79:13, 1976.

45. Verta, M. J., Gross, W. S., van Bellan, B., Yao, J. S. T., and Bergan, J. J.: Forefoot perfusion pressure and minor amputation for gangrene, Surgery 80:729, 1976.

46. Baker, W. H. and Barnes, R. W.: Minor forefoot amputation in patients with low ankle pressure, Am. J. Surg. 133:331, 1977.

47. Ozeran, R. S., Wagner, G. R., Reimer, T. R., and Hill, R. A.: Neuropathy of the sympathetic nervous system associated with diabetes mellitus, Surgery 68:953, 1970.

48. Husni, E. A., and Simeone, F. A.: Results of lumbar sympathectomy in peripheral vascular disease: An evaluation of preoperative laboratory tests, Arch. Surg. 75:530, 1957.

49. Yao, J. S. T. and Bergan, J. J.: Predictability of vascular reactivity relative to sympathetic ablation, Arch. Surg. 107:676, 1973.

50. Strandness, D. E.: *Peripheral Arterial Disease. A Physiologic Approach,* (Boston: Little, Brown and Company, 1969) pp. 212–213.

51. Bone, G. E., Hayes, A. C., Slaymaker, E. E., and Barnes, R. W.: Value of segmental limb blood pressures in predicting results of aorto-femoral bypass, Am. J. Surg. 132:733, 1976.

52. Dean, R. H., Yao, J. S. T., Stanton, P. E., and Bergan, J. J.: Prognostic indicators in femoropopliteal reconstructions, Arch. Surg. 110:1287, 1975.

53. Garrett, W. V., Slaymaker, E. E., Heintz, S. E., and Barnes, R. W.: Intraoperative prediction of symptomatic result of aortofemoral bypass from changes in ankle pressure index, Surgery 82:504, 1977.

54. O'Donnell, T. F., Raines, J. K., and Darling, R. C.: Intraoperative monitoring using the pulse volume recorder, Surg. Gynecol. Obstet., 145:252, 1977.

55. Kamienski, R. W., and Barnes, R. W.: Critique of the Allen test for continuity of the palmar arch assessed by Doppler ultrasound, Surg. Gynecol. Obstet., 142:861, 1976.

56. Sumner, D. S., and Strandness, D. E.: An abnormal finger pulse associated with cold sensitivity, Ann. Surg., 175:294, 1972.

57. Raines, J. K.: Personal communication, 1975.

58. Rutherford, R. B., Fleming, P. W., and McLeod, F. D.: Vascular diagnostic methods for evaluating patients with arteriovenous fistulas, in Diethrich, E. B. (ed.): *Noninvasive Cardiovascular Diagnosis: Current Concepts* (Baltimore, Maryland: University Park Press, 1978).

59. Rittenhouse, E., Maizner, W., Burr, J., and Barnes, R. W.: Directional arterial flow velocity: A sensitive index of changes in peripheral vascular resistance, Surgery 79:350, 1976.

60. Olson, R. M., and Cooke, J. P.: Human carotid artery diameter and flow by a noninvasive technique, Med. Instrum. 9:99, 1975.

61. Thomas, P. A.: Noninvasive estimation of brachial artery flow, Med. Prog. Technol. 4:163, 1977.

62. Brockenbrough, E. C.: Screening for the Prevention of Stroke: Use of a Doppler Flowmeter. Information and Education Research Support Unit of Washington-Alaska Regional Medical Program, 1969.

63. Wise, G., Brockenbrough, E. C., Marty, R., et al.: The detection of carotid

artery obstruction: A correlation with arteriography, Stroke 2:105, 1971.
64. Barnes, R. W., Russel, H. E., Bone, G. E., and Slaymaker, E. E.: Doppler cerebrovascular examination: Improved results with refinements in technique, Stroke 8:468, 1977.
65. Moore, W. S., Bean, B., Burton, R., and Goldstone, J.: The use of ophthalmosonometry in the diagnosis of carotid artery stenosis, Surgery 82:107, 1977.
66. Planiol, T., and Pourcelot, L.: Doppler effect study of the carotid circulation, in de Vlieger, M., White, D. N., McCreedy, V. W. (eds): *Proceedings of the Second World Congress on Ultrasonics in Medicine* (New York: American Elsevier Publishing Co., Inc., 1975).
67. Rutherford, R. B., Hiatt, W. R., and Kreutzer, E. W.: The use of velocity waveform analysis in the diagnosis of carotid artery occlusive disease, Surgery 82:695, 1977.
68. Rutherford, R. B., Hiatt, W. R., and Kreutzer, E. W.: The use of velocity waveform analysis in the diagnosis of carotid artery occlusive disease, in Diethrich, E. B. (ed.): *Noninvasive Cardiovascular Diagnosis: Current Concepts* (Baltimore, Maryland: University Park Press, 1978).
69. David, T. E., Humphries, A. W., Young, J. R., and Beven, E. G.: A correlation of neck bruits and arteriosclerotic carotid arteries, Arch. Surg. 107: 729, 1973.
70. Kartchner, M. M., McRae, L. P., Crain, V., and Whitaker, B.: Oculoplethysmography: An adjunct to arteriography in the diagnosis of extracranial carotid occlusive disease, Am. J. Surg. 132:728, 1976.
71. Kartchner, M. M. and McRae, L. P.: Noninvasive evaluation and management of the "asymptomatic" carotid bruit, Surgery 82:840, 1977.
72. Gee, W., Oller, D. W., Amundsen, D. G., Goodreau, J. J.: The asymptomatic carotid bruit and the ocular pneumoplethysmography, Arch. Surg. 112: 1381, 1977.
73. Gross, W. S., Verta, M. J., van Bellen, B., Bergan, J. J. and Yao, J. S. T.: Comparison of noninvasive diagnostic techniques in carotid artery occlusive disease, Surgery 82:271, 1977.
74. Martinez, S. A., Oller, D. W., Gee, W. and deFries, H. O.: Elective carotid artery resection, Arch. Otolaryngol. 101:744, 1975.
75. Kempczinski, R.: The noninvasive diagnosis of extracranial carotid arterial occlusive disease (manuscript in preparation).
76. Keller, H. M., Meier, W. E., and Kumpe, D. A.: Noninvasive angiography for the diagnosis of vertebral artery disease using Doppler ultrasound (vertebral artery Doppler), Stroke 7:364, 1976.
77. Kaneda, H., Irino, T., Minami, T., and Taneda, M.: Diagnostic reliability of the percutaneous ultrasonic Doppler technique for vertebral arterial occlusive diseases, Stroke 8:571, 1977.
78. Corson, J. D., Menzoian, J. O., and LoGerfo, F. W.: Reversal of vertebral artery blood flow demonstrated by Doppler ultrasound, Arch. Surg. 112: 715, 1977.
79. Haeger, K.: Problems of acute deep venous thrombosis. I. The interpretation of signs and symptoms, Angiology 20:219, 1969.
80. Cranley, J. J., Canos, A. J., and Sull, W. J.: The diagnosis of deep venous thrombosis, Arch Surg. 111:34, 1976.

81. Barnes, R. W., McDonald, G. B., Hamilton, G. W., Rudd, T. G., Nelp, W. B., and Strandness, D. E.: Radionuclide venography for rapid dynamic evaluation of venous disease, Surgery 73:706, 1973.
82. Kakkar, V. V.: The diagnosis of deep venous thrombosis using the I^{125} fibrinogen test, Arch. Surg. 104:152, 1972.
83. Sumner, D. S.: Evaluation of the venous circulation using the ultrasonic Doppler velocity detector, in Rutherford, R. B. (ed.): Vascular Surgery (Philadelphia: W. B. Saunders Co., 1977).
84. Reagan, B., and Folse, R.: Lower extremity venous dynamics in normal persons and children of patients with varicose veins, Surg. Gynecol. Obstet. 132:15, 1971.
85. Folse, R.: The influence of femoral vein dynamics on the development of varicose veins, Surgery 68:974, 1970.
86. Ludbrook, J., and Beale, G.: Femoral venous valves in relation to varicose veins, Lancet 1:79, 1962.
87. Basmajian, J. V.: The distribution of valves in the femoral, external iliac and common carotid femoral veins and their relationship to varicose veins, Surg. Gynecol. Obstet. 95:537, 1952.
88. Barnes, R. W., Collicott, P. E., Mozersky, D. J., Sumner, D. S., and Strandness, D. E.: Noninvasive quantitation of venous reflux in the postphlebitic syndrome, Surg. Gynecol. Obstet. 136:767, 1973.
89. Barnes, R. W., Collicott, P. E., Mozersky, D. J., Sumner, D. S., and Strandness, D. E.: Noninvasive quantitation of maximum venous outflow in acute thrombophlebitis, Surgery 72:971, 1972.
90. Wheeler, H. B., O'Donnell, J. A., Anderson, F. A., and Benedict, K.: Occlusive impedance phlebography: A diagnostic procedure for venous thrombosis and pulmonary embolism, Prog. Cardiovasc. Dis. 17:199, 1974.
91. Hull, R., vanAken, W. G., Hirsch, J., Gallus, A. S., Hoicka, G., Turpie, A. G. G., Walker, I., and Gent, M.: Impedance plethysmography using the occlusive cuff technique in the diagnosis of venous thrombosis, Circulation 53:696, 1976.
92. Wheeler, H. B., Pearson, D., O'Donnell, D., and Mullick, S. C.: Impedance plethysmography: Technique, interpretation and results, Arch Surg. 104: 164, 1972.
93. Rutherford, R. B., Reddy, C. M., Walker, A. G., and Wagner, H. N.: A new quantitative method of assessing the functional status of the leg veins, Am. J. Surg. 122:594, 1971.
94. O'Donnell, J. A., and Hobson, R. W. II.: Evaluation of venous insufficiency, by ambulatory pressure and volume hemodynamics, cine phlebography and clinical assessment (submitted for publication).
95. Bergan, J. J., Darling, R. C., DeWolfe, V. G., Raines, J. K., Strandness, D. E. and Yao, J. S. T.: Medical instrumentation in peripheral vascular disease. Resource and planning guidelines for the hospital and physician, Circulation 54:A-1, 1976.

RELATED READINGS

Dean, R. H., and Yao, J. S. T.: Hemodynamic measurements in peripheral vascular disease, Curr. Probl. Surg. 13:August, 1976.
Strandness, D. E., and Sumner, D. S.: Hemodynamics for Surgeons (New York: Grune and Stratton, 1975).

Hormonal Influences on Gastric Secretion

JAMES C. THOMPSON, M.D.

Department of Surgery, University of Texas Medical Branch,
Galveston, Texas

The normal flow and ebb of acid-peptic juice from the stomach after a meal provides clear evidence of regulatory mechanisms that are designed initially to stimulate and later to suppress gastric secretion. The control of these mechanisms involves complex neurohumoral interrelations between the vagi and various hormones from the upper gastrointestinal tract. Relative emphasis on neural versus hormonal control has shifted back and forth; Pavlov believed that the nervous system was responsible for most of the physiologic actions of the gut. For the past several decades most interest has been focused on hormonal mechanisms, but recent studies suggest that neural mechanisms may be at the center of control and that hormones may play a more supportive role.

This paper will consider some of the physiologic events that occur when a meal is eaten and will summarize recent information on the role of gastrointestinal hormones in those postprandial events.

Physiologic Stimulation of Gastric Secretion

Ingested food is mixed with saliva and swallowed. Saliva functions to initiate carbohydrate digestion by means of salivary amylase, to aid in the formation of a bolus for swallowing and to dissolve solid substances in order to stimulate the taste buds. Perhaps its most important function is to serve as a moistening

0065–3411/78/0012–0053$03.75

and lubricating agent. Swallowed food enters the stomach, where it is mixed with gastric juice and changed into a more liquid form. The amount of digestion carried on in the stomach is slight, mostly proteolysis; and the chief function of the stomach seems to be to prepare food mechanically by churning and mixing with gastric juice for further digestion. There is evidence that the stomach functions as an osmoregulator by slowing the emptying of hyperosmolar fluids until a lower osmolality has been achieved by mixing. Even so, we have found that foods that are distinctly hyperosmolar do normally reach the duodenum.

Fig 1.—Schematic summary of some of the neurohumoral events that occur when a meal is eaten. Acetylcholine *(Ach)* is released from vagal nerve endings. Histamine is apparently released from mucosal mast cells. Gastrin is released by food (by a mechanism which is pH-sensitive) from antral mucosa *(shaded area)*. Food in the small bowel stimulates release of the intestinal phase hormone. Each stimulant acts on the parietal cell (perhaps, as shown, each by means of a separate receptor on the cell membrane) to stimulate secretion of H+. Delivery of acidified chyme into the duodenum evokes a series of events (some probably reflex, some humoral) which inhibit further gastric secretion. Some of the agents involved are listed.

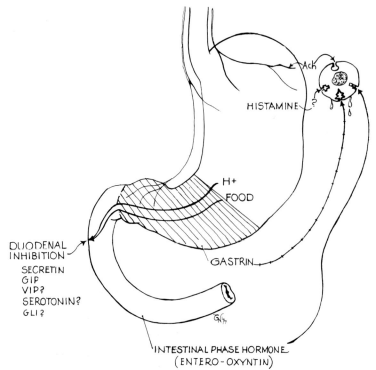

The chief function of the gut is, of course, absorption of food; the main function of the stomach seems to be to mix and churn food so that it is delivered slowly into the duodenum in small particles. The acid gastric contents within the duodenum are neutralized and are mixed with digestive juices from the pancreas, bile and secretions from the duodenal mucosa itself; after this, major digestion and absorption begin.

Pepsin, the proteolytic enzyme of the stomach, is active only in an acid environment (pH<4) so that enzymatic activity of gastric juice is dependent on the amount of acid secreted by parietal cells. Because of this important role of acid in normal digestion (as well as in ulcerogenesis), major attention in gastric physiology has always been placed on the study of acid secretion by the stomach.

Parietal (or oxyntic) cells secrete hydrogen ion (H^+) in a concentration that is more than a million times that of serum. The parietal cell seems to be stimulated by at least four endogenous chemical agents as well as by digested protein, which apparently has the capacity of stimulating the parietal cell without intermediation. The endogenous chemicals are acetylcholine released from the postganglionic vagal fibers in the fundic mucosa, gastrin from G cells in the antrum and duodenum, the intestinal phase hormone (entero-oxyntin) and histamine from fundic mast cells. Grossman and Konturek[1] have proposed that the parietal cell has multiple receptor sites and that maximal stimulation of the cell may be achieved only when each of these sites is occupied. An adaptation of this suggestion is shown schematically in Figure 1. This hypothesis would explain why a blockade of the receptors for any one of these agents (for example, blockade of the acetylcholine receptor by atropine or of the histamine receptor by an H_2-blocking agent [Cimetidine]) will greatly diminish the response to other stimulants.

GASTRIC JUICE

SITES OF SECRETION. — The glands in the gastric fundus contain chief cells that secrete pepsinogen, parietal cells that secrete intrinsic factor and an isotonic solution of HCl (about 165 mM), epithelial cells that probably secrete extracellular fluid (nonparietal secretion) and mucous neck cells that secrete mucus. There are other specialized cells. Gastrin (G) cells within the antral glands synthesize, store and secrete gastrin. Mast cells store heparin, histamine and other vasoactive substances within their granules. A large number of fundic argentaffin cells are present whose function is unknown. Perhaps they synthesize or store enteroglucagon or vasoactive intestinal peptide (VIP) or other hormones. The junction between antral mucosa (shown shaded in Figure 1) and fundic mucosa cannot be seen grossly; application of a pH indicator to the surface of the mucosa after administration of a secretory stimulant will quickly and clearly differentiate the proximal acid-secreting mucosa from the distal neutral antrum.

COMPOSITION. — The daily volume of gastric juice in the adult man varies between 2 and 3 L. According to the two-component theory of Hollander[2, 3] (discussed by Hunt and Wan[4]), gastric juice is composed of parietal and nonparietal components, both of which are iso-osmolar with respect to plasma. The pH of pure parietal cell secretion is about 0.78 (equivalent to 165 mEq of H^+/L). In addition to this H^+, pure parietal cell secretion contains between 165 – 170 mEq Cl^-/L and about 7 mEq K^+/L; the juice is free of sodium.[2, 3] Nonparietal secretion, which is virtually identical with extracellular fluid, has sodium (150 mEq/L) as its chief cation; H^+ is virtually absent. The concentration of acid in gastric juice is dependent, therefore, on the rate of parietal cell secretion and on the degree of admixture with nonparietal secretion as well as the buffering action of ingested food. Gastric juice has a pH of 1 – 2 during fasting. After ingestion of a meal, the pH of the fundus rises to that of the meal mixed with saliva. With secretion of acid, the pH of the mixture gradually falls.

MEASUREMENT OF GASTRIC ACID SECRETION. — Studies on gastric secretion have been made in animals with and without specialized gastric pouches, and in man. The most common experimental preparations are denervated pouches of fundic mucosa (Heidenhain) or simple gastric fistulas that drain the entire stomach. Pavlov pouches are innervated segments of fundic mucosa, which have the advantage of providing juice from innervated pouches that are free from contamination by food. The usefulness of a pouch is its ability to serve as an indicator of what is happening in the main stomach. However, it is not always an accurate indicator since, for example, the secretion from a Heidenhain pouch is responsive only to humoral stimulation. Raising the pH of the main stomach may have the effect of actually prolonging release of gastrin, thereby stimulating release of acid from the Heidenhain pouch.

In man, gastric secretion is measured by collecting gastric juice from a nasogastric tube. Gastric juice is collected for fixed time periods and each sample is titrated to pH 7. Results are expressed in terms of volume for a given period (usually one hour), in acid concentration (mEq/L) and in acid output (usually in mEq/hour). The number of milliequivalents of acid secreted per hour is a valuable index of parietal cell function. The upper limit of normal of basal acid output (BAO) is 6 mEq/hour in men and 4 mEq/hour in women; the upper limit of normal maximal stimulated acid output (MAO) is 40 mEq/hour in men and 30 mEq/hour in women. The MAO seems to be directly related to the number of parietal cells in the fundic mucosa. An MAO of 20 mEq/hour corresponds to a total parietal cell population of one billion cells.[5] The relationship between stimulated acid secretion and parietal cell mass does not hold true under all circumstances; for example, vagotomy causes a diminution in MAO without changing the parietal cell mass.

Acid secretion may be collected overnight, but the difficulties of prolonged collections are so great that shorter periods are preferable. Older studies on acid secretion used terms such as free acid, combined acid, degrees of acidity and clinical unit—these are obsolete and should be abandoned.

Acid secretion should be measured after an overnight fast. The first 30-minute specimen should be discarded and the second 30-minute specimen should be regarded as the basal collection. A secretory stimulus is then administered in a dose that will yield maximal secretory output. Stimulants in standard use and the doses administered for maximal output are shown in

TABLE 1.—DOSAGES OF STIMULANTS FOR
MAXIMAL ACID OUTPUT

STIMULANT	DOSAGE
Pentagastrin	6 μg/kg subcutaneously
	(6 μg/kg/hr intravenously)
Betazole (Histalog)	1.5 to 2.0 mg/kg subcutaneously
Histamine acid phosphate	40 μg/kg subcutaneously
	(40 μg/kg/hr intravenously)
Gastrin (synthetic human gastrin,	2 μg/kg subcutaneously
Imperial Chemical Industries)	(1 μg/kg/hr intravenously)
Insulin (crystalline)	0.2 U/kg/hr intravenously

TABLE 2. – UPPER LIMIT OF NORMAL FOR
ACID OUTPUT (mEq/hr)

	BASAL ACID OUTPUT	MAXIMAL ACID OUTPUT
Women	4	30
Men	6	40

Table 1. It is useful to assign arbitrary values for the upper limit of normal gastric acid output. These values are given in Table 2.

There has been much dissatisfaction with the use of insulin-stimulated gastric secretion, especially as related to the Hollander test for completeness of vagotomy. We no longer use the Hollander test. The reasons for this change in attitude have been summarized:[6] induction of insulin hypoglycemia in older patients, especially those with cardiovascular disease, may be dangerous and several deaths have been reported; gastric secretory tests are of little value in diagnosing recurrent ulcer and insulin tests are no better than any other in separating patients

Fig 2. – Mean gastric acid secretion in response to a 10% amino acid meal (varying in pH) in 9 duodenal ulcer and 12 normal subjects. * = significant increase over basal levels; ** = significant difference between duodenal ulcer and normal subjects; *** = significantly less than peak. (Adapted from Thompson, J. C., and Swierczek, J. S.: Acid and endocrine responses to meals varying in pH in normal and duodenal ulcer subjects, Ann. Surg. 186:541, 1977).

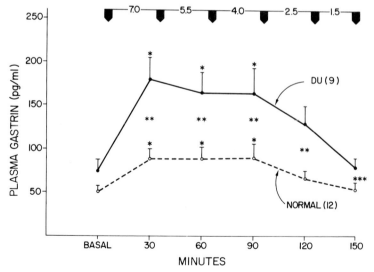

with recurrence from those without recurrence; the notion that insulin-stimulated acid secretion is mediated only by the vagus is unproven (since antrectomy alone may result in a negative Hollander test, the entire anatomic significance of insulin testing must be reassessed); although insulin tests probably detect most incomplete vagotomies, as few as 60% of patients with recurrent ulcer will have a positive response; 10% of patients with positive Hollander tests and 2% of patients with negative Hollander tests will develop recurrent ulceration. Because the test is difficult to interpret, because it is dangerous, and because it provides no better discrimination than does any other secretory test, we have replaced it with determination of maximal acid output using Histalog (betazole) or pentagastrin.

By means of a technique for the intragastric titration of acid secreted in response to the instillation of a meal,[7] it has been possible to show that patients with duodenal ulcer manifest a consistent hypersecretion of acid in response to the more physiologic type of stimulation provided by a meal (Fig 2).[8, 9]

MECHANISMS OF STIMULATION

Gastric secretion may be spontaneous (basal or interdigestive) or may be stimulated (or prandial). Spontaneous secretion occurs without known stimulation in man and in certain other species and may reflect a basal secretion of gastrin or acetylcholine or other agents. Pavlov in 1892 observed that food stimulation of gastric secretion could be brought about by a stimulus from the head or from the stomach (this work was reported in English in 1902[10]); later it was found that stimuli also may arise from the intestine.

The cephalic phase of gastric secretion is stimulated by the sight or smell or chewing of food. The gastric phase is stimulated by the presence of food in the stomach and the intestinal phase is stimulated by food in the small intestine. These co-called phases of gastric secretion originally were thought to be quite separate and distinct and to bring about temporally distinct stimulation of secretion. It is now known that gastrin is released by the vagus and that gastric distention brings about stimulation of vago-vagal reflexes, that gastrin and acetylcholine (and probably the intestinal phase stimuli and perhaps histamine) may potentiate one another and that with minor variations, the periods of secretions stimulated by each of the phases over-lap extensively. Nonetheless, secretion will be discussed here under the three phases because of historical acceptance of this concept.

CEPHALIC PHASE. — The sight or smell of food stimulates the vagal nuclei in the medulla, which intiates impulses that tra-verse the peripheral vagi and terminate in the gastric mucosa with the release of acetylcholine from vagal nerve endings. Re-lease of acetylcholine in fundic mucosa directly stimulates acid secretion by the parietal cell and the release of pepsinogen by chief cells. Release of acetylcholine in the antral mucosa in the region of G cells brings about vagal release of gastrin.

GASTRIC PHASE. — Food in the stomach stimulates gastric se-cretion by direct contact and by distention. Distention of the fundus of the stomach excites the vago-vagal reflex. Distention of the antrum brings about release of the hormone gastrin, first discovered by Edkins in 1905.[11, 12] Gastrin is liberated from the antral mucosa by acetylcholine (released either by long vagal fibers or by local reflexes on antral distention) and on direct con-tact with certain chemicals (for example, 2-carbon alcohols, small peptides, amino acids and calcium).

One of the most important aspects of the mechanisms for gas-trin release is its acid sensitivity. When in the course of gastric secretion the surface pH of the antral mucosa reaches 3.5, out-put of gastrin is diminished. When it reaches about 1.5, further secretion of gastrin is halted completely. As is true with other endocrine organs, there seems to be a closed-loop inverse rela-tionship between the concentration of the hormone and the out-put of the end organ; in this case, the relationship is between gastrin and H^+. Gastrin stimulates secretion of acid and a con-centration of H^+ sufficient to drop the pH of the antral mucosa below 3.5 – 1.5 diminishes and then halts gastrin output.

INTESTINAL PHASE.[13] — The intestinal phase of gastric secretion can be stimulated by food, especially proteins, or acid in the proximal jejunum (see Fig 1). Jejunal distention also appears to stimulate acid secretion from the stomach. The humoral agent of intestinal stimulation of gastric secretion has not been identi-fied, but it does not appear to be either cholecystokinin or gas-trin from extra-antral sources.[14] Portacaval shunting is known to augment the gastric secretory response to a meal. This increase is thought to be due to an "unmasking" of the intestinal phase secretagogue that is normally inactivated on transit of the liver.[13, 15]

MECHANISM OF INHIBITION

Once the flow of gastric juice has been initiated by stimuli evoked by eating, how is secretion halted? Vagal activity ceases when cephalic stimulation is removed, but probably the most important control mechanism is the secretion of acid itself, which acts to block further release of gastrin and to initiate active duodenal suppression of gastric secretion. Acidification of the antrum clearly suppresses further release of gastrin.[16] For years there was a question of whether antral acidification might, in addition, release a separate inhibitory hormone. The evidence for such an antral chalone has been reviewed[17]; the weight of evidence clearly is against existence of a separate agent.

There is clear evidence for the role of the duodenum in the inhibition of gastric secretion.[13, 18] Secretion from the stomach is inhibited by the presence of acid, fat or hypertonic solutions in the duodenum. Acidification of the duodenum inhibits gastric secretion. It also releases secretin, which is known to inhibit gastrin-stimulated gastric secretion and to suppress gastrin release.[14] Secretin has been proposed as the enterogastrone from the duodenum,[19] but gastric inhibitory polypeptide (GIP) is more likely the agent responsible for the humoral inhibition previously ascribed to enterogastrone.[14, 20] Fat in the duodenum in an absorbable form is a highly effective inhibitor of gastric secretion. Gastric inhibitory polypeptide is released by fat and probably mediates this inhibition.[20] Other humoral agents from the duodenum that may be involved in inhibition of gastric secretion are VIP, serotonin (the vasoactive amine produced from enterochromaffin cells) and GLI (the term proposed by Unger for the peptide found in the small intestine that possesses glucagon-like immunoreactivity)[21] (see Fig 1).

Hypertonic solutions of sugars, salts and peptone inhibit gastric secretion, apparently by stimulating a duodenal osmoreceptor that may release an unidentified humoral inhibitor. We have recent (unpublished) evidence showing that hyperosmolar solutions in the duodenum suppress the release of antral gastrin. Whether nervous reflexes play a primary or a permissive role in duodenal inhibition has not been clarified.

Gastrointestinal Hormones Involved in Gastric Secretion

Recent reviews are available on gastrin[22-24] and on other gastrointestinal hormones.[14, 25, 26] A brief summary of the information available on various humoral agents involving gastric secretion will be provided here.

GASTRIN

Although Edkins had reported stimulation of acid secretion from extracts of antral mucosa as early as 1905,[11, 12] it was not until 1964 that the biochemical era in the study of gastrointestinal hormones was initiated when Gregory and Tracy reported the isolation, purification and synthesis of gastrin.[27, 28] The first form of isolated gastrin (later to be known as little gastrin or G-17) was composed of 17 L-amino acids arranged in a linear form with a molecular weight of around 2100 (Table 3). Gastrin was found to exist in two variants, forms I and II which are identical except for an esterified sulfate attached to the tyrosyl residue of gastrin II. The N-terminus of the molecule is blocked by a pyroglutamyl group and the C-terminus is blocked with an amide group. The molecule has no basic amino acids; it is therefore strongly acidic and is only slightly soluble in dilute acid. Gastrin heptadecapeptides, G-17-I and G-17-II, have been isolated and purified from the antral mucosa of man, hog, cow, sheep, dog and cat (see Table 3). The C-terminal four amino acids of the gastrin molecule ($Trp-Met-Asp-Phe-NH_2$) have been shown to possess the full physiologic range of action of the parent molecule. This material is now available (with a prosthetic beta-alanine group attached to the N-terminus) as pentagastrin (see Table 3).

Gastrin exists in a variety of sizes, the larger of which apparently contain the smaller ones (see Table 3).[22, 23] Minigastrin (G-14) contains the 14 C-amino acid residues of G-17. Big gastrin (G-34) has been found to be the predominant form in circulation, whereas little gastrin predominates in tissue. G-17 can be split enzymatically from G-34, which separates it from the ap-

TABLE 3.—THE GASTRIN-CHOLECYSTOKININ FAMILY OF HORMONES*

GASTRIN†	APPROXIMATE MOLECULAR WEIGHT I	APPROXIMATE MOLECULAR WEIGHT II	Sequence (positions 1–17)
Little gastrin (G-17)			
Man	2098	2178	Pyr‡-Gly-Pro-Trp-Leu-Glu-Glu-Glu-Glu-Glu-Ala-Tyr§(SO_3H)-Gly-Trp-Met-Asp-Phe-NH_2
Hog	2116	2196	-Met- (position 5)
Cow and sheep	2026	2106	-Val- (position 5)
Dog	2058	2138	-Met- (position 5) -Ala- (position 8)
Cat	2040	2120	-Ala- (position 9)
Minigastrin (G-14-I, 5-17)			
Man	1833		Trp-Leu-Glu-Glu-Glu-Ala-Tyr-Gly-Trp-Met-Asp-Phe-NH_2
Big gastrin (G-34-I)			
Man	3839		Pyr‡-Leu-Gly-Pro-Gln-Gly-His-Pro-Ser-Leu-Val-Ala-Asp-Pro-Ser-Lys-Lys- ⇒→ Gln-Gly-Pro-Trp-Leu-Glu-Glu-Glu-Glu-Glu-Ala-Tyr-Gly-Trp-Met-Asp-Phe-NH_2
Hog	3883		Pyr‡-Leu-Gly-Leu-Gly-His-Gly-His-Pro-Pro-Leu-Val-Ala-Asp-Leu-Ala-Lys-Lys- ⇒→ Gln-Gly-Pro-Trp-Met-Glu-Glu-Glu-Ala-Tyr-Gly-Trp-Met-Asp-Phe-NH_2
Pentagastrin	768		N-t-butyloxycarbonyl-β-Ala-Trp-Met-Asp-Phe-NH_2
Cholecystokinin (CCK-33)‖	3918		Lys-Ala-Pro-Ser-Gly-Arg-Val-Ser-Met-Ile-Lys-Asn-Leu-Gln-Ser-Leu-Asp-Pro-Ser-His-Arg-Ile-Ser-Arg-Asp-Ala-Tyr(SO_3H)-Met-Gly-Trp-Met-Asp-Phe-NH_2

*Modified from Thompson, J. C.: The Stomach and Duodenum, in Sabiston, D. C. (ed.): Christopher's *Textbook of Surgery* (Philadelphia: W. B. Saunders, 1977), p. 905.
†Except where noted, the amino acid sequences for gastrins of different species are identical.
‡Pyr = pyroglutamyl.
§Gastrin of each species exists in form I and II; in form I, there is no SO_3H attached to Tyr in position 12.
‖Points of cleavage by trypsin.
¶Another form of CCK with 39 amino acid residues [CCK-39] has been isolated; the two forms are equally potent. The larger form is not yet chemically characterized.

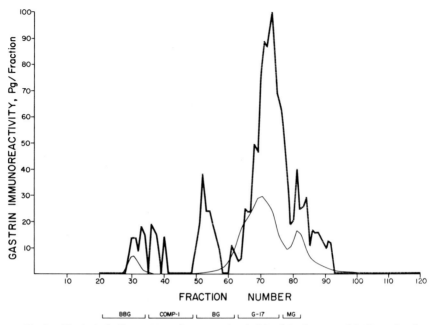

Fig 3. — Typical elution pattern from portal vein blood during acetylcholine stimulation of the antrum of a dog. The fine-line graph on the ordinate depicts, from right to left, the measured radioactivity of first the ^{125}I peak and then the larger labeled G-17 peak. Gastrin immunoreactivity of eluate fractions is determined by gastrin radioimmunoassay. The fractions labeled BBG (big-big gastrin), Comp-1 (Rehfeld's Component 1), BG (big gastrin), G-17 (heptadecapeptide gastrin), and MG (minigastrin) shown at the bottom of the figure are derived from the location occupied by specific markers placed upon the column. This figure demonstrates that the major gastrinlike immunoreactivity in the portal vein is in the G-17 fragment. (Adapted from Thompson et al.: Patterns of release and uptake of heterogeneous forms of gastrin, in Thompson, J. C. (ed.): *Gastrointestinal Hormones* (Austin: University of Texas Press, 1975), pp. 125–151.

parently inactive N-terminal tryptic residue of 17-amino acids. Two larger forms of gastrin (Component I of Rehfeld and big-big gastrin) have been identified by chromatography, but their molecular structure and physiologic functions are unknown. It is possible to demonstrate the various forms of gastrin by Sephadex gel column filtration of serum with subsequent determination of gastrinlike immunoreactivity in the component fractions. Figure 3 shows such a pattern of gel filtration of gastrin in portal vein blood obtained during stimulation of gastrin release by the application of acetylcholine to the antrum of a dog.

The physiologic actions and metabolic functions of gastrin

have been reviewed recently.[22, 23] The most remarkable action of gastrin is its profound ability to stimulate secretion of gastric acid by the parietal cell; G-17 is 30 times more potent than histamine by weight and 500 times more potent on a molar basis. Administered in amounts that are probably supraphysiologic, gastrin seems to have many motor and secretory actions on various target organs in the gut, liver and pancreas. In addition to its effect on acid secretion, the only actions of gastrin that have been shown to be caused by physiologic concentrations of the hormone are stimulation of pepsin secretion and of gastric mucosal blood flow. Gastrin does have a pronounced growth hormonelike effect on the stomach and pancreas and it has been shown to stimulate pancreatic enzyme secretion in man. These latter actions are probably physiologic.

Gastrin appears to be synthesized and is stored by specialized G cells in the pyloric glands of antral mucosa[29] (Fig 4) and in the mucosa of the proximal small intestine.[30] Gastrin is present in fundic mucosa in concentrations of 1×10^{-12} by weight, whereas in antral mucosa the concentration is more than 1,000 times greater.[31] In man, duodenal mucosa contains 10% – 20% as much gastrin as does the antrum.[32]

Gastrin is released by mechanical, neural or chemical stimuli that act on the G cell,[23] and it is carried by the blood to effector sites in various organs. Gastrin, cholecystokinin and secretin all seem to act on the same target organs; because of their structural similarity (see Table 3), gastrin and cholecystokinin probably act upon the same receptor site.[33] Secretin,[34] as well as other members of the secretin family of hormones (glucagon,[35] GIP and VIP[36]), has been shown to block the action of gastrin on the parietal cell, in addition to suppressing the food-stimulated release of gastrin.[34] Calcium given intravenously[37] or orally[38] stimulates gastric secretion by releasing gastrin. Cyclic AMP may be involved as an intraparietal cell second messenger in the stimulation of acid secretion, but the current evidence that gastrin works by this pathway is, at best, inconclusive.[39]

Gastrin has been shown to disappear rapidly from circulation[40] and the kidney has been thought to be the main organ of catabolism.[41] There are recent studies[42] which indicate that gastrin may be picked up by nearly all tissues.

The Zollinger-Ellison syndrome[43] of massive gastric hypersecretion and peptic ulceration was shown by Gregory and

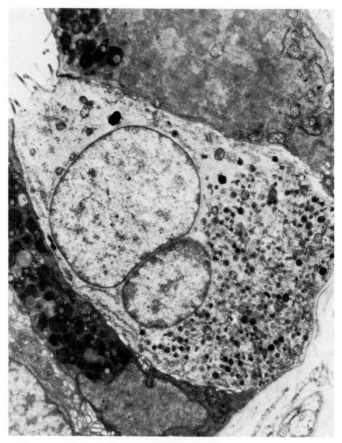

Fig 4.—Electronmicrograph of a G (gastrin) cell in antral mucosa (×3000). Dark granules contain gastrin. Note that microvilli at apex of cell reach into lumen of antral gland, providing opportunity for direct contact with stimulants and inhibitors of gastrin release. (Courtesy of J. Lechago, M.D.)

colleagues[44, 45] to be caused by high levels of circulating gastrin elaborated by gastrinomas of the pancreas or duodenum. Hypergastrinemia is also seen in patients with pernicious anemia (due to loss of acid inhibition of antral gastrin release), in patients with the antral exclusion operation (which results in permanent sequestration of antral mucosa in the alkaline environment of the duodenum), in chronic renal failure (thought to be due to loss of normal renal catabolism)[46] and occasionally in patients with pyloric outlet obstruction.

Detailed studies on the metabolism of gastrin have been made possible by the development of specific and highly sensitive radioimmunoassay methods. Normal values for the concentration of gastrin in serum vary according to technique. Most basal values in man are under 100 pg/ml and the upper limit of normal in our assay is 200 pg/ml. Many patients with the Zollinger-Ellison syndrome have serum gastrin levels that are greater than 1,000 pg/ml and some have values as high as 100,000 pg/ml.

We recently have reviewed the relationship between gastrin and peptic ulcer disease.[23] Since gastrin stimulates secretion of gastric acid and since the duodenal ulcer diathesis is associated with hypersecretion of acid, it was common, before the days of radioimmunoassay, to assume that patients with duodenal ulcer would have high levels of circulating gastrin. Such is not the case.[47, 48] Only in the Zollinger-Ellison syndrome (and in rare patients with antral exclusion) is acid hypersecretion caused by hypergastrinemia. Basal gastrin levels in duodenal ulcer patients are normal. Duodenal ulcer patients do release more gastrin in a more rapid fashion in response to a standard meal than do normal individuals[9, 48-50] (Fig 5). Because duodenal ulcer pa-

Fig 5. – Plasma gastrin levels in response to stimulation of a 10% amino acid meal in 9 duodenal ulcer patients and 12 normal subjects. * = an increase above basal values; ** = significant difference between duodenal ulcer and normal subjects; *** = significantly less than peak *and* significant difference between duodenal ulcer and normal subjects. (Reprinted with permission from Thompson, J. C., and Swierczek, J. S.: Acid and endocrine responses to meals varying in pH in normal and duodenal ulcer subjects, Ann. Surg. 186:541, 1977).

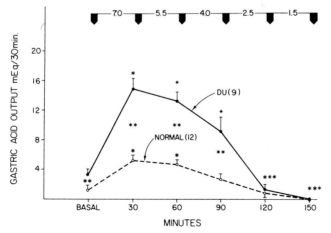

tients do seem to release more gastrin in spite of acid hypersecretion, the effectiveness of the biofeedback mechanism for inhibition of gastrin release in ulcer patients has been questioned[8]; we found no evidence of defective feedback inhibition of gastric secretion or of gastrin release in duodenal ulcer subjects.[9]

After truncal vagotomy and drainage, gastric acid secretion is diminished but gastrin values increase, presumably because of the loss of acid inhibition. We found that all types of vagotomy currently in practice cause an increase of basal and of postprandial levels of serum gastrin.[6]

Patients with gastric ulcer have higher concentrations of serum gastrin than do patients with duodenal ulcer, presumably because of lower acid output. In patients with gastric achlorhydria, serum gastrin levels are apt to be very high and the instillation of acid into the stomach causes an abrupt fall in serum gastrin levels.

It is now possible, in most clinical settings, to obtain radioimmunoassay measurement of serum gastrin concentrations. Gastrin levels should be measured in any patient in whom the Zollinger-Ellison syndrome is suspected, and specifically in patients with recurrent peptic ulcers or recurrent peptic ulcer symptoms after an acid-reducing operation; in patients with a duodenal ulcer and massive hypersecretion of acid (>15 mEq/hour basal); in patients with duodenal ulcer and diarrhea; in patients with duodenal ulcer and hypercalcemia; in ulcer patients with relatives who have the Zollinger-Ellison syndrome or the multiple endocrine adenoma I syndrome; in patients who have postbulbar or jejunal peptic ulcers; in patients whose upper gastrointestinal radiologic studies are suggestive of the Zollinger-Ellison syndrome; in patients under 20 years of age with duodenal ulcers; and in postoperative patients in whom inadvertent exclusion of antral mucosa is suspected.

CHOLECYSTOKININ

Cholecystokinin is a 33-amino acid straight-chain peptide with a molecular weight of 3918 (see Table 3). The C-terminal 5-amino acids of gastrin and of cholecystokinin are identical; because of this shared group, cholecystokinin and gastrin have similar physiologic actions. I have reviewed the structure-function interrelations between gastrin and cholecystokinin.[51]

The main action of cholecystokinin is to stimulate contraction of the gallbladder and to stimulate secretion of enzymes by the pancreas.[14]Acting alone, cholecystokinin is a stimulant of gastric acid secretion, about one third as potent as gastrin. In the presence of the gastrin, however, cholecystokinin acts as a competitive inhibitor of gastric secretion. Since cholecystokinin is released physiologically after a meal[52] as is gastrin, the physiologic role of cholecystokinin is probably that of a competitive inhibitor of gastric secretion.[51]

SECRETIN

In 1902 Bayliss and Starling[53] demonstrated that introduction of hydrochloric acid into an isolated loop of small intestine elicited the brisk secretion of pancreatic juice. They understood the implications of this observation immediately and suggested that some unidentified blood-borne chemical messenger was released from the acidified intestine to mediate this response. The entire field of endocrinology began with this observation.

The amino acid sequence of secretin was provided in 1966 by Mutt and Jorpes,[54] who described a 27-amino acid peptide with a molecular weight of 3055 (Table 4). Secretin, glucagon, GIP and

TABLE 4.—THE SECRETIN-GLUCAGON FAMILY OF HORMONES*

Secretin (molecular weight, 3055; 27 amino acids)

His-Ser-Asp-Gly-Thr-Phe-Thr-Ser-Glu-Leu-Ser-Arg-Leu-Arg-Asp-Ser-Ala-Arg-Leu-
   Gln-Arg-Leu-Leu-Gln-Gly-Leu-Val-NH₂

Glucagon (molecular weight, 3485; 29 amino acids)

His-Ser-Gln-Gly-Thr-Phe-Thr-Ser-Asp-Tyr-Ser-Lys-Tyr-Leu-Asp-Ser-Arg-Arg-Ala-
   Gln-Asp-Phe-Val-Gln-Trp-Leu-Met-Asp-Thr

GIP (Gastric Inhibitory Polypeptide) (molecular weight, 5104; 43 amino acids)

Tyr-Ala-Glu-Gly-Thr-Phe-Ile-Ser-Asp-Tyr-Ser-Ile-Ala-Met-Asp-Lys-Ile-Arg-Gln-Gln-
   Asp-Phe-Val-Asn-Trp-Leu-Leu-Ala-Gln-Gln-Lys-Gly-Lys-Lys-Ser-Asp-Trp-Lys-
   His-Asn-Ile-Thr-Gln

VIP (Vasoactive intestinal peptide) (molecular weight, 3326; 28 amino acids)

His-Ser-Asp-Ala-Val-Phe-Thr-Asp-Asn-Tyr-Thr-Arg-Leu-Arg-Lys-Gln-Met-Ala-
   Val-Lys-Lys-Tyr-Leu-Asn-Ser-Ile-Leu-Asn-NH₂

*Modified from Thompson[26] with minor corrections of molecular weights; all sequences listed are from porcine species.

VIP share many structural similarities (for example, of the 27 amino acids in secretin, 14 occupy the same position as in glucagon) and for this reason, the four agents are grouped together into the so-called secretin-glucagon family of hormones. Secretin is a strongly basic molecule. The amino acids between position 5 and position 13 form a helix (it has been suggested that the helix is necessary for full biologic activity[55]).

Secretin is widely distributed in the mucosa of the small intestine, with maximal concentration in the proximal duodenum. We have shown that there is considerable secretin immunoreactivity in ileal mucosa.[56] Since the degree of acidification required to release secretin is never achieved in these distal locations, the role played by these secretin stores in the jejunoileum

Fig 6.—Electronmicrograph of a portion of an S cell in transitional area of duodenal mucosa (×7000). Dark granules contain secretin. (Courtesy of E. Solcia, M.D.)

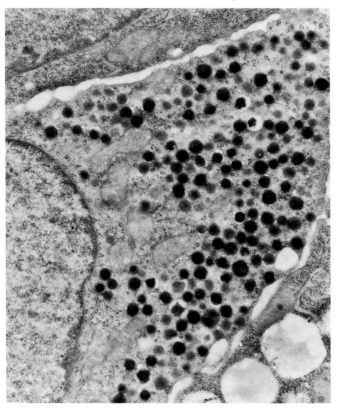

is unknown. Secretin immunoreactivity is localized to specialized S-cells (Fig 6) which are present between the crypts and villi of small bowel mucosa where a maximal concentration of secretin has been extracted.[57, 58]

Secretin is released by H^+ and concentrations of acid sufficient to lower the pH below 5.5 are required for release. Secretin is not released by vagal stimulation or irrigation of the duodenal mucosa with acetylcholine.[59] The amount of secretin released depends on the amount of acid bathing the mucosa and the linear extent of mucosa exposed to acidification. Once the release of secretin has begun, continued stimulation is pH-dependent, and raising the pH above 4.5 will suppress further release of secretin.[60] A typical endocrine closed-loop relationship exists between secretin and HCO_3^-. Secretin stimulates pancreatic secretion of HCO_3^- into the duodenum and the HCO_3^- neutralizes the H^+ from the stomach, raises the pH and eventually halts release secretin in dogs or cats.[62]

Alcohol has been suggested as a releasing agent for secretin,[61] but we have provided evidence that the alcohol probably acts by

Fig 7.—Plasma secretin response to a 10% amino acid meal adjusted to pH 7.0–1.5. * = significant increase above basal level. (Reprinted with permission from Thompson, J. C., and Swierczek, J. S.: Acid and endocrine responses to meals varying in pH in normal and duodenal ulcer subjects, Ann. Surg. 186:541, 1977)

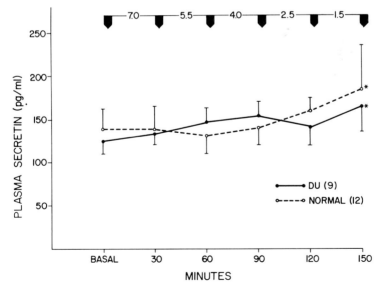

stimulating acid secretion from the stomach, which in turn releases secretin. Direct duodenal irrigation with alcohol does not release secretin in dogs or cats.[62]

Contrary to an early suggestion,[63] a defect in the mechanism for secretin release in duodenal ulcer patients has not been confirmed[9, 64] (Fig 7). It appears unlikely, then, that a defect in the mechanism for the release of secretin is involved in the pathogenesis of duodenal ulcer.

The primary action of secretin is to stimulate pancreatic secretion of water and bicarbonate.[65] Bicarbonate secretion from the pancreas is roughly equivalent to the secretion of acid by the stomach; and neutralization of acid by bicarbonate occurs in the crucible of the duodenum. In the stomach, secretin stimulates pepsin secretion, stimulates the pyloric sphincter, inhibits gastrin-stimulated acid secretion, inhibits food-stimulated gastrin release and inhibits motility.[14] In the pancreas, secretin stimulates the secretion of water and bicarbonate and also some enzyme secretion, largely due to a washout phenomenon. It stimulates the release of insulin and inhibits the release of glucagon. Secretin inhibits contraction of the lower esophageal sphincter. Stimulation of pancreatic bicarbonate secretion by secretin is mediated by the cyclic AMP system. Secretin causes a dose-dependent increase in cyclic AMP content in pancreatic tissue and pancreatic juice.[66] Administration of exogenous secretin has been shown to suppress the release of gastrin in man and dogs. Hansky, Soveny and Korman[67] showed that secretin suppressed the release of gastrin in man in the basal state and we[34] observed that secretin suppressed food-stimulated release of gastrin but had no effect on basal gastrin in man and in dogs. Interestingly, secretin stimulates gastrin release in patients with Zollinger-Ellison tumors.[34, 68] In these patients, secretin infusion causes a brisk increase in circulating levels of gastrin as compared to a depression of postprandial levels in normal patients and patients with peptic ulcer disease. The mechanism underlying this gastrin release from Zollinger-Ellison tumors remains unclear, but it appears to be due to a direct action of secretin on gastrinoma cells.[69]

Because secretin acts to neutralize acid produced by the stomach (by stimulating flow of bicarbonate into the duodenum) and because it blocks gastrin-stimulated gastric secretion and appears to interfere with release of gastrin, it has been proposed as nature's antacid. There were suggestions that it might be the long sought-after enterogastrone from the duodenum, but since it is not released by fat, this seems unlikely and GIP appears to be a more likely candidate.

GIP

Gastric inhibitory polypeptide was isolated by Brown and colleagues from mucosa of the upper small intestine in 1969.[70] Because of its inhibitory activity, the material was called gastric inhibitory polypeptide.[71] Gastric inhibitory polypeptide has 43 amino acids with a molecular weight of 5104 (see Table 4). Fifteen of the first 26 amino acids are in the same position as glucagon and 9 of the first 26 are in the same position as secretin. The material has been localized to specialize cells in the duodenum and in lesser number in the jejunum of man and dog.[72] Circulating levels of GIP show a biphasic response to food with an initial peak stimulated by glucose and a late plateau in response to fat.[20] Gastric inhibitory polypeptide inhibits secretion of gastric acid in pepsin and strongly suppresses the food-stimulated release of gastrin.[36] As a stimulant for the release of insulin, the time-course of release of GIP after administration of glucose orally suggests that the former may play an important physiologic role in insulin release.[20, 73] The role of GIP in inhibition of acid secretion in man is not clear-cut, and the physiologic significance of GIP in inhibition of acid secretion remains to be established.

VIP

Vasoactive intestinal polypeptide was first isolated from the mucosa of the upper small bowel by Said and Mutt in 1972.[74] The material is a 28-amino acid peptide with a molecular weight of 3326 (see Table 4). There is recent evidence that VIP, like secretin, exists in a helical configuration.[75]

Vasoactive intestinal polypeptide is widely distributed in the gut with especially high concentrations in the colon. Concentrations in many areas of the gut are higher in the muscular wall than in the mucosa. It is a potent vasodilator, it relaxes the muscles of the trachea and it is a strong inhibitor of histamine and gastrin-stimulated acid secretion. It stimulates the electrolyte and water secretion by the pancreas and increases flow of bile. The physiologic role of the hormone and its mechanisms of release are unknown.[14] Many now believe that it may have its most important function as a neurotransmitter. Considerable evidence has been accumulated that VIP may be the agent responsible for the pancreatic-cholera syndrome (watery diarrhea, hypokalemia and achlorhydria)[76]; a more recent report, however, has implicated prostaglandin E_1.[77]

GLUCAGON

Pancreatic glucagon is the hormone of energy release, as insulin is the hormone of energy storage. Pancreatic glucagon is responsible for glycogenolysis, gluconeogenesis and lipolysis. Glucagon inhibits gastric secretion, and we have shown that it is a powerful inhibitor of gastrin release.[35] Glucagon has 29 amino acids and has a molecular weight of 3484 (see Table 4). There is a peptide in the intestinal tract of man and animals that is identical with pancreatic glucagon. In addition, there is a peptide with a smaller molecular weight (2900) which has less biologic activity than pancreatic glucagon, but which cross-reacts exactly with specific glucagon antiserum. Unger's group[21] has proposed that the terms pancreatic glucagon and gut glucagon (or enteroglucagon) be restricted to the two compounds with a molecular weight of about 3500, and that the material of 2900 molecular weight be referred to as GLI (glucagonlike immunoreactivity).

Alimentary hyperglycemia in patients after gastric operations may be caused by loss of signals to the intestine from the antrum.[78] Patients studied had abnormally high levels of plasma GLI and insulin. Infusion of secretin diminished the hyperglycemia and lowered the GLI and insulin levels, which suggests that postgastrectomy hyperglycemia may be due to elevated GLI levels and that the beneficial action of secretin is due to suppression of GLI release.[79]

OTHER ACTIVE AGENTS

There are several other agents – some of them peptide hormones, some of them candidate hormones – that are known or are thought to influence gastric secretion. Some certainly will be accepted as members of the group of agents known to stimulate or inhibit gastric secretion; others probably will be rejected.

BOMBESIN. — Erspamer and colleagues[80, 81] isolated a 14-amino acid peptide from the skin of certain European frogs. When infused, this material causes stimulation of gastric acid secretion, contraction of the gallbladder, pancreatic secretion and the release of gastrin and cholecystokinin.[14] There is recent evidence that a bombesinlike compound may exist in the stomach and duodenum in man and other mammals which acts as a local releasing agent for gastrin.[14]

INTESTINAL PHASE HORMONE. — Gregory and Ivy[82] observed in 1941 that introduction of protein into the small intestine of dogs resulted in stimulation of gastric acid secretion. Portacaval shunting is known to augment the acid secretory response to a meal[83]; this increase probably is caused by an unmasking of the intestinal phase secretagogue which is normally inactivated by the liver.[15] Postprandial levels of serum gastrin are not increased after portacaval shunting[84] and jejunal acidification stimulates acid secretion without stimulating gastrin release[85]; these findings disqualify gastrin as the agent responsible for postshunt hypersecretion. The name "entero-oxyntin" has been proposed for the agent.[86] The major site of origin probably is the jejunum.[87]

SOMATOSTATIN. — Somatostatin is a 14-amino acid peptide (originally isolated from the hypothalamus) which has the property of suppressing the release of growth hormone.[88, 89] Bloom and colleagues[90] showed that somatostatin inhibits both fasting and stimulated levels of gastrin. This effect is independent of the suppression of growth hormone release, since it has been shown to occur in a hypophysectomized patient.[91] In addition, somatostatin directly inhibits the secretory processes of the parietal cell[92] and also suppresses the release of secretin.[93]

Bombesin and somatostatin may well function as local agents to stimulate and suppress the release of various gastrointestinal hormones.

SEROTONIN. — Serotonin, or 5-hydroxytryptamine, differs from all the previous agents mentioned in that it is not a peptide. It is a vasoactive amine secreted into the portal circulation. Its release from duodenal mucosa is stimulated by acidification. Jaffe and colleagues[94] recently have suggested that serotonin may be one of the physiologic messengers of duodenal inhibition of gastric secretion. They have shown by radioimmunoassay that serotonin is released after duodenal acidification. This rise in serotonin was found to be related closely to suppression of acid secretion from innervated, but not denervated, gastric pouches. They further demonstrated that, contrary to previous belief, much serotonin escapes hepatic deactivation, so that peripheral as well as portal concentrations of serotonin are raised after duodenal acidification.[94]

PROSTAGLANDINS. — Prostaglandins are 20-carbon fatty acids with molecular weights around 340.[94] There are at least three major groups (PGE, PGA and PGF) and each group contains a number of subdivisions which depend on the number of unsaturated double bonds in the side chain. For example, PGE_2 is a member of the "E" group of prostaglandins that has two double bonds in the side chain. Prostaglandins inhibit gastric secretion[96, 97] without suppressing release of gastrin.[96] There is abundant evidence that prostaglandins may be involved in at least two endocrine diarrheogenic syndromes, originally

Fig 8. — Agents that directly or indirectly stimulate or inhibit H^+ secretion from the parietal cell. CCK acting alone stimulates acid secretion; in the presence of gastrin (which is almost always the case under physiologic conditions), it is an inhibitor. (Adapted and modified from Baker, R. D.: *Teaching Syllabus*, Vol. V, [Department of Physiology and Biophysics, The University of Texas Medical Branch, Galveston].)

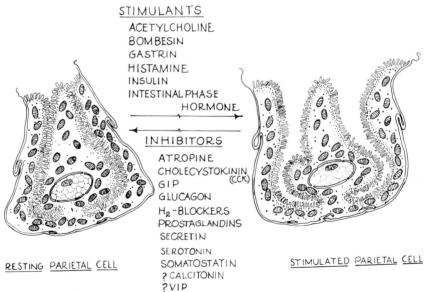

STIMULANTS
ACETYLCHOLINE
BOMBESIN
GASTRIN
HISTAMINE
INSULIN
INTESTINAL PHASE
    HORMONE

INHIBITORS
ATROPINE
CHOLECYSTOKININ (CCK)
GIP
GLUCAGON
H_2-BLOCKERS
PROSTAGLANDINS
SECRETIN
SEROTONIN
SOMATOSTATIN
? CALCITONIN
? VIP

RESTING PARIETAL CELL   STIMULATED PARIETAL CELL

thought to be caused by other agents.[77] The first of these is the Werner-Morrison syndrome of pancreatic cholera; the other is the carcinoid syndrome.

CALCITONIN. — Gastrin is known to release calcitonin. This has been used in tests for patients with possible calcitonin-secreting medullary carcinoma of the thyroid in the so-called multiple endocrine adenoma II syndrome.[98] Calcitonin is a potent inhibitor of basal or pentagastrin-stimulated gastric secretion in man.[99] We studied the effect of calcitonin infusions in patients with peptic ulcer and found that calcitonin produced significant depression of gastric secretion as well as food-stimulated release of gastrin.[100] These findings suggest that calcitonin may have a regulatory function in the release of gastrin.

Summary

Gastric secretion in response to a meal is stimulated by a variety of neurohumoral agents. Acidified chyme flowing into the duodenum evokes a series of events that bring about the neutralization of H^+ or suppression of further acid secretion. The actions of several proven and putative stimulatory and inhibitory agents are summarized in Figure 8.

REFERENCES

1. Grossman, M. I., and Konturek, S. J.: Inhibition of acid secretion in dog by metiamide, a histamine antagonist acting on H_2 receptors, Gastroenterology 66:517, 1974.

2. Hollander, F.: Gastric secretion of electrolytes, Fed. Proc. 11:706, 1952.

3. Hollander, F.: The significance of sodium and potassium in gastric secretion: A review, Gastroenterology 40:477, 1961.

4. Hunt J. N., and Wan, B.: Electrolytes of mammalian gastric juice, in American Physiological Society: Handbook of Physiology, Vol. II, Code, C. F. (ed.), (Baltimore: Williams & Wilkins Company, 1967), pp. 781–804.

5. Card, W. I., and Marks, I. N.: The relationship between the acid output of the stomach following "maximal" histamine stimulation and the parietal cell mass, Clin. Sci. 19:147, 1960.

6. Thompson, J. C., Fender, H. R., Watson, L. C., and Villar, H. V.: The effects on gastrin and gastric secretion of five current operations for duodenal ulcer, Ann. Surg. 183:599, 1976.

7. Fordtran, J. S., and Walsh, J. H.: Gastric acid secretion rate and buffer content of the stomach after eating, J. Clin. Invest. 52:645, 1973.

8. Walsh, J. H., Richardson, C. T., and Fordtran, J. S.: pH dependence of acid secretion and gastrin release in normal and ulcer subjects, J. Clin. Invest. 55:462, 1975.

9. Thompson, J. C., and Swierczek, J. S.: Acid and endocrine responses to meals varying in pH in normal and duodenal ulcer subjects, Ann. Surg. 186:541, 1977.

10. Pavlov, I. D.: *Lectures on the Work of the Digestive Glands* (London: Charles Griffin and Company, 1902).

11. Edkins, J. S.: On the chemical mechanism of gastric secretion, Proc. R. Soc. Lond. [Biol.] 76:376, 1905.

12. Edkins, J. S.: The chemical mechanism of gastric secretion, J. Physiol. 34:133, 1906.

13. Thompson, J. C., and Peskin, G. W.: The intestinal phase of gastric secretion, Am. J. Med. Sci. 241:253, 1961.

14. Rayford, P. L., Miller, T. A., and Thompson, J. C.: Secretin, cholecystokinin and newer gastrointestinal hormones, N. Engl. J. Med. 294: 1093; 1157, 1976.

15. Thompson, J. C.: Alterations in gastric secretion after portacaval shunting, Am. J. Surg. 117:854, 1969.

16. Woodward, E. R.: The role of the gastric antrum in the regulation of gastric secretion, Gastroenterology 38:7, 1960.

17. Thompson, J. C.: Antral chalone, in Grossman, M. I. et al.: Candidate hormones of the gut, Gastroenterology 67:730, 1974.

18. Andersson, S.: Gastric and duodenal mechanisms inhibiting gastric secretion of acid, in American Physiological Society: *Handbook of Physiology,* Vol. II, Code, C. F. (ed.) (Baltimore: Williams & Wilkins Company, 1967), pp. 865–877.

19. Johnson, L. R., and Grossman, M. I.: Secretin: The enterogastrone released by acid in the duodenum, Am. J. Physiol. 215:885, 1968.

20. Brown, J. C., Dryburgh, J. R., Moccia, P., and Pederson, R. A.: The current status of GIP, in Thompson, J. C. (ed.): *Gastrointestinal Hormones* (Austin: University of Texas Press, 1975), pp. 537–547.

21. Sasaki, H., Rubalcava, B., Srikant, C. B., Baetens, D., Orci, L., and Unger, R. H.: Gut glucagonoid (GLI) and gut glucagon. In: Thompson, J. C. (ed.): *Gastrointestinal Hormones* (Austin: University of Texas Press, 1975), pp. 519–528.

22. Walsh, J. H., and Grossman, M. I.: Gastrin, N. Engl. J. Med. 292: 1324; 1377, 1975.

23. Rayford, P. L., and Thompson, J. C.: Gastrin, Surg. Gynecol. Obstet. 145: 257, 1977.

24. Thompson, J. C.: Gastrin and gastric secretion, Ann. Rev. Med. 20:291, 1969.

25. Chey, W. Y. and Brooks, F. P. (eds.): *Endocrinology of the Gut* (Thorofare, N. J.: Charles B. Slack, 1974).

26. Thompson, J. C. (ed.): *Gastrointestinal Hormones* (Austin: University of Texas Press, 1975).

27. Gregory, R. A.: Memorial lecture: The isolation and chemistry of gastrin, Gastroenterology 51:953, 1966.

28. Gregory, R. A., and Tracy, H. J.: The constitution and properties of two gastrins extracted from hog antral mucosa, Gut 5:103, 1964.

29. McGuigan, J. E., and Greider, M. H.: Correlative immunochemical and

light microscopic studies of the gastric cell of the antral mucosa, Gastroenterology 60:223, 1971.

30. Watson, L. C., Reeder, D. D., Becker, H. D., LaGrone, L., and Thompson, J. C.: Gastrin concentrations in upper gastrointestinal mucosa in dogs, Surgery 76:419, 1974.

31. Jackson, B. M., Reeder, D. D., Hirose, F., and Thompson, J. C.: Correlation of the surface pH, histology, and gastrin concentration of gastric mucosa, Ann. Surg. 176:727, 1972.

32. Rehfeld, J. F., Stadil, F., Malmstrøm, J., and Miyata, M.: Gastrin heterogeneity in serum and tissue: A progress report, in Thompson, J. C. (ed.): *Gastrointestinal Hormones* (Austin: University of Texas Press, 1975), pp. 43–58.

33. Grossman, M. I.: Gastrin and its activities, Nature 228:1147, 1970.

34. Thompson, J. C., Reeder, D. D., Bunchman, H. H., Becker, H. D., and Brandt, E. N., Jr.: Effect of secretin on circulating gastrin, Ann. Surg. 176:384, 1972.

35. Becker, H. D., Reeder, D. D., and Thompson, J. C.: The effect of glucagon on circulating gastrin, Gastroenterology 65:28, 1973.

36. Villar, H. V., Fender, H. R., Rayford, P. L., Bloom, S. R., Ramus, N. I., and Thompson, J. C.: Suppression of gastrin release and gastric secretion by gastric inhibitory polypeptide (GIP) and vasoactive intestinal polypeptide (VIP), Ann. Surg. 184:97, 1976.

37. Reeder, D. D., Becker, H. D., and Thompson, J. C.: Effect of intravenously administered calcium on serum gastrin and gastric secretion in man, Surg. Gynecol. Obstet. 138:847, 1974.

38. Reeder, D. D., Conlee, J. L., and Thompson, J. C.: Effect of calcium carbonate antacid on serum gastrin concentrations in duodenal ulcer patients, Surg. Forum 22:308, 1971.

39. Jacobson, E. D., and Thompson, W. J.: Cyclic AMP and gastric secretion: The illusive second messenger, in *Advances in Cyclic Nucleotide Research* (New York: Raven Press, 1976), pp. 199–224.

40. Villar, H. V., Reeder, D. D., Rayford, P. L., and Thompson, J. C.: Rate of disappearance of circulating endogenous gastrin in dogs, Surgery 81:404, 1977.

41. Thompson, J. C., Rayford, P. L., Ramus, N. I., Fender, H. R., and Villar, H. V.: Patterns of release and uptake of heterogeneous forms of gastrin, in Thompson, J. C. (ed.): *Gastrointestinal Hormones* (Austin: University of Texas Press, 1975), pp. 125–151.

42. Strunz, U. T., Walsh, J. H., and Grossman, M. I.: Removal of gastrin by various organs in dogs, Gastroenterology 74:32, 1978.

43. Zollinger, R. M., and Ellison, R. H.: Primary peptic ulcerations of the jejunum associated with islet cell tumor of pancreas, Ann. Surg. 142:709, 1955.

44. Gregory, R. A., Grossman, M. I., Tracy, H. J., and Bentley, P. H.: Nature of the gastric secretagogue in Zollinger-Ellison tumors, Lancet 2:543, 1967.

45. Gregory, R. A., and Tracy, H. J.: A note on the nature of the gastrin-like stimulant present in Zollinger-Ellison tumours, Gut 5:115, 1964.

80   JAMES C. THOMPSON

46. Hansky, J., King, R. W., and Holdsworth, S.: Serum gastrin in chronic renal failure, in Thompson, J. C. (ed.): *Gastrointestinal Hormones* (Austin: University of Texas Press, 1975), pp. 115–124.
47. Petersen, H., Schrumpf, E., and Myren, J.: Fasting serum gastrin and basal gastric acid secretion, Scand. J. Gastroenterol. 10:721, 1975.
48. Walsh, J. H., and Grossman, M. I.: Circulating gastrin in peptic ulcer disease, Mt. Sinai J. Med. 40:374, 1973.
49. Reeder, D. D., Jackson, B. M., Ban, J. L., Davidson, W. D., and Thompson, J. C.: Effect of food on serum gastrin concentrations in duodenal ulcer and control patients, Surg. Forum 21:290, 1970.
50. Chayvialle, J. A., Lambert, R., Touillon, C., and Moussa, F.: Antral acidification and gastrin release in man, in Thompson, J. C. (ed.): *Gastrointestinal Hormones* (Austin: University of Texas Press, 1975), pp. 447–459.
51. Thompson, J. C.: Chemical structure and biological actions of gastrin, cholecystokinin and related compounds, in Holton, P. (ed.): *The International Encyclopedia of Pharmacology and Therapeutics* (Oxford: Pergamon Press Ltd., 1973), pp. 261–286.
52. Thompson, J. C., Fender, H. R., Ramus, N. I., Villar, H. V., and Rayford, P. L.: Cholecystokinin metabolism in man and dogs, Ann. Surg. 182:496, 1975.
53. Bayliss, W. M., and Starling, E. H.: The mechanisms of pancreatic secretion, J. Physiol. (Lond.) 28:325, 1902.
54. Mutt, V., and Jorpes, J. E.: Secretin: Isolation and Determination of Structure. Paper presented at the Fourth International Symposium on the Chemistry of Natural Products, Stockholm, June 26–July 2, 1966.
55. Grossman, M. I.: Structure of secretin, Gastroenterology 57:610, 1969.
56. Miller, T. A., Llanos, O. L., Swierczek, J. S., Rayford, P. L., and Thompson, J. C.: Concentrations of gastrin and secretin in the alimentary tract of the cat, Surgery 83:90, 1978.
57. Krawitt, E. L., Zimmerman, G. R., and Clifton, J. A.: Localization of secretin in dog duodenal mucosa, Am. J. Physiol. 211:935, 1966.
58. Solcia, E., Polak, J. M., Buffa, R., Capella, C., and Pearse, A. G. E.: Endocrine cells of the intestinal mucosa, in Thompson, J. C. (ed.): *Gastrointestinal Hormones* (Austin: University of Texas Press, 1975), pp. 155–168.
59. Sum, P. T., Schipper, H. L., and Preshaw, R. M.: Canine gastric and pancreatic secretion during intestinal distention and intestinal perfusion with choline derivatives, Can. J. Physiol. Pharmacol. 47:115, 1969.
60. Meyer, J. H., and Grossman, M. I.: Release of secretin and cholecystokinin, in Thompson, J. C. (ed.): *Gastrointestinal Hormones* (Austin: University of Texas Press, 1975), pp. 43–55.
61. Straus, E., Urbach, H. J., and Yalow, R. S.: Alcohol-stimulated secretion of immunoreactive secretin, N. Engl. J. Med. 293:1031, 1975.
62. Llanos, O. L., Swierczek, J. S., Teichmann, R. K., Rayford, P. L., and Thompson, J. C.: Effect of alcohol on the release of secretin and pancreatic secretion, Surgery 81:661, 1977.
63. Bloom, S. R., and Ward, A. S.: Failure of secretin release in patients with duodenal ulcer, Br. Med. J. 1:126, 1975.
64. Cano, R., Bloom, S. R., and Isenberg, J. I.: Pancreatic bicarbonate secretion and serum secretin in response to graded amounts of duodenal acidi-

fication in duodenal ulcer and normal subjects, Gastroenterology 68:870, 1975.
65. Hubel, K. A.: Secretin: A long progress note, Gastroenterology 62:318, 1972.
66. Domschke, S., Konturek, S. J., Domschke, W., Dembinski, A., Thor, P., Krol, R., and Demling, L.: Cyclic-AMP and pancreatic bicarbonate secretion in response to secretin in dogs, Proc. Soc. Exp. Biol. Med. 150:773, 1975.
67. Hansky, J., Soveny, C., and Korman, M. G.: Effect of secretin on serum gastrin as measured by immunoassay, Gastroenterology 61:62, 1971.
68. Isenberg, J. I., Walsh, J. H., Passaro, E., Jr., Moore, E. W., and Grossman, M. I.: Unusual effect of secretin on serum gastrin, serum calcium, and gastric acid secretion in a patient with suspected Zollinger-Ellison syndrome, Gastroenterology 62:626, 1972.
69. Thompson, J. C., Reeder, D. D., Villar, H. V., and Fender, H. R.: Natural history and experience with diagnosis and treatment of the Zollinger-Ellison syndrome, Surg. Gynecol. Obstet. 140:721, 1975.
70. Brown, J. C., Pederson, R. A., Jorpes, E., and Mutt, V.: Preparation of highly active enterogastrone, Can. J. Physiol. Pharmacol. 47:113, 1969.
71. Brown, J. C.: A gastric inhibitory polypeptide. I. The amino acid composition and the tryptic peptides, Can. J. Biochem. 49:255, 1971.
72. Polak, J. M., Bloom, S. R., Kuzio, M., Brown, J. C., and Pearse, A. G. E.: Cellular localization of gastric inhibitory polypeptides in the duodenum and jejunum, Gut 14:284, 1973.
73. Makhlouf, G. M.: The neuroendocrine design of the gut: The play of chemicals in a chemical playground, Gastroenterology 67:159, 1974.
74. Said, S. I., and Mutt, V.: Isolation from porcine-intestinal wall of vasoactive octacosapeptide related to secretin and to glucagon, Eur. J. Biochem. 28:199, 1972.
75. Bodanszky, M.: The secretin family and evolution, in Thompson, J. C. (ed.): *Gastrointestinal Hormones* (Austin: University of Texas Press, 1975), pp. 507–518.
76. Said, S. I., and Faloona, G. R.: Elevated plasma and tissue levels of vasoactive intestinal polypeptide in watery-diarrhea syndrome due to pancreatic, bronchogenic and other tumors, N. Engl. J. Med. 293:155, 1975.
77. Jaffe, B. M., and Condon, S.: Prostaglandins E and F in endocrine diarrheagenic syndrome, Ann. Surg. 184:516, 1976.
78. Breuer, R. I., Moses, H., III, Hagen, T. C., and Zuckerman, L.: Gastric operations and glucose homeostasis, Gastroenterology 62:1109, 1972.
79. Breuer, R. I., Zuckerman, L., Hauch, T. W., Green, W., O'Gara, P., Lawrence A. M., Foà P. P., and Matsuyama, T.: Gastric operations and glucose homeostasis. II. Glucagon and secretin, Gastroenterology 69:598, 1975.
80. Bertaccini, G., Erspamer, V., Melchiorri, P., and Sopranzi, N.: Gastrin release by bombesin in the dog, Br. J. Pharmacol. 52:219, 1974.
81. Erspamer, V., and Melchiorri, P.: Actions of bombesin on secretions and motility of the gastrointestinal tract, in Thompson, J. C. (ed.): *Gastrointestinal Hormones* (Austin: University of Texas Press, 1975), pp. 575–589.

82. Gregory, R. A., and Ivy, A. C.: The humoral stimulation of gastric secretion, Q. J. Exp. Physiol. 31:111, 1941.
83. Lebedinskaja, S. I.: Über die Magensekretion bei Eckschen Fistelhunden, Z. Gesamte Exp. Med. 88:264, 1933.
84. Clendinnen, B. G., Reeder, D. D., Jackson, B. M., Miller, J. H., and Thompson, J. C.: Effect of portacaval shunting on postprandial serum gastrin levels in dogs, Surg. Forum 21:339, 1970.
85. Way, L. W., Cairns, D. W., and Deveney, C. W.: The intestinal phase of gastric secretion: A pharmacological profile of entero-oxyntin, Surgery 77:841, 1975.
86. Grossman, M. I.: Entero-oxyntin, in: Grossman, M. I. et al.: Candidate hormones of the gut, Gastroenterology 67:730, 1974.
87. Orloff, M. J., Villar-Valdes, H., Abbott, A. G., Williams, R. J., and Rosen, H.: Site of origin of the hormone responsible for gastric hypersecretion associated with portacaval shunt, Surgery 68:202, 1970.
88. Brazeau, P., Vale, W., Burgus, R., Butcher, M., Rivier, J., and Guillemin, R.: Hypothalamic polypeptide that inhibits the secretion of immunoreactive pituitary growth hormone, Science 179:77, 1973.
89. Coy, D. H., Coy, E. J., Arimura, A., Schally, A. V.: Solid phase synthesis of growth hormone-release inhibiting factor, Biochem. Biophys. Res. Commun. 54:1267, 1973.
90. Bloom, S. R., Mortimer, C. H., Thorner, M. O., Hall, R., Gomez-Pon, A., Roy, V. M., Russel, R. C. G., Coy, D. H., Kastin, A. J., and Schally, A. V.: Inhibition of gastrin and gastric-acid secretion by growth-hormone release-inhibiting hormone, Lancet 2:1106, 1974.
91. Raptis, S., Dollinger, H. C., von Berger, L., Schlegel, W., Schroder, K. E., and Pfeiffer, E. F.: Effects of somatostatin on gastric secretion and gastric release in man, Digestion 13:15, 1975.
92. Barros D'Sa, A. A. J., Bloom, S. R., and Baron, J. H.: Direct inhibition of gastric acid by growth-hormone release-inhibiting hormone in dogs, Lancet 1:886, 1975.
93. Boden, G., Sivitz, M. C., Owen, O. E., Landor, J. H.: Somatostatin suppresses secretin and pancreatic exocrine secretion, Science 190:163, 1975.
94. Jaffe, B. M., Kopen, D. F., and Lazan, D. W.: Endogenous serotonin in the control of gastric acid secretion, Surgery 82:156, 1977.
95. Jaffe, B. M., and Behrman, H. R.: Prostaglandins E, A, and F. in Jaffe, B. M., and Behrman, H. R. (eds.): Methods of Hormone Radioimmunoassay (New York: Academic Press, 1974), pp. 19–34.
96. Becker, H. D., Reeder, D. D., and Thompson, J. C.: Effect of prostaglandin E_1 on the release of gastrin and gastric secretion in dogs, Endocrinology 93:1148, 1973.
97. Konturek, S. J., Oleksy, J., Biernat, J., Sito, E., and Kwiecien, N.: Effect of synthetic 15-methyl analog of PGE_2 on gastric acid and serum gastrin response to peptone meal, pentagastrin, and histamine in duodenal ulcer patients, Am. J. Dig. Dis. 21:291, 1976.
98. Wells, S. A., Jr., Ontjes, D. A., Cooper, C. W., Hennessey, J. F., Ellis, G. J.: McPherson, H. T., and Sabiston, D. C., Jr.: Early diagnosis of medullary carcinoma of the thyroid gland in patients with multiple endocrine neoplasia type II, Ann. Surg. 182:362, 1975.

99. Hesch, R. D., Hufner, N., Schmidt, H., Winkler, K., Hasenjager, M., Paschen, K., Becker, H. D., Fuchs, K., and Creutzfeldt, W.: Gastrointestinal effects of calcitonin in man, in Demling, L. (ed.): *Gastrointestinal Hormones* (Stuttgart: Georg Thieme Verlag, 1972), p. 94.
100. Becker, H. D., Reeder, D. D., Scurry, M. T., and Thompson, J. C.: Inhibition of gastrin release and gastric secretion by calcitonin in patients with peptic ulcer, Am. J. Surg. 127:71, 1974.

Treatment of Perforated Diverticular Disease of the Colon

E. JOHN HINCHEY, M.D., F.R.C.S.(C.), F.A.C.S.;
P. G. H. SCHAAL, M.D., F.R.C.S.(C.); AND G. K.
RICHARDS, M.B., M.R.C. (PATH.)

McGill University and Montreal General Hospital, Montreal, Canada

Colonic diverticula have been shown to be unusual if they appear before the age of 40. However, their frequency increases in direct proportion to age thereafter, so that by the ninth decade of life they are present in two-thirds of the population.[1] The majority of patients with colonic diverticula have no symptoms. Although advances have been made in the understanding of the pathogenesis of diverticular disease of the colon, the natural history of this disorder is poorly understood.[2] It is now recognized that recurring attacks of left lower quadrant pain and tenderness in a patient with diverticular disease are not necessarily associated with inflammation, but rather represent a functional abnormality of the sigmoid musculature. Inflammation, if it occurs, takes the form of a peridiverticulitis, usually involving only a single diverticulum. This may be an isolated clinical episode and may resolve permanently without any therapy. A small group of patients, however, may develop life-threatening complications as a result of perforation of a diverticulum. The management of such patients is the subject of this review.

Pathogenesis

Diverticula appear between the mesenteric and antimesenteric tenia at the points of entry of blood vessels through the mus-

85

0065–3411/78/0012–0085$03.75

cular layers of the bowel wall. Although they may be present throughout the large bowel, the sigmoid colon is the site that is usually involved. Colonic diverticula were recognized as a curiosity in the 19th century; Cruveilhier[3] in 1849 was among the first to recognize their potential as sites of inflammation and infection. Beer[4] in 1904 suggested that inflammation is initiated by fecal masses in diverticula and that this may progress to peridiverticulitis, perforation and fistula formation. Telling and Gruner,[5] in an extensive review in 1917, suggested that factors in pathogenesis include increased intraluminal pressure, localized areas of weakness in the bowel wall and increased tonic contraction of the tenia. They also believed that fecal masses filling imperfectly drained diverticular sacs were responsible for inflammation and drew attention to the peridiverticulitis that occurred in the tissue adjacent to a diverticulum. Recent observations support these factors, with increasing emphasis on the muscle component. The occurrence of mucosal herniation is now thought to be due to abnormal muscle contraction leading to uneven thickness of the muscle coat and increased intraluminal pressure. Painter et al.[6] used both intraluminal open-tipped catheters and simultaneous cineradiography to record pressure patterns resulting from various stimuli and to correlate these with radiographic changes. They described segmentation, which is associated with small waves of positive pressure superimposed on a close-to-atmospheric basal resting pressure, as a normal physiological occurrence in the sigmoid colon. Segmentation causes the colon to act as a series of little bladders with outflow obstruction on both sides. Although this is a normal phenomenon, it can be accentuated in patients with diverticula by the administration of morphine and neostigmine (Prostigmin), which can stimulate pressures in excess of 90 mm Hg, distending diverticula to an alarming degree. Arfwidsson[7] showed that higher pressures occurred in colons of patients with the prediverticular state than in normal patients, suggesting that muscle changes and alterations in pressure precede the development of diverticula. Diverticula, therefore, seem to be secondary phenomena; the primary problem is a muscle abnormality. It is this primary motility disturbance which has led some surgeons to suggest myotomy either as treatment for symptomatic disease or as an adjunct to operation.[8, 9] Painter and Burkitt[10] suggest that highly refined low-residue diets contribute to increased segmentation and that high fiber diets decrease segmentation by producing a larger volume of feces and, hence, wider diameter of the colon along with the more rapid passage of a less viscous fecal stream. Morson[11] studied 155 resected specimens of sigmoid colon from patients with a clinical diagnosis of diverticulitis and found inflammation in only 103. Inflammation even of a very slight or focal character was absent in one-third of the specimens. Muscle changes were present in all specimens. The teniae coli were thick and almost cartilagenous in consistency in some specimens. The circular muscle was much thicker than normal with a corrugated or concertinalike appearance. The bowel appeared markedly shortened as a result of muscle contraction and the lumen was filled with redundant folds of mucosa. When inflammation was found it usually began in the apex of a single diverticulum, was related to the presence of hard inspissated feces and spread directly into the soft pericolic or mesenteric fat. A growing abscess could then spread up and down the bowel wall, deeper into the mesocolon, perforate into the peritoneal cavity or more chronically erode into a neighboring viscus. Ming and Fleischner[12] reported almost identical findings in 62 specimens resected for a clinical diagnosis of diverticulitis. Berman et al.[13] reported similar findings in 54 specimens. In nearly all, induration and some congestion were noted in the pericolic fatty tissues along with gross thickening of the intestinal wall. Microscopically the most constant alterations were within the serosa and pericolic fat, with some degree of chronic nonspecific inflammation and occasionally small foci of granulation tissue. Nodular aggregates of lymphoid tissue and foreign body granulomas were not unusual and rare microabscesses were recognized in the pericolic tissue. In most instances, however, the specimens were totally devoid of any inflammatory component. The gross impression of hypertrophy of the muscle generally was corroborated microscopically.

To summarize, diverticular disease of the sigmoid colon is due primarily to a functional muscular abnormality in the colon wall which leads to marked shortening of the bowel, abnormal segmentation and increased intraluminal pressures. This leads to mucosal herniation, usually at the point of penetration of the colonic wall by a blood vessel. If inflammation occurs it usually results from the involvement of a single diverticulum and is related to the presence of a fecalith. Extension of the inflammatory process may lead to any of the many complications of the disease.

Surgery in Diverticular Disease

The traditional indications for operation in patients with diverticular disease are recurrent diverticulitis, perforation, abscess, obstruction, fistula, hemorrhage and the inability to rule out carcinoma. The literature dealing with the operative management of patients with perforated diverticular disease has stimulated a great deal of controversy. Part of the confusion results from failure to differentiate patients with perforation from those with less emergent reasons for operation. When this is done the experience with perforation in any given institution tends to be limited. The result of perforation of a diverticulum varies from a small pericolic abscess to fecal peritonitis – conditions with a marked difference in mortality. These and other variables such as age and associated disease in other organ systems make the comparison of the results of various series difficult. In an attempt to more accurately classify perforated diverticular disease, we reviewed the records of 95 patients from our hospital with the disease and have been able to identify four reasonably distinct stages (Fig 1). This classification is very similar to that suggested by Hughes et al. in 1963.[14]

STAGE I. – This is a pericolic abscess confined by the mesentery of the colon. It may enlarge by spreading either deeper into the mesentery or along the outer layer of the bowel wall. The abscess may resorb with conservative therapy or may drain spontaneously into the lumen of the colon. It may, however, progress either to stage II or stage III.

STAGE II. – This is a pelvic abscess resulting from local perforation of a pericolic abscess. The abscess may be walled off by colon, mesocolon, omentum, small bowel, uterus, fallopian tubes and ovaries, and pelvic peritoneum.

STAGE III. – This is generalized peritonitis resulting from the rupture of either a pericolic or pelvic abscess into the general peritoneal cavity. Free communication between the abscess and the lumen of the bowel does not exist because of obliteration of the neck of the diverticulum by the inflammatory process. This has also been called acute noncommunicating diverticulitis.[15]

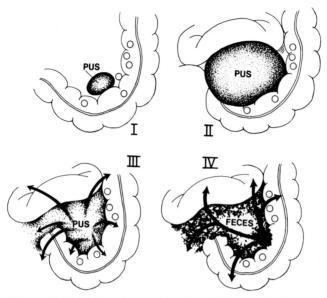

Fig 1. — The four clinical stages of perforated diverticular disease.

STAGE IV. — Fecal peritonitis results from the free perforation of a diverticulum. Its evolution usually is rapid and feces escape from the lumen of the colon through the perforated diverticulum and are present in the free peritoneal cavity. This also has been called acute communicating diverticulitis.[15]

Microbiologic Aspects

The bacteria isolated from abscesses and peritonitis complicating diverticular disease of the large bowel are the same bacteria that form the normal flora of the colon content and feces.[16, 17] Anaerobes are the predominant organisms. These form at least 99% of the total bacterial content of normal flora and are present in the order of $10^{10.5}$ organisms per gm, exceeding the coliform *(Enterobacteria)* content by approximately 10,000-fold.[18] A recent study of normal fecal flora isolated 113 separate and named species; when ranked in order of frequency *Bacteroides fragilis* placed first and the familiar coliforms *(Escherichia coli, Klebsiella-enterobacteria*, etc.) ranked 76th – 113th.[19]

With improved culture techniques this predominance of anaerobes now is seen increasingly in the qualitative examination of pus from intra-abdominal infections.[20] Anaerobic *Bacteroides* is almost always present and indeed may be the only isolate from purulent material or from circulating blood.[16]

The suspicion, therefore, is that anaerobes may be the most important determinants of clinical infection.[20] Studies on prophylactic regimens for large bowel surgery in which the antibiotics chosen were effective against anaerobes support this view, in that not only are postoperative infections with anaerobes decreased, but also all forms of gut-derived bacterial infections are decreased; i.e., the main pathogens are anaerobes and they probably play a complex synergistic role in the development of infection.[16, 20-24]

It is therefore desirable, when planning antibiotic therapy for this class of complex infection, to direct the main thrust of the antibiotics chosen against the expected anaerobic bacterial content. Antibiotics may be grouped into three families, although there is considerable overlap in their activities (Table 1). The penicillin-erythromycin group is especially effective against gram-positive aerobes (staphylococci, enterococci). The aminoglycoside group is especially effective against gram-negative aerobes (coliforms, *E. coli*, etc.). The anaerobic group has agents particularly effective against anaerobes (*Bacteroides, Clostridia,* anaerobic cocci).

It can be assumed that in perforated diverticular disease that enterococci, coliforms (*E. coli*, etc.) and *Bacteroides* are all pres-

TABLE 1.—CLASSES OF ANTIBIOTICS USED TO TREAT
PATIENTS WITH PERFORATED DIVERTICULAR DISEASE

PENICILLIN-ERYTHROMYCIN GROUP	AMINOGLYCOSIDE GROUP	ANAEROBIC GROUP
Penicillin	Streptomycin	Metronidazole
Cloxacillin	Kanamycin	Clindamycin
Ampicillin	Gentamicin	Chloramphenicol
Carbenicillin	Tobramycin	(Erythromycin)*
Cephalosporins	Amikacin	(Tetracycline)*
Cephalothin	Sisomycin	(Rifampicin)*
Cefazolin	Netilmycin	
Cephradine	(Chloramphenicol)*	
Erythromycin		
Lincomycin		
Clindamycin		
(Chloramphenicol)*		

*Parentheses indicate variable effect, antibiotic not of first choice.

ent. Such polymicrobial infections should be treated with a multiple antibiotic regimen directed against each of the three bacterial groups.[16, 25] With regard to the treatment of the aerobes (enterococci and coliforms), members of the penicillin group are synergistic with the aminoglycosides. Both groups therefore should be used in combination in view of the limitation of dosage of the aminoglycosides because of their inherent toxicity. The choice of which penicillin and which aminoglycoside for initial blind therapy can be made best by examining laboratory antibiotic susceptibility patterns for the preceding year. Our laboratory currently recommends ampicillin plus gentamicin for the initial management of the aerobes, thereby avoiding the potential nephrotoxic effect of combining cephalothin with gentamicin and additionally holding the cephalosporins in reserve against need. In a different geographic locale, however, cephalothin plus tobramycin or amikacin may be more appropriate. Irrespective of the initial choice, the results of culture of specimens obtained at operation are available 18 hours later and will allow the correction of antibiotics for optimal coverage.

Chloramphenicol is held in reserve. In a patient with a severe or life-threatening infection, particularly with intra-abdominal abscess formation, in whom the initial cultures reveal coliforms resistant to cephalosporins (e.g., Keflin) but sensitive to chloramphenicol, then the latter would be prescribed in full dosage as a replacement for the ineffective penicillins. It would be combined with an appropriate aminoglycoside and an additional antibiotic effective against anaerobes.

The antibiotic of choice for the anaerobic bacterial component is of major importance; clinical experience and a study of the current anaerobic sensitivity patterns in the regional laboratory are again the best guides. Clindamycin has been well studied and is regarded by many as the current initial agent of choice, in combination with cephalothin and gentamicin.[16, 25]

In our laboratory, due to a high incidence of clindamycin-resistant organisms, metronidazole currently is favored, since in the past 18 months no anaerobes resistant to an arbitrary concentration of 2 μg/ml have been isolated from clinical material, and this level in tissue fluid is readily exceeded in vivo. Our initial therapy for abscess or peritonitis for this geographic area is, therefore, metronidazole plus ampicillin plus gentamicin.[24-30]

Clinical Presentation

There is considerable variation in the evolution of symptoms in patients with perforating diverticular disease of the colon. The usual presentation is the rather sudden onset of left lower quadrant pain which may be preceded by or associated with abdominal cramps, nausea, vomiting and obstipation. The signs are those of an intra-abdominal septic process and include tenderness, muscle guarding and rigidity; these may be localized to the lower quadrants or they may be generalized. Rectal examination usually reveals pelvic tenderness, sometimes a tender fullness and occasionally a tender mass. Sigmoidoscopic examination may be particularly painful when the end of the instrument contacts the inflammatory mass. Fever, tachycardia and leukocytosis are present. There may be signs of hypovolemia and altered mentation. Patients with small localized perforations may look quite well. X-ray films of the abdomen may reveal free air in some patients either on the upright or lateral decubitus views, but this is uncommon unless the perforation is free (stage IV). More often, however, abdominal x-ray films show nonspecific signs which consist of a few gas-filled loops of small bowel and perhaps separation of these loops by fluid. In a few patients a homogeneous density may be recognized in the left lower quadrant or pelvis.

Differential diagnosis includes perforated appendix, obstructing perforating carcinoma, perforation of the cecum, strangulation obstruction, mesenteric vascular insufficiency and leaking aneurysm of aorta or common iliac artery.

Treatment

Initial treatment consists of nasogastric suction, salt solutions administered intravenously (either sodium chloride or Ringer's lactate), antibiotics as previously described and careful observation. Most patients will improve on this regimen and as long as the inflammatory process remains localized to the left lower quadrant, observation is continued. We have become more conservative in recent years, persisting with conservative therapy as long as there is no evidence of increase in the degree or extent of abdominal findings and as long as systemic signs are not increasing. Frequent repeat examination of the patient, however, is absolutely necessary. Sudden resolution may occur in some patients and may be associated with the passage of a bloody liquid bowel movement which represents spontaneous drainage of the abscess into the lumen of the colon. If the patient improves on conservative therapy, barium enema examination is carried out two to three weeks after symptoms subside. If no mucosal abnormality is identified and carcinoma is ruled out, the patient is discharged on a high-residue diet and undergoes repeat barium enema examination four to six months after discharge. We generally follow the criteria of Rodkey and Welch[1] to select patients in whom a resection might be required. These are:

1. Recurrent attacks of local inflammation;
2. Persistent tender mass;
3. Narrowing or marked deformity of the sigmoid on x-ray examination;
4. Dysuria associated with diverticular disease;
5. Rapid progression of symptoms from time of onset;
6. Relative youth of the patient (younger than age 50); and
7. Clinical x-ray signs equivocal in ruling out carcinoma.

If the patient's condition does not improve, if signs of spreading peritonitis are present at the time of admission or develop during conservative therapy, immediate operation is carried out. The usual operative findings are purulent fluid in the peritoneal cavity with an inflammatory mass involving the sigmoid colon and mesocolon. The site of perforation usually is not seen, although in some patients a small opening is seen in the mesosigmoid a short distance from the edge of the bowel.[15] This represents the site of perforation of a pericolic abscess and does not communicate with the lumen of the bowel. Less commonly, fecal peritonitis is present with obvious perforation of the bowel wall. In some cases the sigmoid and mesosigmoid may be thickened and inflamed, with the perforation near the junction of the mesocolon with the bowel wall. In others the colon may be quite mobile with a near-normal mesocolon with a free perforation on the antemesenteric border between the two antimesenteric teniae.

Operative Approach

The operations in current use for the management of perforated diverticular disease of the sigmoid colon are shown in Fig 2.

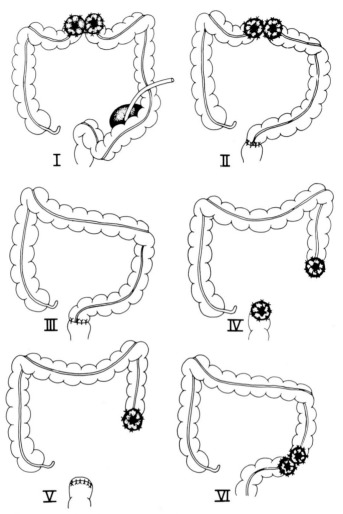

Fig 2.—Operations: I—colostomy and drainage; II—primary resection anastomosis colostomy; III—primary resection anastomosis; IV—primary resection colostomy mucous fistula; V—Hartmann procedure; VI—exteriorization resection.

The choice of operation has been the subject of ongoing controversy for the past twenty years. The three basic operations are:

1. Three-stage resection (this leaves the diseased segment in the abdominal cavity at the first operation);
2. Primary resection with anastomosis; and
3. Primary resection without anastomosis.

THREE-STAGE RESECTION

Mayo in 1907[31] advised free drainage for perforated diverticulitis with the addition of proximal colostomy if obstruction coexisted. This was later followed in some cases by resection of the diseased segment. Rankin and Brown in 1930[32] were among the first to suggest the routine use of three-stage resection with an interval of two to four months between colostomy and drainage and resection of the diseased sigmoid colon. Smithwick in 1942[33] suggested that primary transverse colostomy be performed in all cases in which resection of the colon is contemplated and that the period of delay before resection should be from three to six months. He felt that resection should be avoided in the acute stage of the disease. Although a number of authors supported three-stage resection for the various complications of diverticular disease,[34-37] mortality was high when perforation and peritonitis were present.[36] MacLaren,[38] in a large series, reported a mortality rate of 50% when colostomy and drainage was used as the primary operation for perforated diverticulitis. The mortality rate, in a collected series, for colostomy and drainage was 30% (Table 2). The mortality rate for three-stage resection is 6–11% in series which include both abscess formation and generalized peritonitis as indications for operation.[39, 40] This difference emphasizes the need for accurate reporting of the stage of disease present when comparing the results of different operations. Morbidity and complications for three-stage resection as measured by number of hospitalized days are high. For these reasons some authors who earlier supported three-stage resection have more recently suggested a reappraisal of its role in the management of these patients.[39, 41, 42] Rodkey and Welch[39] summarized the arguments for primary removal of the perforated segment as follows:

1. The removal of a septic focus or continued source of peritoneal contamination may be tolerated better than continued local sepsis or recurrent peritoneal soiling.
2. Defunctioning of a segment of colon does not necessarily result in subsidence of acute diverticulitis.
3. Excision of the involved segment of colon does not seem to promote extension of infection to the retroperitoneal tissues.
4. The mixed enteric bacterial flora present in these cases may not be very responsive to antibiotic therapy.

TABLE 2. – MORTALITY WITH GENERALIZED PERITONITIS AND VARIOUS OPERATIONS

AUTHOR	COLOSTOMY AND DRAINAGE		RESECTION NO ANASTOMOSIS		RESECTION ANASTOMOSIS		EXTERIORIZATION	
	PATIENTS	DEATHS	PATIENTS	DEATHS	PATIENTS	DEATHS	PATIENTS	DEATHS
Present series	20	4	8	1				
Himal et al.[44]	20	6	6	1				
Eng et al.[42]			8	0				
Nahrwold and Demuth[45]			10	1				
Laimon[46]			15	1				
Ryan[47]	3	0			12	0		
Endrey-Walder and Judd[48]	22	8	1	1	5	1		
Miller and Wichern[49]	9	1	4	0			1	1
Byrne and Garick[50]	13	4	2	0				
Whelan, Furcinitti and Lavarreda[51]	14	4	4	1				
Tagart[52]	13	3	16	0	5	0		
Watkins and Oliver[53]					8	1	12	0
Roxburgh, Dawson and Yeo[54]			16	2				
Smiley[55]	16	9	3	0				
Large[56]					13	2		
Hartley[57]	11	3						
Staunton[58]	5	2					5	0
Madden[59]	6	2			7	1		
Total	152	46 (30%)	93	8 (8.6%)	50	5 (10%)	18	1 (6%)

5. The duration of hospitalization and disability may be shortened significantly by this choice of treatment.

PRIMARY RESECTION

Although there were sporadic reports of primary resection of
the perforated segment of colon in the literature in the first half
of this century, Crile in 1954[43] stimulated considerable interest
with an editorial on the dangers of conservative surgery in abdominal emergencies. Crile suggested that it was not the operation that caused death of the critically ill patient, but the disease for which the operation was performed. If the operation did
not correct the pathologic condition by removal of the diseased
segment, the patient was doomed and might as well have had no
operation at all. This concept of definitive operation in perforated diverticular disease was embraced by a number of surgeons
over the next 20 years and a collected series from the literature
would suggest that this approach does, in fact, reduce the mortality rate (see Table 2). The management of the bowel ends after primary resection remains a controversy. Although there are
many options the fundamental difference is whether or not a
primary anastomosis should be performed.

Resection with Anastomosis

Gregg in 1955[60] was among the first to report planned primary
resection and anastomosis in seven patients having perforating
diverticular disease of the colon with no deaths or anastomotic
leaks. If the bowel was empty of fecal content, free of edema and
if the distal segment was well above the peritoneal reflection he
did not add proximal colostomy. If there was any question concerning the integrity of the anastomosis and particularly if the
lower segment was near or below the peritoneal reflection, he
added a proximal complementary transverse colostomy. Belding
in 1957[61] reported three primary resections with anastomosis
with no mortality and uneventful recoveries. Ryan in 1958[62] reported primary resection and anastomosis in 4 patients with
perforated diverticulitis who were relatively well, who had a
mobile sigmoid colon and who had no intestinal obstruction.
Ryan updated his experience in 1974.[47] He treated 12 of 23 patients with immediate resection and anastomosis, which is his

preferred method unless contraindicated by the presence of a large pericolic abscess, severe concurrent disease or advanced general peritonitis. All 12 patients survived; however, 8 had postoperative complications which included 5 wound abscesses, 1 fecal fistula and a left ileac fossa abscess, presumably from anastomotic leak. Madden[59] reported on 16 patients who had primary resection and anastomosis for perforated diverticular disease, 2 of whom had a complementary transverse colostomy. One patient died of persisting shock in the immediate postoperative period. Four patients developed fecal fistula, 2 developed wound dehiscence and 1 developed wound infection. Fecal fistula was observed only in those patients in whom the rectum was mobilized from the hollow of the sacrum and in this situation the author recommended a complementary transverse colostomy. Large[56] reported 18 patients with peritonitis treated by primary resection and anastomosis. Five subsequently proved to be perforated carcinomas. There were 2 deaths. Roxburgh[54] treated 8 patients with peritonitis by resection with anastomosis, adding transverse colostomy in 1 and cecostomy in another. One patient died and no patient developed an anastomotic leak. Dandekar and McCann[63] carried out primary resection and anastomosis in 7 patients with 1 death, 1 fecal fistula and 1 pelvic abscess.

Although these reports suggest that in selected cases resection and primary anastomosis can be carried out with low mortality, most surgeons of experience remain skeptical and advise extreme caution in the widespread application of this approach. Although primary resection of the diseased bowel is gaining increasing support, the wisdom of doing a primary anastomosis using unprepared bowel in the presence of peritonitis is strongly questioned.[64] Even with elective operation on prepared bowel the anastomotic leak rate can be as high as 40% with low anastomosis.[65] Leaks were the major cause of preventable death in patients undergoing elective one-stage resection in one large series.[66]

Exteriorization Resection (Resection without Anastomosis)

Wheeler and de Courcy in 1930[67] reported the successful treatment of a perforated diverticulum with generalized peritonitis by bringing out the diseased sigmoid loop through a left grid-iron incision. Guy and Werelius in 1952[68] stated that the dangers of resection in the acute phases of diverticulitis had been overemphasized and did not hesitate to perform a resection for acute perforation, even in the presence of small abscess formation or peritonitis if it was obvious that simple closure of the perforation was not feasible. They did feel, however, that primary anastomosis in such cases was decidedly unwise even with a complementary colostomy. Smithwick,[69] a strong proponent of three-stage resection, stated he had no objection to exteriorizing a freely mobile loop of perforated sigmoid colon providing one proposed to resect it later and perform end-to-end anastomosis. Gilchrist and Economous[70] and Boyden[71] used resection without anastomosis for free perforation of diverticulitis with general or spreading peritonitis. Staunton in 1962[58] used exteriorization in 5 of 14 patients with no deaths. He felt that it would have been possible to carry out exteriorization in 12 of the 14 patients. Watkins and Oliver in 1966[72] reported on 7 patients treated by exteriorization with no deaths. Extensive mobilization frequently was necessary but opening of retroperitoneal tissue planes to accomplish this did not result in invasive infection. Definitive resection was carried out 5 – 6 weeks later. The average hospital stay for the first operation was 10.3 days and for the second stage 13 days. For free perforation Colcock in 1968[73] recommended either a Mikulicz exteriorization resection or a Hartmann procedure. For a large pelvic abscess he recommended drainage and transverse colostomy. Roxburgh, Dawson and Yeo[54] in 1968 reported on 16 patients, 8 with a Mikulicz exteriorization resection and 8 with a Hartmann's procedure. There was one death in each group. Rodkey and Welch[39] in 1969 concluded that primary resection without anastomosis merited a more general trial. They based this conclusion not on mortality but rather on the extensive period of hospitalization involved with a three-stage resection. Watkins and Oliver[53] updated their experience in 1970 with a total of 12 patients and no deaths. Miller and Wichern[49] carried out 6 resections without anastomosis, 4 for peritonitis and 2 for abscess. In 4 patients the distal loop was brought out as a mucous fistula and in 2 patients it was oversewn as a Hartmann procedure. All patients enjoyed a smooth, short hospital course and the second stage was carried out three to six weeks later. Tagart's recommendations in 1973,[52] based on his own experience and a review of the literature, established the following guidelines for the management of the patient with perforation and peritonitis:

1. Very aggressive medical treatment, surgery with minimum delay as soon as the patient is fit;
2. Removal of the inflamed bowel at the first operation taking less rather than more when in doubt;
3. Thorough peritoneal cleaning;
4. Mikulicz, Hartmann or two-stoma procedure; and
5. Restoration of bowel continuity at a second stage.

This approach is a compromise between the policy of immediate resection and anastomosis without colostomy and the overcautious attitude that advocates a three-stage procedure with colostomy only at the first stage. Laimon[46] carried out emergency Hartmann resection in 15 patients with diffuse fecal peritonitis. There was one death. The colostomy was considered to be permanent in 3 patients and 11 patients were re-explored and in 10 coloproctostomy was carried out. Important technical factors included identification of the left ureter above the site of the main area of disease and blunt finger dissection of the ureter away from the diseased colon. He felt it important to avoid excessive resection at the initial operation and stressed that it is only necessary to get just above and just below the affected portion of bowel. Initial overenthusiasm might result in unnecessary mobilization, possible stenosis of a colostomy placed under tension or an excessively short rectal stump, making future coloproctostomy more difficult. The seromuscular sutures of silk used to close the distal segment should be left long in order to identify more easily the rectal stump at a subsequent operation. There is increasing support and enthusiasm in the literature for primary resection of the diseased segment without anastomosis.[40, 42, 44, 45, 74-80]

Montreal General Hospital Experience

We reviewed the charts of 95 patients with perforated diverticular disease of the sigmoid colon in an attempt to assess more precisely the optimal staging of the disease, to define the causes of increased mortality and to establish the optimal treatment in a variety of clinical situations.

Twenty-nine patients had a pericolic abscess (Table 3). The

TABLE 3.—STAGE I: PERICOLIC ABSCESS

OPERATION	PATIENTS	DEATHS	MORTALITY
Colostomy	15	1	7%
Resection — no anastomosis	4	0	0
Resection plus anastomosis*	10	0	0
TOTAL	29	1	3%

*Three had complementary colostomy.

TABLE 4.—STAGE II: PELVIC ABSCESS

OPERATION	PATIENTS	DEATHS	MORTALITY
Colostomy	23	2	9%
Resection — no anastomosis	6	0	0
Resection plus anastomosis*	9	1	9%
TOTAL	38	3	8%

*2 had complementary colostomy

only death occurred in a patient undergoing colostomy and drainage. There were no deaths in the 4 patients treated by resection without anastomosis and no deaths in the 10 patients treated by resection and anastomosis.

Thirty-eight patients had a pelvic abscess (Table 4). Two deaths occurred in the 23 patients treated by colostomy and drainage and 1 death occurred in 9 patients treated by resection and anastomosis. There were no deaths in 6 patients treated by resection without anastomosis.

Twenty-one patients had purulent peritonitis with 1 death in 15 patients treated by colostomy and drainage (Table 5). There were no deaths among 6 patients treated by resection without anastomosis.

Seven patients had fecal peritonitis (Table 6). Four of these patients died, 3 following colostomy and drainage and 1 follow-

TABLE 5.—STAGE III: PURULENT PERITONITIS

OPERATION	PATIENTS	DEATHS	MORTALITY
Colostomy	15	1	7%
Resection — no anastomosis	6	0	0
Resection plus anastomosis	0	0	0
TOTAL	21	1	5%

TABLE 6.—STAGE IV: FECAL PERITONITIS

OPERATION	PATIENTS	DEATHS	MORTALITY
Colostomy	5	3	60%
Resection — no anastomosis	2	1	50%
Resection plus anastomosis	0	0	0
TOTAL	7	4	57%

ing resection without anastomosis. No patients were treated by resection and anastomosis.

Our data suggest that the mortality rate varies between 5 and 10% for stage I, II, and III disease. The mortality rate for stage IV, on the other hand, is 57%. For all stages of the disease the mortality rate was not affected significantly by the type of operative procedure carried out. There were no deaths as the result of subsequent operations in those patients who had staged procedures. The most important determinant of mortality in this series was the stage of the disease process. The number of patients with fecal peritonitis is too small to allow comparison of the effects of staged versus primary resection with regard to mortality rate.

Morbidity was assessed by complication rate and by number of days spent in the hospital. The most frequent complications were wound infection, atelectasis and pneumonia, wound dehiscence, pelvic abscess and fistula formation. Since a single patient could develop more than one complication, the total number of complications per group was divided by the number of patients in the group. For the initial operation the complication rate for colostomy and drainage was 90%, for resection without anastomosis, 130%, and for primary resection with anastomosis, 55%. For those completing the various stages the total complication rate was 150% for the three-stage procedure, 220% for the two-stage procedure and 55% for the one-stage procedure. The complication rate is lowest in those patients who had a one-stage resection; however, these patients were selected in that all had either stage I or II disease. It is of interest that the classic three-stage resection approach had a lower total complication rate than did primary resection without anastomosis. This difference was due largely to a higher incidence of both wound infection and dehiscence in the latter group.

The length of hospital stay increased as the severity of the

TABLE 7.–AVERAGE LENGTH OF HOSPITAL STAY

	PERICOLIC ABSCESS	PELVIC ABSCESS	PURULENT PERITONITIS	FECAL PERITONITIS
3-Stage resection	(14) *57 days	(21) 75 days	(14) 66 days	(2) 88 days
Resection – no anastomosis	(4) 46 days	(6) 35 days	(6) 60 days	(1) 76 days
Resection plus anastomosis	(10) 22 days	(8) 32 days	–	–

*Number of patients indicated in parentheses.

disease increased (Table 7). Total length of hospital stay was shorter for patients undergoing primary resection than for those treated by the three-stage procedure. As with mortality rate, however, the major determinant of hospital stay was the stage of the disease process.

Proposed Plan of Management

Our present operative management of patients with perforated diverticular disease has been influenced by the following:
1. Recognition of the importance of staging the disease;
2. Increasing experience with primary resection in selected patients;
3. Advances in intensive care for the general support of an ill patient undergoing major surgery;
4. Advances in the pharmacologic support and treatment of the septic patient; and
5. Selection of an operative procedure at the first operation that seems most appropriate to the patient and to the stage of the disease present.

For stage I disease we carry out primary resection of the diseased colon and abscess. The decision to do a primary anastomosis is made at operation and depends on the local condition of the bowel and its content. A protective right transverse colostomy is recommended particularly if the pelvic peritoneum has been opened. The addition of a protective colostomy is an operative decision that should always be considered and frequently done.

For stage II disease the factors to be considered are the acuteness of the disease process and the extent of distal involvement of the bowel. The mature, well walled-off abscess probably is treated best by extraperitoneal drainage and right transverse colostomy. A more acute process with minimal walling off can be treated by primary resection without anastomosis, especially if the distal segment can be brought to the skin as a mucous fistula. This may require dividing the bowel through a partially diseased segment in order to achieve sufficient length. A Hartmann-type procedure which leaves a short rectal stump should be avoided because of the technical difficulties this may cause when reanastomosis is performed. In two of our patients with short distal segments who had this operation it was impossible to re-establish continuity of the colon at a second operation. On occasion a primary resection with anastomosis can be carried out in this stage of the disease, but if it is done a protective colostomy should always be considered.

Stage III disease is treated by primary resection without anastomosis in most cases. In some patients in whom the bowel is mobile, unobstructed, relatively empty and when the bowel ends are relatively free of inflammation, primary anastomosis with a protecting right transverse colostomy is the procedure of choice. If a surgeon so elects, however, a colostomy with drainage of the perforated segment is a safe operation.

We feel that resection or exteriorization of the perforated segment is mandatory for stage IV disease. We would not carry out primary anastomosis in the presence of fecal peritonitis. If the distal segment cannot be brought to the skin as a mucous fistula it is oversewn and left in the pelvis after being anchored near the promontory of the sacrum for later identification.

Summary

Diverticular disease of the colon now is recognized to be a functional disease resulting from altered neuromuscular activity in the colon. Inflammatory complications, when they occur, usually result from inflammation around a single diverticulum. This may lead to the formation of a pericolic or pelvic abscess. Free perforation of these leads to purulent peritonitis. The original communication with the lumen of the bowel usually is obliterated. More rarely, with either rapid evolution or failure of the diverticular neck to obliterate, a free communication develops between the bowel lumen and the peritoneal cavity, leading to fecal peritonitis. Fecal peritonitis results in an extremely high mortality rate. The operative approach for a patient with perforated diverticular disease should be individualized and depends on the stage of the disease present, the general condition of the patient, the experience of the surgeon in colon surgery and the availability of facilities and personnel to provide intensive care. In larger institutions when these conditions are optimal, primary resection of the diseased bowel with or without anastomosis is becoming the procedure of choice. In smaller institutions or if conditions are not optimal, right transverse colostomy with drainage of the perforated segment can be relied on to control the disease with a mortality rate compared to that of primary resection. If free perforation and fecal peritonitis are present, exteriorization or primary resection of the perforated segment must be carried out. We would not recommend primary anastomosis under these circumstances.

REFERENCES

1. Rodkey, G. V., and Welch, C. E.: Diverticulitis of the colon: Evolution in concept and therapy, Surg. Clin. North Am 45:1231, 1965.
2. Larson, D. M., Masters, S. S., and Spiro, H. M.: Medical and surgical therapy in diverticular disease: a comparative study, Gastroenterology 71:734, 1976.
3. Cruveilhier, J.: *Traite d'Anatomie Pathologique Generale*, Vol. I (Paris: Bailliere, 1849), p. 593.
4. Beer, E.: Some pathological and clinical aspects of acquired (false) diverticula of the intestine, Am. J. Med. Sci. 128:135, 1904.
5. Telling, W. H. Maxwell, and Gruner, O. C.: Acquired diverticula, diverticulitis, and peridiverticulitis of the large intestine, Br. J. Surg. 4:468, 1917.
6. Painter, N. S., Truelove, S. C., Ardran G. M., et al.: Segmentation and the localization of intraluminal pressures in the human colon, with special reference to the pathogenesis of colonic diverticula, Gastroenterology 49: 169, 1965.
7. Arfwidsson, S.: Pathogenesis of multiple diverticula of the sigmoid colon in diverticular disease, Acta Chir. Scand. 34 (suppl 342)321, 1964.
8. Reilly, M.: Sigmoid myotomy, Proc. R. Soc. Med. 57:556, 1964.
9. Veidenheimer, M. C., and Lawrence, D. C.: Anastomotic myotomy: an adjunct to resection for diverticular disease, Dis. Colon Rectum 19:310, 1976.
10. Painter, N. S., and Burkitt, D. P.: Diverticular disease of the colon, a 20th century problem, Clin. Gastroenterol. 4:3, 1975.
11. Morson, B. C.: The muscle abnormality in diverticular disease of the sigmoid colon, Br. J. Radiol. 36:385, 1963.
12. Ming, Si-Chun, and Fleischner, F. G.: Diverticulitis of the sigmoid colon: reappraisal of the pathology and pathogenesis, Surgery 58:627, 1965.

13. Berman, L. G., Burduk, D., Heitzman, R., et al.: A critical reappraisal of sigmoid diverticulitis, Surg. Gynecol. Obstet. 127:481, 1968.
14. Hughes, E. S. R., Cuthbertson, A. M., and Carden, A. B. C.: Surgical management of acute diverticulitis, Med. J. Aust. 1:780, 1963.
15. Hughes, L. E.: Complications of diverticular disease: inflammation, obstruction and bleeding, Clin. Gastroenterol. 4:147, 1975.
16. Wilson, W., Martin, W., Wilkowske, C., et al.: Anaerobic Bacteremia, Mayo Clin. Proc. 47:639, 1972.
17. Moore, W., Cato, E., Holdeman, L.: Anaerobic bacteria of the gastrointestinal flora and their occurrence in clinical infections. J. Infect. Dis. 119: 641, 1969.
18. Drasar, B. S., Shiner, M., and McLeod, G. M.: Studies on the intestinal flora, Gastroenterology 56:71, 1969.
19. Moore, W., and Holdeman, L.: The human fecal flora of 20 Japanese-Hawaiians, Appl. Microbiol. 27:916, 1974.
20. Zabransky, R. J.: Isolation of anaerobic bacteria from clinical specimens, Mayo Clin. Proc. 45:256, 1970.
21. Brass, C., Richards, G., Ruedy, J., et al.: The effect of metronidazole on the incidence of post-operative wound infections in elective colon surgery, Am. J. Surg. 135:1, 1978.
22. Washington, J. A., Dearing, W., Judd, E., et al.: Effect of preoperative antibiotic regimen on development of infection after intestinal surgery, Ann. Surg. 180:567, 1974.
23. Goldring, V., McNaught, C., Scott, A., et al.: Prophylactic oral antimicrobial agents in elective colon surgery, Lancet 2:997, 1975.
24. Willis, A. J., Ferguson, I., Jones, P., et al.: Metronidazole in the prevention and treatment of bacteroides infections in elective colonic surgery, Br. Med. J. 1:607, 1977.
25. Pass, R., Scholand, J. F., Hodges, G. R., et al: Clindamycin in the treatment of serious anaerobic infections, Ann. Intern. Med. 78:853, 1973.
26. Willis, A., Bullen, C., Ferguson, I., et al.: Metronidazole in the prevention and treatment of bacteroides infections in gynecological patients, Lancet 2:1540, 1974.
27. Eykyn, S., Phillips, I.: Metronidazole and anaerobic sepsis, Br. Med. J. 2: 1418, 1976.
28. Willis, A. T., Ferguson, I. R., and Jones, P.: Metronidazole in prevention and treatment of bacteroides infections after appendicectomy, Br. Med. J. 1:318, 1976.
29. Willis, A. T., Ferguson, I., Jones, P., et al.: An evaluation of metronidazole in the prophylaxis and treatment of anaerobic infections in surgical patients, J. Antimicrob. Chem. 1:393, 1975.
30. Tally, F., Sutter, V., and Finegold, S.: Treatment of anaerobic infections with metronidazole, Antimicrob. Agents Chemother. 7:672, 1975.
31. Mayo, W. J.: Acquired diverticulitis of the large intestine, Surg. Gynecol. Obstet. 5:8, 1907.
32. Rankin, F. W., and Brown, P. W.: Diverticulitis of the colon, Surg. Gynecol. Obstet. 30:836, 1930.
33. Smithwick, R. H.: Experiences with surgical management of diverticulitis of sigmoid, Ann. Surg. 115:969, 1942.

34. Pemberton, J. de J., Black, B. M., and Maino, C. R.: Progress in the surgical management of diverticulitis of the sigmoid colon, Surg. Gynecol. Obstet. 85:523, 1947.

35. Bacon, H. E.: Surgical management of diverticulitis of the sigmoid, J. Int. Coll. Surgeons 11:560, 1948.

36. Welch, C. E., Allen, A. W., and Donaldson, G. A.: An appraisal of resection of the colon for diverticulitis of the sigmoid, Ann. Surg. 138:332, 1953.

37. Colcock, B. P.: Surgical management of diverticulitis, Surg. Gynecol. Obstet. 102:721, 1956.

38. MacLaren, I. F.: Perforated diverticulitis. A survey of 75 cases, J. R. Coll. Surg. Edinb. 3:129, 1957.

39. Rodkey, G. V., and Welch, C. E.: Surgical management of colonic diverticulitis with free perforation or abscess formation, Am. J. Surg. 117:265, 1969.

40. Classen, J. N., Bonardi, R., O'Mara, C. S., et al.: Surgical treatment of acute diverticulitis by staged procedures, Ann. Surg. 184:582, 1976.

41. Lacalio, S. A., and Stahl, W. M.: Diverticular disease of the alimentary tract, Part I, Curr. Probl. in Surg. 4:December, 1967.

42. Eng, K., Ranson, J. H., and Localio, S. A.: Resection of the perforated segment. A significant advance in treatment of diverticulitis with free perforation or abscess. Am. J. Surg. 133:67, 1977.

43. Crile, G.: Dangers of conservative surgery in abdominal emergencies, Surgery 35:122, 1954.

44. Himal, H. S., Ashby, D. B., Duignan, J. P., et al.: Management of perforating diverticulitis of the colon, Surg. Gynecol. Obstet. 144:225, 1977.

45. Nahrwold, D. L., and Demuth, W. E.: Diverticulitis with perforation into the peritoneal cavity, Ann. Surg. 185:80, 1977.

46. Laimon, H.: Hartmann resection for acute diverticulitis, Rev. Surg. 31:1, 1974.

47. Ryan, P.: Emergency resection and anastomosis for perforated sigmoid diverticulitis, Aust. N.Z. J. Surg. 44:16, 1974.

48. Endrey-Walder, P., and Judd, E. S.: Acute perforating diverticulitis: Emergency surgical treatment, Minn. Med. 56:27, 1973.

49. Miller, D. W., and Wichern, W. A.: Perforated sigmoid diverticulitis: appraisal of primary vs delayed resection, Am. J. Surg. 121:536, 1971.

50. Byrne, J. J., and Garick, E. I.: Surgical treatment of diverticulitis, Am. J. Surg. 121:379, 1971.

51. Whelan, C. S., Furcinitti, J. F., and Lavarreda, C.: Surgical management of perforated lesions of the colon with diffusing peritonitis, Am. J. Surg. 121:374, 1970.

52. Tagart, R. E. B.: General peritonitis and hemorrhage complicating colonic diverticular disease, Ann. R. Coll. Surg. Engl. 55:175, 1973.

53. Watkins, G. L., and Oliver, G. A.: Surgical treatment of acute perforative sigmoid diverticulitis, Surgery 69:215, 1970.

54. Roxburgh, R. A., Dawson, J. L., and Yeo, R.: Emergency resection in treatment of diverticular disease of colon complicated by peritonitis, Br. Med. J. 3:465, 1968.

55. Smiley, D. F.: Perforated sigmoid diverticulitis with spreading peritonitis, Am. J. Surg. 111:431, 1966.

56. Large, J. M.: Treatment of perforated diverticulitis, Lancet 1:413, 1964.
57. Hartley, R. C.: Dangers of diverticulitis coli: an estimation of the place of resection in avoidance of complications, Br. J. Surg. 51:45, 1964.
58. Staunton, M. D. M.: Treatment of perforated diverticulitis coli, Br. Med. J. 1:916, 1962.
59. Madden, J. L.: Primary resection and anastomosis in the treatment of perforated lesions of the colon, Am. Surg. 31:781, 1965.
60. Gregg, R. O.: The place of emergency resection in the management of obstructing and perforating lesions of the colon, Surgery 37:754, 1955.
61. Belding, H. H.: Acute perforated diverticulitis of the sigmoid colon with generalized peritonitis, Arch. Surg. 74:511, 1957.
62. Ryan, P.: Emergency resection and anastomosis for perforated sigmoid diverticulitis, Br. J. Surg. 45:611, 1958.
63. Dandekar, N. V., McCann, W. J.: Primary resection and anastomosis in the management of perforation of diverticulitis of the sigmoid flexure and diffuse peritonitis, Dis. Colon Rectum 12:172, 1969.
64. Hunt, T. K., and Howley, P. R.: Surgical judgement and colonic anastomosis, Dis. Colon Rectum 12:167, 1969.
65. Garnjobst, W., Hardwick, C.: Further criteria for anastomosis in diverticulitis of the sigmoid colon, Am. J. Surg. 120:264, 1970.
66. Botsford, T. W., Zollinger, R. M., and Hicks, R.: Mortality of the surgical treatment of diverticulitis, Am. J. Surg. 121:702, 1971.
67. Wheeler, W. I. de Courcy: Perforative diverticulitis of the colon, Br. Med. J. 1:5, 1930.
68. Guy, C. C., Werelius, C. Y.: Complications of diverticulitis of the colon, Surg. Clin. North Am. 32:91, 1952.
69. Smithwick, R. H.: Surgical treatment of diverticulosis of the sigmoid, Am. J. Surg. 99:192, 1960.
70. Gilchrist, R. K., and Economous, S.: Surgical treatment of diverticulitis of colon, Arch. Surg. 70:276, 1955.
71. Boyden, A. M.: Two-stage (obstructive) resection of the sigmoid in selected cases of complicated diverticulitis, Ann. Surg. 154:210, 1961.
72. Watkins, G. L., and Oliver G. A.: Management of perforative sigmoid diverticulitis with diffusing peritonitis, Arch. Surg. 92:928, 1966.
73. Colcock, B. P.: Surgical management of complicated diverticulitis, Surg. Clin. North Am. 48:543, 1968.
74. Graves, H. A., Franklin, R. M., Robbins, L. B., et al.: Surgical management of perforated diverticulitis of the colon, Am. Surg. 39:142, 1973.
75. Rugtiv, G. M.: Diverticulitis: selective surgical management, Am. J. Surg. 130:219, 1975.
76. Tolins, S. H.: Surgical treatment of diverticulitis: experience at a large municipal hospital, JAMA 232:830, 1975.
77. Lubbers, E. J., Crutzen, J. J., and Hesp, W. L.: Findings in patients with diverticulosis and diverticulitis of the colon, Arch. Chir. Neerl. 28:179, 1976.
78. Griffen, W. O., Jr.: Management of the acute complications of diverticular disease: acute perforation of colonic diverticula, Dis. Colon Rectum 19:293, 1976.

79. Stevens, L. W.: Surgical management of colonic diverticulitis and complicated diverticulosis, Postgrad. Med. 60:122, 1976.
80. Sweatman, C. A., Jr., Aldrete, J. S.: The surgical management of diverticular disease of the colon complicated by perforation, Surg. Gynecol. Obstet. 144:47, 1977.

Hemorrhoids, Fistulae and Fissures: Office and Hospital Management — A Critical Review

JAMES A. FERGUSON, M.D., F.A.C.S. AND
JOHN M. MacKEIGAN, M.D., F.R.C.S.(C)

Colon and Rectal Surgery, Ferguson Clinic, Grand Rapids, Michigan

Anorectal conditions such as hemorrhoids, fissures, and fistulae present some of the commonest management problems in a family physician's or surgeon's practice. The variety of treatment modalities is confusing. Because the anus is the anus, the significance of patients' symptoms may not be appreciated and treatment may be compromised. Many physicians are unaware of the disabilities that hemorrhoids, fissures or fistulae can generate. Appropriate management is attended by an appreciative patient. Inappropriate management may be attended by continuation and even intensification of symptoms. This paper will attempt to put the management of such common problems in proper perspective.

Hemorrhoids

The nature, pathogenesis and treatment of hemorrhoids are of continuing controversy. There is little agreement on the anatomic or physiologic derangement that allows symptomatic hemorrhoids to develop. There are no satisfactory methods to compare symptoms and results of treatment. Symptoms are widely divergent and discomfort is difficult to assess objectively.

111

0065–3411/78/0012–0111$03.75

There are numerous forms of therapy, all having some degree of success. Effective treatment often depends on the degree of reconstruction of the normal anatomic form and function.

The size of hemorrhoids or the degree of prolapse cannot always be correlated with symptoms. Small, actively bleeding hemorrhoids that do not prolapse may be equally or more troublesome than large, prolapsing hemorrhoids that become reduced spontaneously. Large, internal hemorrhoids with no prolapse but marked friability may be seen in male patients with hypertonic anal sphincters. Small internal hemorrhoids with a large ring of perianal skin tags and significant mucosal prolapse may be seen in female patients with anal sphincter hypotonia. Such diversity of anatomy and symptoms requires judgment in choosing the appropriate course. A well conceived, properly executed anatomic operation may correct most forms of hemorrhoidal symptoms but may represent overtreatment. Forms of therapy such as sclerosing injection, rubberbanding, dilatation and cryotherapy may be appropriate but their limitations and applications must be appreciated.

ANATOMY AND PHYSIOLOGY

Hemorrhoidal veins comprise a normal communication system between the caval and portal venous systems. This fact is apparently of academic interest only and we have never noted any important clinical significance. Should these veins dilate, become tortuous, enlarge, protrude or bleed clinically, significant hemorrhoids or piles are present.

Stelzner[77] in Germany has demonstrated arterial venous communications in hemorrhoids. Although this may account for the bright red bleeding noted from hemorrhoids, it does not explain their cause. Congestion and dilatation do not explain the solitary enlarged hemorrhoid or the relatively infrequent occurrence of hemorrhoids in portal hypertension. Thomson,[79] in a recent analysis of cadavers, noted that dilated veins are a normal and constant finding. He confirmed the arterial venous communications discovered by Stelzner and noted that histologically, hemorrhoids do not differ significantly from normal anal submucosa. Thomson postulated that hemorrhoids are normal, anal "cushions" that are prolapsed or displaced. The reason for displacement, however, is not apparent. Heredity, straining, constipation, diarrhea, increased anal sphincter tone, decreased anal sphincter tone, obstruction to portal flow or pelvic congestion are factors in symptomatic hemorrhoidal development.

There usually are three main hemorrhoidal cushions which commonly occur in the right posterior, right anterior and left lateral positions. These anatomic positions have been attributed by Miles[56] to branching of the superior hemorrhoidal artery. Thomson, with his cadaver and arterial injection studies, could not confirm this theory.

Goligher[29] has classified hemorrhoids into four categories according to their degree of prolapse. This is useful in the comparison of treatment regimens and occasionally in the choice of appropriate therapy. It does not suggest that there is a natural progression of hemorrhoids to prolapse, nor does it suggest degrees of severity of symptoms.

External hemorrhoids often are given undue significance in producing symptoms. There are no easily identifiable, distinct, external hemorrhoids. What are commonly called external hemorrhoids are redundant tags of skin at the anal verge which result from displacement of the mucocutaneous junction. They rarely cause significant symptoms. Their importance lies in surgical correction of the prolapsing internal hemorrhoids. With surgery, every attempt should be made to reduce the anoderm into the anal canal and, thereby, to obliterate the skin tags. Only rarely do the plexuses of veins at the anal verge dilate significantly unless there is associated internal hemorrhoidal enlargement. Isolated small thrombosis of the external venous plexus at the anal verge commonly occurs but cannot always be equated with the presence of significant internal hemorrhoids.

The role of the anal sphincter in the pathogenesis of hemorrhoids probably is minor. Hemorrhoids occur with both a clinically tonic or lax sphincter. Lord[51] advocates anal dilatation for the treatment of hemorrhoids on the basis that hemorrhoids result from a chronically contracted anal sphincter. This is not the case in most patients. Whereas some studies[35] suggest that hemorrhoids are associated with high resting anal pressure, others[45] suggest that there is no difference between controls and patients with hemorrhoids.

Hemorrhoids are best identified by anoscopy with an instru-

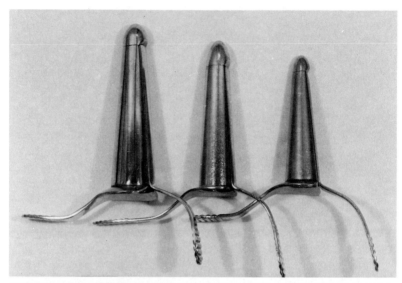

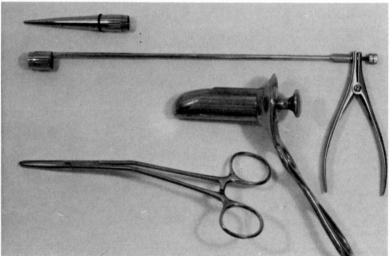

Fig 1 (top). – Brinkerhof anoscopes (V. Mueller, Chicago).
Fig 2 (bottom). – McGivney hemorrhoidal ligator (Fort Dixon Co., Dallas), Hirschman anoscope and angulated forceps.

ment that creates little distortion of the anal canal and permits segmental inspection. The Brinkerhof speculum, with its slide-controlled fenestrum, is ideal (Fig 1). Obturator anoscopes, such as the Hirschman type (Fig 2) allow all anal tissue to roll into view as the scope is withdrawn.

Symptoms

Bleeding and prolapse are the predominant symptoms of hemorrhoids. Bright red, painless, intermittent bleeding is characteristic of internal hemorrhoids and may be mild or severe enough to saturate clothing. It may be well tolerated and it may cause serious anemia. Prolapsing hemorrhoids are accompanied by constant mucus discharge, which softens and excoriates. Hemorrhoids alone do not cause pruritus ani but are one of many factors. Pain is not characteristic of hemorrhoids unless there is associated thrombosis. Usually, significant pain with defecation results from an associated anal fissure or ulcer.

Management

In general, hemorrhoids need no treatment at all. Most patients need a thorough examination and a good opinion more than they need treatment. Although hemorrhoids have nothing to do with cancer, the two diseases do imitate each other by bleeding. It is more important to rule out cancer than to rule in hemorrhoids. Therefore, any hemorrhoidal treatment must be preceded by sigmoidoscopy and barium enema. Hemoccult tests without sigmoidoscopy and x-ray are grossly inadequate. If treatment is indeed indicated, standards against which all modalities of treatment must compare are those of a well-conceived, well-executed, anatomic and physiologic surgical operation.

Nonsurgical management of hemorrhoids includes topical applications, injection therapy, galvanic electric current therapy, application of constricting bands, dilatation and cauterization by cryotherapy. Recent advocates of "conservative" therapy have suggested that such therapies offer an equal alternative to surgical therapy. Many times such enthusiasm for nonoperative or conservative therapy is influenced by the lack of operating room facilities or hospital beds. Surgeons treating hemorrhoidal disease should have several alternatives of therapy with which they are familiar. In some patients, surgery may represent "too much, too soon," and in others nonsurgical treatment may represent "too little, too late."

Topical Applications

Topical applications are generally of great value in controlling mild anal and perianal skin irritation, as well as in their placebo effect. They usually are over-the-counter preparations that are used in direct proportion to the intensity of their sales presentation. Obviously, no externally applied medication will eradicate hemorrhoids but it may eradicate symptoms by its soothing and astringent effects.

Injection Therapy

Injection of sclerosing solutions submucosally is good treatment for internal hemorrhoids only. Such therapy is time-tested and a valuable clinical adjunct. Commonly used solutions are 5% quinine and urea hydrochloride or 5% phenol in almond oil. We can find no comparative studies of these two agents. Graham-Stewart[32] in 1962 reported the comparative histologic changes from injecting 5% phenol and oil vs those from oil injected alone. He could find no difference and attributed the changes to the oil. This is in contrast to Goligher's improved results with phenol and oil over oil alone.[15]

The reaction to sclerosing injections is apparent from histologic studies of Duke in 1924 and Graham-Stewart in 1962.[32] The injections cause submucosal fibrosis, which constricts and obliterates hemorrhoidal veins. This decreases the congestion and results in reduced tendency for bleeding. Fixation of the hemorrhoids by the reaction to the underlying musculature may afford some relief of mild prolapse.

Injection therapy may be impermanent but can be repeated as necessary. Usually, 2 cc of reagent is injected submucosally above the mucocutaneous junction in each of three quadrants. Ample time is allowed for maximum effect and the patient is reexamined in two months. Re-injection can be done then, if indicated. An 18-gauge spinal needle with or without an extending adapter is useful (Fig 3). No attempt to enter or avoid the actual lumen of the vein is made.

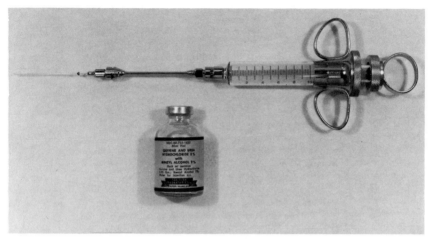

Fig 3. – Syringe with extension for hemorrhoidal injection.

Mild hypotensive reactions to injection occur rarely; we have never seen an allergic or anaphylactoid reaction of any significance. We have had no local complications of injection though submucosal abscess, stricture, hematoma formation or oleogranuloma, and prostatic abscess has been reported.

Injection treatment is intended for internal hemorrhoids only and may need to be repeated, but it has the tremendous advantages of painlessness, economy, facility, nonhospitalization, no anesthesia and no disability; and it is very effective in controlling symptoms.

Elastic Band Ligation

Inelastic ligation of hemorrhoids has a long history dating back to the middle ages. Involving some dissection and ligation with a nonabsorbable suture material such as linen or cotton, it should not be confused with the technique of ligation described by Blaisdell in 1958.[10] Barron modified Blaisdell's technique and developed his special instrument for placing an elastic band around the prominent internal hemorrhoid.[5] The technique and instruments have been modified by others (see Fig 2).[71, 73]

Ligation, also restricted to internal hemorrhoids, destroys by ischemia in the same way that injection destroys by fibrosis. The internal hemorrhoidal mass needs to be rather polypoid in shape and of moderate size. Sessile masses of great volume do not strangulate well.

Exposure of the internal hemorrhoid by Brinkerhof, Hirschman or other anoscope or retractor is a matter of patient comfort and personal preference. The hemorrhoid is grasped through the ring of the ligator and the ring is advanced over the hemorrhoid, maintaining traction with the forceps. The angulated forceps allow good visualization of the area to be ligated. The lower edge of the ring must be above the mucocutaneous junction. Two bands are applied by the banding instrument and three internal hemorrhoids may be treated at the same time. The bands usually are sloughed in ten days and patients should be re-examined then. Figure 2 depicts the McGivney bander, Hirschman anoscope and angulated forceps, which is our banding kit.

The complications of banding are few. Thrombosis of the external venous complexes, slippage and breakage of the bands and late bleeding, requiring hospital admission, may occur. The resulting ulceration may be slow to heal and may be a source of continued discomfort or drainage. Even with proper application, the procedure is not without discomfort.

In a comparative study of a variety of treatment modalities, surgical hemorrhoidectomy gave overall superior results.[44] Steinberg, Leigois and Alexander-Williams in a long-term evaluation of elastic banding, reported that less than one-half of patients were symptom-free up to six years after the procedure.[76]

The disadvantages of ligation treatment are few; the advantages are the same as for injection treatment. Ligation, however, is not as broadly applicable as is injection. The combination of elastic ligation and cryotherapy is a sophisticated modification of ligation and is subject to the same observations and limitations.

Anal Dilatation

Anal dilatation has become widely used in Great Britain for treatment of hemorrhoids after Lord's description in 1958.[51] According to Lord, there is a constriction of the lower rectum and anus in patients with hemorrhoids. He feels that anal dilatation releases the constriction and resulting congestion of the hemorrhoids and holds that the nature of the constriction has not been determined.

We have no experience with avulsion as the primary treatment of hemorrhoids and cannot imagine its challenging or supplanting more accurate means of control.

Cryotherapy

Destruction of hemorrhoids by cauterization has been advocated since the hot irons of Hippocrates' day. Since 1969 cryodestruction of hemorrhoids has been possible with technical developments.[50]

There appear to be no contraindications to freezing hemorrhoids or skin tags. Various instruments are available using nitrous oxide or liquid nitrogen. The latter allows a colder temperature but generally is more expensive. The procedure is performed either with application of a probe to the prominent area or while squeezing the prominent hemorrhoid. Although the freezing process is not associated with pain, the pressure of the probe may cause sufficient discomfort to warrant local anesthesia or even general anesthesia for good access to the anal canal. Following cryotherapy, there is initially a significant edema. A foul discharge ensues and persists for six weeks. Goligher states that despite previous reports, 60 of his 68 patients had significant postoperative pain.[30]

The results of therapy are variously reported. We could find no comparative studies of cryotherapy. O'Conner reports 96% satisfactory results. Goligher reports 70% satisfactory results and he notes that postoperative pain is the main disadvantage. This was enough to "mitigate against a repetition" of cryotherapy in the remaining 30%.[30]

We have no experience with cryotherapy and have little interest in it for the same reasons as for sphincter muscle avulsion.

SURGICAL MANAGEMENT

There are few procedures in anorectal surgery that cause more disagreement than the advantages and disadvantages of various forms of surgical therapy for hemorrhoids. The results of different forms of therapy naturally depend on the expertise of the operator. No procedure is comfortably performed by all surgeons. Even comparative studies of techniques are weighted in significance by the usual procedure performed by the surgeon seeking the result.

The goal of any surgical procedure must be to re-establish normal anatomy in a well-functioning anal canal. This involves excising completely the prominent internal hemorrhoidal tissue while preserving as much of the anal lining as possible, thus maintaining pliancy and preventing stenosis. The resulting anus must be skin-lined and pliant to be dry and comfortable. Ectropion of mucosa such as that seen in an improperly done Whitehead operation produces the "wet anus" of constant mucus secretion. The wound should heal within reasonable time, with minimal pain, discomfort and scar formation. The operative procedures are all excisional methods with various treatment of pedicles or various forms of closure of the wound. The common procedures are simply classified as open, radical and closed techniques by noting various treatments of the wound.

Open Hemorrhoidectomy (St. Mark's Hospital)

There are a number of different "open" techniques and modifications. In all procedures, the hemorrhoidal area is excised and the pedicle is either clamped, ligated or oversewn. The pedicle is either sutured high or low and the wounds are left open to varying degrees to heal by secondary intention. This treatment of the wound is assumed to be necessary for drainage or to prevent infection.

Salmon, of St. Mark's Hospital in London, is credited with describing an excision and open technique with high ligation of the pedicle.[4] Miles described a similar technique in 1919 with low ligation to prevent the excess of scarring in the upper anal canal.[56] Milligan et al.[59], in 1937, described a modification of Miles' technique with ligation of the pedicle, suturing it low in the anal canal. This perhaps is the commonest hemorrhoidectomy performed in Great Britain. The advantage is its simplicity; however, it has definite disadvantages. The procedure is bloody and good visualization of the internal sphincter is not always possible. The anatomy is distorted by traction. A portion of the sphincter may be included in the ligation of the pedicle. It leaves only 1/4 inch of mucosa between the excised areas with resultant wide, bare areas. The ligated portion often slips, causing the mucosa to retract upward and increasing the bare area.

The displaced anoderm is not reduced back into the anal canal. The wounds are large and take a long time to heal. At St. Mark's Hospital, approximately 25% of patients are required to use anal dilators postoperatively.[73] Despite these obvious disadvantages, it is surprising that anal stenosis and a "wet anus" do not occur with greater frequency than is reported.

Mitchell[60] in 1903 introduced a similar method, with clamping of the pedicle and oversewing of the pedicle afer amputation. This was popularized by Earl[18] in the United States.

Fansler[23] and Buie[70] are credited with emphasizing the need to relocate the anoderm into the anal canal. Despite common belief to the contrary, Whitehead[83] described a total hemorrhoidal excision but emphasized the need to preserve the squamous epithelium.

Parks[63] in 1956 introduced the technique of submucosal hemorrhoidectomy, a modification of the technique of Petit described in 1774.[69] Operating within the anal canal so as to prevent its distortion, the surgeon infiltrates the mucosa with epinephrine. A small portion of the anoderm is excised, the mucosa is incised and two flaps of mucosa are developed over the hemorrhoidal complex. Hemorrhoids are dissected free and the hemorrhoidal pedicle is ligated. Two flaps of mucosa are sutured at their lower ends, with fixation to the underlying sphincter. The upper and lower portions are left open or partially closed.

The advantages of submucosal hemorrhoidectomy are the preservation of the mucosa and the high ligation of pedicles. The disadvantages of the technique are noteworthy. First, it is performed in an anal canal that is stretched by the special retractor. This tends to shorten the anal canal and, subsequently, flatten the area to be operated on. Second, it broadens the hemorrhoidal area and probably accounts for less complete hemorrhoidal excision and the high recurrence rate reported by Watts et al.[81] Third, the operation creates a dead space under the mucosal flap. The mucosa is excessively bruised and handled by the procedure. It is difficult to perform and therefore has not been adopted by all surgeons at St. Mark's Hospital.

Bekhit[6] compared the high ligation technique of Parks and the low ligation technique of Milligan in a small series with 50 cases in each group. He discovered that the submucosal technique of Parks was less painful but had a higher incidence of submucosal abscess. Advocates of the low ligation technique feel there is a lessened incidence of postoperative bleeding due to placement of the pedicle within the anal canal. Bleeding occurred in one case of low ligation and two cases of high ligation in Bekhit's series. Since the series is small, too much should not be deduced. The closer approximation of the anatomy is the major credit of Parks' technique but possibly has a higher infection and recurrence rate.

Radical Hemorrhoidectomy (Whitehead)

Complete excision of the entire hemorrhoidal area was described by Whitehead[83] in 1882, whose technique has been much maligned due to modification by others. Whitehead excised the mucosa and veins of the anal canal, stressing the need to preserve the skin portion. The mucosa was then sutured to the skin at the mucocutaneous junction. Because the suture line is under tension, it may separate, leaving large, bare areas. A long, circumferential scar is created, leading to possible stenosis. The mucocutaneous junction is displaced toward the anal verge because of prolapsing hemorrhoids. This leads to exteriorization of the glandular mucosa and increased drainage postoperatively. With time, other operators adopted this technique, suturing the mucosa to the anal verge and excising the skin portion. This caused a severe deformity with mucus discharge, soiling and, often, disproportionate pain. This has been called the "Whitehead deformity." Because the technique is badly performed by most surgeons, resulting in severe disability, we feel that the Whitehead procedure has limited general applicability.

Closed Hemorrhoidectomy (Ferguson Clinic)

This procedure, described in 1959 by Ferguson and Heaton,[24] involves the excision of the hemorrhoidal tissue with total anatomic reconstruction of a normal anal canal. The principles of hemorrhoidal surgery are exemplified in the closed technique. Vascular pads or hemorrhoids are removed with preservation of the anal mucosa and skin. The internal hemorrhoidal pedicle is always in the lower rectal ampulla, while the anal canal is entirely lined by glandular and squamous epithelium. All incisions are primarily closed, heal more quickly and the resulting anal canal is smooth and pliable.

We perform the procedure in the modified Sims position. It is equally adaptable to the jacknife or the lithotomy position. Although widely accepted today, closed hemorrhoidectomy was a complete departure from standard practice less than 20 years ago.

Hemorrhoids are operated on in situ with no distortion of the anatomy and no eversion of the lining. A Hill-Ferguson retractor is used to approximate the normal size of the anal canal. The hemorrhoidal complex is outlined with elliptical incision down to the internal sphincter (Fig 4), from which it is dissected upward well into the submucosal space of the lower rectal ampulla. The hemorrhoidal complex is then amputated distal to a clamp (Fig 5). Amputation without the clamp is feasible, safe and preferred by some surgeons. The pedicle is oversewn with 3-0 chromic or 5-0 Dexon above the anorectal ring (Fig 6). Adjacent varices are dissected out from under the edges of the incision but no effort to undermine the edges for their own sake is made. The ellipses thus are narrow and easily closed with a continuous suture under no tension (Fig 7). Dead space is prevented and the

Fig 4 (left). – Excision of hemorrhoidal complex with sharp dissection.
Fig 5 (right). – Amputation of the hemorrhoid distal to clamp.

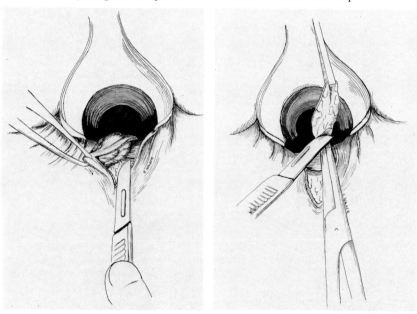

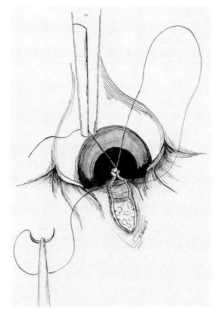

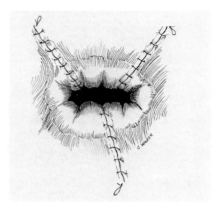

Fig 6 (left). – Suture ligation of the pedicle.
Fig 7 (above). – Closure of hemorrhoidectomy incisions.

anal skin is returned to its normal location. Closure of the incision with the medium sized Hill-Ferguson retractor in place closely approximates the size of the anal canal. If there is associated stenosis or anal ulcer, superficial internal anal sphincterotomy is performed in all three quadrants. This decreases postoperative pain as stated by Eisenhammer and creates a normal, funnel-shaped anal outlet.[19] The closed technique is probably the most versatile of surgical techniques as we have no reluctance to fit, trim, reposition, realign and, above all, reapproximate anal and perianal skin.

The results of closed hemorrhoidectomy are gratifying and we continue its use because of its great versatility, dependability and minimal morbidity in many thousands of patients.

Results of Surgery

We are aware of only one small study comparing various techniques. Watts et al.[81] in 1954 reported the results of common techniques of hemorrhoidectomy in 100 patients. Five different techniques were analyzed with only 5–38 patients in each group. Patients were not randomly allocated. The results can be expected to be influenced by the familiarity of the operator with the various techniques. The group reporting the results normally performed a Milligan type of low-ligation hemorrhoidectomy.

When wounds were examined at ten days following the low ligation technique, patients showed wounds extending to the top of the anal canal and one-third had coalescence of the excised areas. Submucosal hemorrhoidectomy showed many mucosal wounds closed with others with only narrow, 6-mm bare areas. Closed technique showed that 50% of the skin wounds had united primarily but that mucosal wounds often were separated. This has not been our experience when viewing patients 5–14 days postoperatively. Most of the skin in these patients or mucosal wounds were united or showed only thin lines. This is in a group presenting with postoperative bleeding in which it would be expected that most of the wounds would have healed less satisfactorily than normal.

With the three techniques — low ligation, submucosal and closed — at six months the closed technique had the least incidence of recurrent hemorrhoids and skin tags. A higher incidence of stenosis was reported with the closed technique but this may be due to technical differences and postoperative care. We have found no incidence of stenosis unless the patient was taking cathartics or had long-standing diarrhea. Both conditions cause stenosis in the unoperated anal canal. We use no laxatives or stool softeners following discharge from the hospital and have found that the best anal dilator is a well-formed stool. Watts' series found a higher incidence of pain with the closed technique, which has not been our experience.

In general, the operative excision of hemorrhoids is the standard and most reliable means of ablation of hemorrhoidal veins. It also is the most versatile and permanent treatment of anal disease associated with hemorrhoids such as fissure, ulcer, stenosis and even fistulae. If one is willing to close anal wounds, there is no limit to plastic relocation and repair of anal skin and mucous membrane. If one is unwilling to close anal wounds, the limitations are great.

Thrombosed Hemorrhoids

Treatment of a small, acute, thrombosed, external hemorrhoidal venous plexus offers no controversy. If left alone or treated

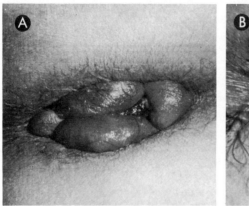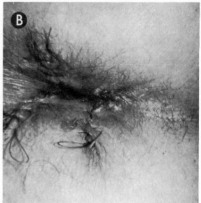

Fig 8. – Acute thrombosis of hemorrhoids treated with surgical excision and primary closure.

symptomatically, it will resolve spontaneously. If persistent, painful or bothersome, it can be excised in the office under local anesthesia.

If there is acute thrombosis and prolapse of internal hemorrhoids, attempts at evacuation of the clot are futile. The clots usually are multiloculated and edema is extensive. Conservative management of acute, severe, thrombosed hemorrhoids is the usual practice at most centers and is attended by tedious hospitalization, much discomfort, slow resolution and ultimate hemorrhoidectomy. Urgent hemorrhoidectomy is indicated and we have found no increase in complications. Long morbidity is avoided and definitive solution of the problem is achieved within 4 – 5 days (Fig 8).

An analysis of conservative treatment of prolapsed and thrombosed hemorrhoids showed a high incidence of continuing symptoms.[31] Only 13% of patients had no further symptoms after resolution of the problem. History of previous prolapsed hemorrhoids or a three-year history of symptoms prior to the episode seemed to be strong indication for urgent hemorrhoidectomy.

For many years it was feared that hemorrhoidectomy for acute thrombosed hemorrhoids was dangerous. Fears of pylephlebitis, gangrene, secondary hemorrhage or stricture are unfounded. Ackland,[1] in reviewing the literature, found only one case of pylephlebitis, which occurred after routine hemorrhoidectomy. Gangrene was reported in the literature in three cases, once each after routine hemorrhoidectomy, emergency hemorrhoidectomy and conservative treatment. Laurence and Murray[48] showed that any infection in acutely thrombosed hemorrhoids usually is superficial and confined to the areas of ulceration.

It has been reported in a number of series that an urgent hemorrhoidectomy can be performed with no increased complications over routine hemorrhoidectomy. Mazier[53] analyzed 400 cases treated in the acute state by closed hemorrhoidectomy and found results favorably comparable to elective procedures.

Anal Fissures and Ulcers

Anal fissures are disruptions of the anoderm of the anal canal which cause more pain than the pathologic condition would seem to justify. Chronic anal fissures, commonly called anal ulcers, can occur in any age group and are equal in sex distribution. The anal fissures are distinguished from the anal ulcers by their superficial nature and thin, linear appearance in the undilated anal canal, as well as by the lack of visible internal sphincter muscle in the base of the lesion. They may be of primary or secondary etiology.

ETIOLOGY

Although we are impressed by the frequent association of anal ulcers and hemorrhoids, the presence of hemorrhoids cannot be implicated in causation. Trauma appears to be the currently accepted etiology. This is the explanation most commonly mentioned by patients who relate onset either following a firm stool or an episode of diarrhea. The predisposing causes are purely a matter of conjecture. The predominately posterior midline locations of fissures have encouraged theories of a posterior angulation of the anal canal, the relative fixation of the anal canal posteriorly, the divergence of the fibers of the external sphincter muscle posteriorly, and the elliptical shape of the anal canal. The frequency with which most fissures heal with minimum of therapy while others become chronic seems unexplainable. Nor do theories explain the increased frequency of anterior ulcers in women or the occasional lateral ulcer that looks and behaves like a typical posterior ulcer. The frequency of surgically induced "fissures" with operative incisions would be expected to precipitate a higher incidence of ulcer if trauma and anal sphincter spasm were the main etiologic agents.

The triad of ulcer, hypertrophied anal papilla and sentinel skin tag is even more an enigma. Although the lack of support of the anoderm at the anal verge distal to the ulcer may contribute to a sentinel tag, we can conjecture no reasonable explanation for the often-prominent anal papilla.

Recently, there has been increasing interest in the internal sphincter muscle and its role in either the pathogenesis or treatment of anal fissures or ulcers. It has been shown that the resting pressures of the internal sphincter muscle are essentially the same in controls and patients with anal fissures.[45] This is contrary to what clinical judgment would seem to dictate when viewing the patient who may be virtually impossible to examine because of apparent spasm. Nothmann and Schuster[61] demonstrated that following rectal distention there is a normal reflex relaxation of the internal sphincter. In addition, they found an abnormal "overshoot contraction" following the initial relaxation.

Secondary causes of anal fissures or ulcers commonly are grouped as curiosities. Unless a high index of suspicion is maintained for nonspecific inflammatory causes such as mucosal ulcerative colitis or Crohn's disease, or for specific inflammatory diseases such as syphilis or tuberculosis, disastrous results can follow. Other than their atypical location, the lesions of anal Crohn's disease often present a typical surrounding edema and rubor. The symptoms of anal Crohn's disease are often less than would be anticipated by the extent and nature of the ulcerative lesion. Unfortunately, biopsy or excision may not always support the clinical impression and subsequent course. Contrary to popular and perhaps prudent teaching, selective, quiescent and symptomatic anal Crohn's disease can be surgically treated satisfactorily in highly selected patients. With increasing frequency, the patient with a syphilitic chancre, with or without associated gonorrheal proctitis, is misdiagnosed. Contrary to common belief, the syphilitic chancre may typify a common anal ulcer and may be painful as well. Anal tuberculosis is exceedingly rare and we suspect that many cases of pathologic and clinical examination may have represented anal Crohn's disease. Primary squamous cell carcinoma or cloacogenic carcinoma may cause severe pain and bleeding, mimicking an anal ulcer, and in all respects may appear like a benign lesion. The disproportionate firmness of the lesion on palpation usually denotes the etiology. Postsurgical anal fissures develop with varying frequency, depending on the degree of subsequent anal fibrosis or stenosis.

Occasionally, even though symptoms may suggest acute anal fissure or even a chronic, recurring fissure or ulcer, no lesion can be demonstrated. This may just represent a healed fissure at the time of examination but an intermuscular abscess must be ruled out, particularly in the obviously painful and spastic anal canal. Deliberate palpation of the anal canal itself may reveal a localized deep induration or tenderness with suspicion of an intermuscular abscess. A short anal sinus or pea-sized nodule may be felt deep in the musculature.

Symptoms

Pain following defecation variously described as sharp, lancing, biting or burning is the hallmark of anal fissures and ulcers. Not uncommonly, such pain is incorrectly attributed to hemorrhoids. In most instances of hemorrhoidal disease uncomplicated by thrombosis, the pain can be assumed to be related to an undiagnosed ulcer. Occasionally the pain of an acute fissure may result in urinary retention or fecal impaction. The bleeding of anal fissures or ulcers is variable but usually occurs as streaks on the outside of the stool or spots noted on toilet tissue.

Patients with pruritus ani may have superficial perianal excoriation and fissuring which extend into the anal canal. Such fissures are a part of and not a cause of the dermatitis. Only rarely should surgical correction of anal fissures or ulcers be undertaken as a specific cure for anal pruritus.

Diagnosis

Inspection is the only means of diagnosis of fissures and ulcers. In a patient with a history of pain or bleeding or both, possibly with anal sphincter spasm, the lesion can be missed easily by palpation and anoscopy. The lesion can be identified by spreading the radiating perianal skin folds and inverting the anoderm by traction of the perianal skin. Once its presence is known, localized subtle induration or dimpling in the anal canal may be detected by palpation. Localized tenderness to palpation is not very reliable. Palpation of the perianal skin must be performed carefully to rule out any induration suggesting an abscess. If anal spasm and discomfort are severe, instillation of an anesthetic ointment (1% cyclomethycaine sulfate) followed by a 5–10-minute wait usually will allow digital examination. This must be done with deliberate and slow pressure on the anal margin with the index finger and with pressure away from the site of the ulcer.

It may be difficult to visualize an anal fissure or ulcer with an anoscope despite its known presence. Most anoscopes have an obturator and visualization is expected on its withdrawal. The presence of the linear folds of the canal or hemorrhoids may obscure the lesion. A Brinkerhof anoscope allows the use of varying diameters and allows inspection of a limited portion of the anal canal while dilating the canal itself. With this instrument and similar anoscopes it is noted that most "fissures" are, in fact, superficial, ovoid or round lesions and not at all linear. Progressing to an anal ulcer by repeated trauma, the lesion develops a punched-out, circular, fibrotic rim with visible muscle fibers at its base. The presence of a large sentinel tag and hypertrophied papilla (Lane's polyp) is further evidence of chronicity. Conservative treatment of such ulcers usually is a futile effort. Superficial healing may occur temporarily or patients may become accustomed to a less than optimal situation of anal stenosis, with the chronic use of stool softeners.

If muscle is visible in the base of the ulcer, operative intervention is likely. By identifying the chronic lesion, an early decision may be made for a trial of either conservative or operative treatment. If there is any question of the chronicity, by history or by appearance of the lesion, little is lost by a trial of conservative management.

MANAGEMENT

Many fissures of a superficial nature and short history will heal spontaneously with a minimum of supportive care. This is particularly true in the pediatric age group, where healing almost inevitably results from nonoperative treatment. This occurs despite a relatively long and recurrent history. The patient with a short history may be writhing in the agony of anal spasm. Such a patient may be afforded relief by anal sphincterotomy. While preferably performed with good exposure and control in the operating room, individual community access to operative facilities may dictate the necessity of performing the procedure in the office.

If the examiner is satisfied with the examination and his ability to visualize the lesion sufficiently to rule out any associated abscess or secondary cause of fissures, then a trial of nonoperative treatment is appropriate. If pain partially limits the examination, re-examination is necessary in 7–10 days. If pain or apprehension is such that no satisfactory examination is possible, then examination with the patient under general anesthesia is desirable.

The armamentarium for nonoperative treatment is limited to pain pills, stool softeners, soothing ointment and sitz baths. Oral pain medication should be taken preferably before any anticipated bowel movement. Stool softeners should be hydrated to provide a soft, formed stool. Agents such as psyllium-containing products mixed with juices or with artificial cocktail mixers provide a palatable means of administering the softener. Under no circumstances can we see the need for oil aperients, with their possible short-term complications of aspiration and long-term complications of promoting vitamin deficiency. This is particularly true of pediatric patients. The dosage of the softener should be reduced gradually after the patient has been symptom free for a week. Any treatment modality, nonsurgical or surgical, will fail if long-term cathartics are permitted.

There are many soothing ointments available with probably little difference in efficacy. Whether the ointments or creams promote healing or only allow some lubrication of the anal canal is unknown. Anesthetic ointments are generally for use in the most painful cases but should be used for a short term only as they may cause dermatitis. Any ointment is administered preferably before and after a bowel movement.

Suppositories and injection foams have no rational appeal to us in the treatment of anal fissures. Inserted above the lesion, they cannot be expected to provide anything but psychologic support. Self-dilatation may be curative but, as mentioned previously, the best anal dilator is a well-formed stool. Any anal stenosis in a patient with superficial fissure usually is of a reflex muscular origin and resolves with healing of the fissure. Injection of long-acting anesthetic solutions promotes little relief and has significant complications. Applications of silver nitrate to the fissure site have not been of proven value.

SURGICAL MANAGEMENT

There are various operative procedures for anal ulcers, with varying reported results. The common denominator in all procedures is the division of a portion of internal sphincter muscle. Unfortunately, there are few comparative studies of results of treatment. The association of other anal disease present at the time of discovery of the anal canal may make comparison difficult. The choice of procedure may be modified by the accessibility of the patient to a hospital bed. This probably accounts for the more recent appeal of anal dilatation and lateral anal sphincterotomy.

Anal Dilatation

Anal dilatation is a method of performing anal sphincter disruption with the use of 4, 6 or 8 fingers. Watts, Bennett and Goligher[82] report a failure rate of 16% with dilatation with 4 fingers in patients with idiopathic anal ulcers. This is with a rate of soiling of 20% postoperatively. As well, there is an aggravation of associated hemorrhoids and creation of mucosal prolapse and decreased anal sensation. With results such as these, we can see no justification for dilatation to 6 or 8 fingers to try to lessen the failure rate.[17] In the rare patient with painful anal Crohn's disease and stenosis, a limited dilatation to 1 or 2 fingers may afford some pain relief without the danger of creating a slow-healing wound.

Anal Sphincterotomy

Internal anal sphincterotomy is an essential part of any operative therapy for anal ulcers. Little has changed in the operative treatment over the past 40 years. Blaisdell (1937),[11] Milligan and Morgan (1934)[58] and Gabriel (1948)[27] advocated sphincter division. They unknowingly described division of the internal sphincter muscle, although they thought it was the "subcutaneous external sphincter." Miles[57] in 1939 stated that any essential part of the treatment of anal ulcers was the division of "pecten band" in the lower portion of the anal canal. This was divided radially in the posterolateral quadrant. It is probably safe to assume that these surgeons were describing and dividing the firm, sometimes fibrotic and prominent edge of the internal sphincter muscle. Eisenhammer[20] is credited with demonstrating the true nature and importance of the internal sphincter muscle in anal fissure disease.

Posterior Sphincterotomy

The method favored by Eisenhammer in 1953 and followed by others was the use of a posterior midline sphincterotomy, usually through the base of the ulcer.[20] This usually involved division of the distal third to half of the internal sphincter through its entire thickness. This method unfortunately has the obvious disadvantage of causing a significant "keyhole" defect of the anal outlet, allowing continued fecal soiling and incontinence of flatus. Goligher[29] reports a disappointing 34% incidence of impaired control of flatus and a 15% incidence of impairment of fecal control with this method. This impairment tends to improve with time but the overall results are disappointing, with 28% of patients having fecal soiling.

This full-thickness division of the sphincter has not been shown to be necessary and consequently any posterior sphincterotomy becomes suspect as an appropriate treatment modality. We have had considerable success for a number of years with a sphincterotomy which is rarely of full thickness. The prominent distal edge of the sphincter and ulcer bed is well visualized at the time of surgery by para-anal infiltration of 50 cc of 0.5% xylocaine with 1:200,000 epinephrine. If excision of the ulcer is chosen because of the ulcer's rather deep and fibrotic edge and associated papilla and skin tag, then a superficial division of the internal sphincter and prominent distal margin is performed (Fig 9). This re-creates a normal smoothed and rounded outlet with a funnel shape and no keyhole deformity. On occasion, if there is associated stenosis, this is performed in more than one quadrant to preserve the integrity of the greatest length of muscle. This re-creates the funnel shape of the normal

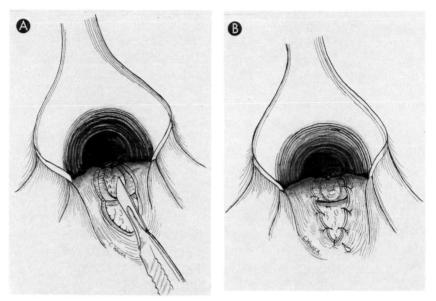

Fig 9.—Distal margin of internal sphincter muscle lightly incised to obliterate the distal margin.

anal outlet and minimizes soiling. The superficial nature of this sphincterotomy has been referred to by one of us as a "five-fiber anal sphincterotomy" to emphasize its superficial nature. The firmness or prominence of the muscle can be felt easily by the examining finger. Sphincterotomy sufficient to give a smooth and free margin to the outlet is all that is usually necessary. This may be accomplished with 4 or 5 light strokes of the scalpel. Sphincterotomy usually is complete when the firm edge of the internal sphincter is felt to disappear. Often the remaining uninvolved sphincter is felt to "give," allowing return of the normal-sized anus. In the case of severe anal stenosis, which often accompanies the anal ulcer, the sufficient nature of the sphincterotomy at the time of surgery is judged easily by the insertion of the medium Hill-Ferguson retractor. This retractor approximates the size of the normal and comfortably dilated anal canal (Fig 10). Thus, the device is of assistance at any time the anal sphincter muscle is being divided or repaired as a gauge of the anal outlet during the operation.

A review of 1,000 patients treated in such fashion showed a 4.4% recurrence rate in follow-up of up to four years, with only

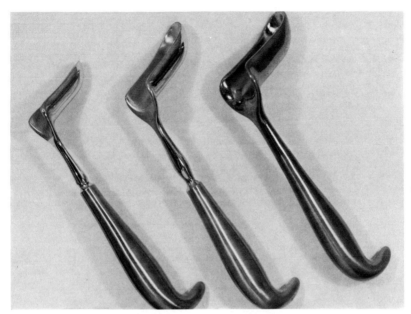

Fig 10. – Hill-Ferguson anal retractors (V. Mueller, Chicago).

1.2% complaining of the opening being "too tight" and less than 1% with frequent soiling or drainage.[54] It must be emphasized that superficial internal sphincterotomy may be all that is necessary and that it certainly approximates the normal situation.

Lateral Anal Sphincterotomy

Because of exceedingly disappointing results with a full-thickness posterior sphincterotomy, Eisenhammer[21] in 1959 and Bennett and Goligher[9] in 1962 first advocated lateral internal anal sphincterotomy. Parks[64] in 1967 suggested this could be accomplished with a short, curcumferential perianal incision so that incision in the anal canal was not necessary. Notaras[62] in 1969 suggested this could be performed with a small stab wound in the perianal region, using a cataract knife. The advantage of this method is its obvious simplicity and relatively decreased time off work. It is not, however, without some disadvantages. Hematoma formation, fistula, abscess formation and prolapse of hemorrhoids have been reported. Unfortunately, its recent publicity in some centers may stem in part from a deficiency of hospital beds or operating facilities in those centers. It has never been demonstrated that full-thickness internal sphincterotomy is necessary for the cure of anal ulcers. Although the occasional postsurgical recurrent anal ulcer may require a full-thickness sphincterotomy, this simple procedure may represent overtreatment of the sphincter at the time of initial surgery.

The simplicity of the procedure does not equate well with the postoperative complications, which can be significant. While Hoffman and Goligher[40] in 1970 showed improved results with the lateral sphincterotomy over that of full-thickness posterior sphincterotomy, 12% of patients still showed one or more minor defects of anal control such as fecal soiling or impaired control of stool or feces. Hardy and Cuthbertson[36] could find no difference in impairment between patients undergoing full-thickness posterior or lateral sphincterotomy. Three of 17 patients developed recurrent ulcers. Hoffman and Goligher reported a persistence or recurrence rate of 3% as opposed to 7% for posterior sphincterotomy.

Lateral internal anal sphincterotomy does not deal with associated symptomatic hemorrhoidal disease or prominent sentinel tags or papillae. Separate biopsy or excision of the ulcer should be performed for pathologic examination in all persistent or recurrent ulcers and all ulcers of suspicious nature at the time of surgery. For these reasons it is desirable that this procedure be done under good anesthesia with good visualization of the disease process and not just as a "blind stab" in an office situation.

Lateral anal sphincterotomy generally appears to have a lessened incidence of postoperative sequelae than does full-thickness posterior sphincterotomy. This could almost be expected since there is a slight, natural increase in the anterior-posterior diameter of the anal canal at rest. It is only accentuated by the posterior sphincterotomy. Although not as exaggerated with a lateral sphincterotomy, there is often a visible or palpable keyhole defect after any full-thickness internal sphincterotomy. This defect apparently accounts for the complaints of fecal soiling or drainage and incontinence.

As stated previously, it has never been shown that full-thickness internal anal sphincterotomy is necessary as a first choice in the treatment of anal ulcer. What is obviously needed is a comparative study between superficial and full-thickness sphincterotomy. Even if full-thickness sphincterotomy is proven to be necessary for persistent or recurrent anal ulcer, the obviously lessened morbidity in terms of control perhaps could be anticipated by initial use of a superficial sphincterotomy. The obvious disadvantage of superficial anal sphincterotomy is the necessity of anal incision. This does not seem to be a deterrent to good healing and logically would seem to result in lessened problems of control with a comparable recurrence rate.

Hemorrhoidectomy and Anal Ulcers

Symptomatic hemorrhoidal disease and anal ulcer often coexist. In such circumstances it is important to detail the history to be certain that symptoms are not incorrectly attributed to the anal ulcer or vice versa. If hemorrhoids are present and symptomatic, they must be treated concurrently with the anal ulcer. When sphincterotomy alone — whether posterior or lateral — is performed for treatment of the anal ulcer without dealing with

Fig 11. — Three-quadrant hemorrhoidectomy with superficial "five-fiber anal sphincterotomy" in three quadrants with anal ulcer left in situ.

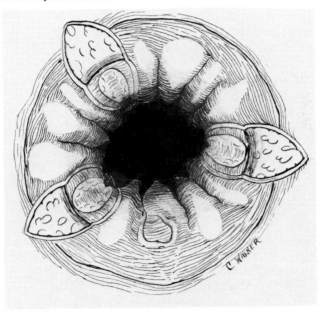

the hemorrhoids, hemorrhoidal symptoms of prolapse and drainage usually are accentuated. Asymptomatic hemorrhoids may become symptomatic following sphincterotomy.

For these reasons, we often recommend a formal, three-quadrant, closed hemorrhoidectomy along with superficial anal sphincterotomy in each quadrant.[26] This has the advantage not only of dealing with the hemorrhoids, but also of correcting the internal sphincter. If there is significant anal stenosis, hemorrhoidectomy incisions may be narrow ellipses or linear incisions so as to preserve the anoderm. The stenosis is corrected and a uniform, funnel-shaped outlet established with no keyhole defect. The anal ulcer may be excised separately and the incision closed, or the ulcer may be ignored (Fig 11).

Excision of Anal Ulcer

The recent popularity of lateral internal sphincterotomy has incorrectly put the treatment of anal ulcer by incision and sphincterotomy in an unfavorable light. It is wrongly stated that there is rarely a place for such therapy, except for the occasional ulcer that is resistant to other forms of therapy. Certainly, the excisional method of Gabriel[27] with wide excision of a triangular portion of external skin does little but prolong the healing time. The method of Hughes,[42] with excision and skin graft of the ulcer site, would seem to have limited general application. But surgical excision with a narrow, short ellipse – usually with a superficial sphincterotomy – still seems to have a place. In all circumstances, treatment should be individualized.

Several circumstances in which excisional therapy may be of value can be outlined. Some anal ulcers are associated with long-standing anal stenosis with contraction and thickening of the anoderm alone. Chronic irritation or lack of dilatation by formed stool in cases of chronic diarrhea, laxative abuse, or following surgical procedures, results in a cicatricial contraction of the anoderm. Contracture of the anal skin following long-term conservative management may occur insidiously, causing symptoms accepted by the physician and tolerated by the patient. In such circumstances, excision of the ulcer releases the contracted anoderm and the underlying internal sphincter seems to fall back from its position of being tethered to the thickened skin. On occasion, sphincterotomy is unnecessary if the process is primarily in the anoderm or, at most, only a superficial sphincterotomy is indicated. The anal outlet is seen to be of normal size. Leaving the area open will usually result in epithelialization.

Healing time can be shortened and the lack of anoderm can be corrected easily using a small triangular portion of skin distal to the anal ulcer site as a full thickness advancement flap. This has been called a "V-Y anoplasty."[74] The triangular portion of skin based posteriorly is advanced forward to the pectinate line and both sides are sutured closed. This heals quickly, with less pain and discomfort than when the area is left open. Hematoma, infection or sloughing of the skin flap is a surprisingly rare occurrence.

Occasionally, an anal ulcer is present in an otherwise normal anal canal. While spastic and apparently stenotic at the time of clinical examination, under anesthesia it appears normal and easily accepts the large Hill-Ferguson retractor. A large, full-thickness sphincterotomy seems rather illogical in this case. As the ulcer is excised, the internal sphincter muscle seems to be adherent to or part of the ulcer itself. After excision of the ulcer, the muscle and the size of the anal canal appear normal. There is no palpable abrupt edge of the muscle and no palpable firmness to indicate fibrosis in the muscle. In such circumstances, closure of the defect within tension is possible. A completely satisfactory result is obtained without injury to the sphincter.

If there is an anal ulcer with associated anal fistula or sinus originating in the base or free edge of the ulcer, surgical treatment of the fistula usually will necessitate surgical excision of at least a portion of the anal ulcer, if not the entire ulcer itself. At a minimum, incision through the ulcer base down through the fistula is necessary for treatment of the fistula itself.

It is obvious that there is no one satisfactory treatment modality for all cases of anal ulcer disease. Proper therapy usually dictates that surgical therapy be undertaken after evaluation of the entire process with the advantage of good anesthesia. Lateral anal sphincterotomy performed in an office environment has the initial appeal of simplicity and lack of hospitalization. Full-thickness sphincterotomy, with its sequelae, often is unnecessary and has the added dangers of missing associated processes or aggravating the hemorrhoidal disease.

Operation is an important part of the treatment of fissure and anal ulcer but will invariably fail if cathartics and laxatives of all types are not prohibited in the immediate and long-range postoperative period.

Anal Fistulae

As with hemorrhoids and fissures, the etiology and treatment of primary anal fistulae are confusing and controversial. Terminology and anatomic descriptions are not uniform. The etiology and classification of fistula sometimes cloud the practical aspects of surgical treatment. What is common to all opinions is that total drainage of the fistula, with clear delineation of its internal opening and all its ramifications, is necessary for cure.

An anal fistula generally is considered to be a chronic abscess. In its simplest form, a fistula is a fibrous tube lined by granulation tissue with an internal opening in the anal canal and external perianal opening. There may be multiple tracts or openings. The internal opening may originate at any level of the anal canal but commonly originates in an anal crypt at the mucocutaneous junction or at the base of an anal ulcer. Sinus tracts originating in the anal canal with no external opening are considered blind fistulae because of similar etiology and presentation.

Diagnosis

An anal fistula may occur with or without symptoms, or as an acute abscess. Usually there is a history of intermittent swelling, discomfort or discharge in the perianal region. The patient with a high intermuscular fistula or abscess may have painful bowel movements or tenesmus. Anteriorly in the female, a similar fistula may be associated with dyspareunia. A high postanal abscess or early intermuscular abscess may occur with acute pain, simulating an anal fissure. The history is of importance in eliminating contributing factors such as diabetes. A high index of suspicion is necessary to rule out subtle causes of fistulae such as inflammatory bowel disease or specific granulomata.

Inspection and palpation usually delineate the course and nature of the fistula. After discovery of an external opening, it is possible to palpate a fibrous cord subcutaneously leading toward the anal canal. If the tract is not palpable because of obesity or its high origin, superficial insertion of a probe may indicate its

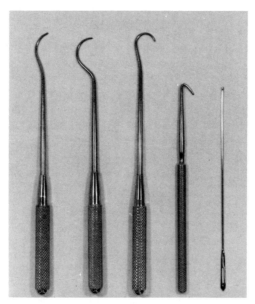

Fig 12. — Fistula probes of Ferguson Clinic.

general direction (Fig 12). Palpation with the thumb and index finger often will discover a postanal fistula or a high fistula. It is equally important to palpate the uninvolved side of the perianum for blind fistulae. Light palpation of the anal canal may suggest the origin of the fistula. The internal opening can be palpated as a pit at the mucocutaneous junction or base of the anal ulcer. Anoscopy may indicate the internal anal opening by discovery of an anal ulcer or a small amount of pus exuding from the site. Sigmoidoscopy is mandatory in the office or operating room to rule out "proximal disease," be it inflammatory, neoplastic or otherwise. In every instance a barium enema should be performed — if not possible preoperatively, then postoperatively. A recurrent fistula, history of diarrhea or any other suspicion of Crohn's disease requires upper gastrointestinal and small bowel x-ray examination. Chest x-ray films must be on hand for obvious reasons.

DIFFERENTIAL DIAGNOSIS. — The unusual causes of anal fistulae include trauma, foreign body, specific granulomas, lymphopathia venereum and carcinoma. The latter are rare and will not be diagnosed unless suspected and biopsied. Para-anal hidradenitis suppurativa and maverick pilonidal sinuses also confuse the issue. Fistula extending anteriorly must be distinguished from chronic Bartholin cyst infection in the female and urethral fistula in the male.

PATHOGENESIS

Anal fistulae occasionally heal spontaneously after drainage of an abscess. Their persistence as fistulae has plausible explanations, but still theoretical ones. Chiari[14] 100 years ago noted the presence of anal crypts and glands as the principal causes of fistulae. Eisenhammer[22] in 1958 pointed out that anal gland infection may cause intermuscular abscess formation between sphincters. The fistulae were thought to develop by extension from the intermuscular region. Parks[66] in 1961 pointed out the existence of anal glandular epithelium lining the inner aspect of the fistula tract. He postulated the fistulae might close spontaneously if the epithelium were not present.

Although many fistulae may originate or persist in this fashion, one theory cannot explain the existence of all fistulae. An intermuscular abscess is discernible in a minority of fistulae. It does not explain fistulae originating in an anal ulcer base. Excision of the glandular epithelium and intermuscular abscess advocated by Parks is not always followed by healing of the fistula.[66]

CLASSIFICATION

Classification of fistulae has been confused by misunderstanding of anatomy and lack of common terminology. There has been confusion about the relationship of the internal and external sphincters to one another. Milligan and Morgan[58] in 1934 helped to delineate the anatomic relationship of the sphincters. They particularly called attention to the role of the "anorectal ring" in maintaining continence. This is the puborectalis muscle felt at the uppermost portion of the anal canal posteriorly and posterolaterally. They classified fistula in relation to this anorectal ring. Goligher[29] in 1961 modified the classification with categories of subcutaneous, low anal, high anal, anorectal and submucosal (or high intermuscular) fistulae. The anorectal group included ischiorectal fistulae occupying the ischiorectal fossa and pelvirectal fistulae, which extend through the levator muscle to occupy a pararectal location. Terminology may have been more precise as ischioanal and pararectal.

High and low are imprecise terms as to location of the opening and extension of the tracts. The low anal fistula originating at the mucocutaneous junction and draining in the intermuscular plane may not have the same significance as a similar fistula that passes through both of the sphincter muscles.

Stelzner[78] in 1959 classified fistulae as intermuscular, trans-sphincteric and extrasphincteric. Intermuscular fistulae extend between the internal and external sphincter; trans-sphincteric fistulae extend through the sphincters to the ischiorectal fossa; extrasphincteric fistulae extend through and around the sphincters to re-enter the rectum. Parks, Gordon and Hardcastle[67] recently prepared a classification of anal fistula modified from the work of Stelzner. This was based on a unifying theory that most fistulae originate as intermuscular abscesses from anal gland infection. Classification includes four major groups and 12 subgroups. Five different categories of high fistula are included. Fistulae are classified in relation to the external sphincter as intersphincteric (between internal and external sphincter), trans-sphincteric (through the external sphincter to the ischioanal fossa), suprasphincteric (passes from intersphincteric region above both sphincter and puborectalis and extrasphincteric (passes from rectum to perianal region).

Such classification is excellent, if somewhat confusing. It ignores the fistula arising in anal ulcer. The relatively common subcutaneous fistula and the small, asymptomatic, squamous-lined fistula distal to anal ulcer are not included. Classification is based on a selected series of patients and is not representative of the incidence of the disease in the population at large.

From a practical viewpoint, classifications are of limited help. The surgeon still must have a good working knowledge of the anatomy and must constantly be aware of the relationship of fistulae to the puborectalis or upper portion of the sphincter. Straightforward trans-sphincteric fistulae in the female anteriorly may cause significantly more problems than a high anal fistula posteriorly. Presence or absence of history of preoperative diarrhea or incontinence should always be documented.

CONSERVATIVE MANAGEMENT OF FISTULAE

Spontaneous or surgical drainage of an abscess may be followed by healing of a fistula. This is uncommon, occurring usually after recent infection and not representing a chronic fistula. Long-standing anal ulcers may be associated with short, squamous-lined fistulae originating at the distal margin of the ulcer. These are called subtegumentary fistulae and are often asymptomatic. They are discovered as incidental findings at the time of surgery for anal ulcer.

Aside from these two incidences, most fistulae persist as chronic draining tracts. If there is an underlying cause, such as inflammatory bowel disease, fistulae may heal or become quiescent by treatment of the systemic disease process. Surgery for anal lesions in inflammatory bowel disease can be performed without incident and with good healing when the inflammatory bowel disease is quiescent. Generally, surgery in the presence of inflammatory bowel disease is reserved for treatment of abscesses, with simple drainage alone.

Long-standing anal fistulae are associated with a small incidence of carcinoma developing in the tracts. The true incidence is unknown due to early surgical treatment of most fistulae.

Injection of fistula with solutions to precipitate scarring or healing has been advocated in the past. The rare success probably has represented spontaneous healing or decreased drainage. A solution of quinine and urea has been used. This is mentioned only for purposes of condemnation. Turnbull at the Cleveland Clinic has tried injection of residual fistula tracts following proctocolectomy for inflammatory bowel disease. He uses a solution of nitrogen mustard but the procedure has not been adopted by others at the same institution.

SURGICAL MANAGEMENT

Primary methods of treating fistulae are fistulotomy and the use of a seton or thread passed around the fistula site. Accounts of fistulotomy date back to the 14th century; and the use of a seton, to Hippocrates. Although little has changed, there is now an improved concept of the anatomy, which allows a rational approach to treatment. With the knowledge of the anatomy, good exposure of the anal region is mandatory for delineating fistulae. Too often, exposure is obscured by lack of proper position of the patient, excessive bleeding or the lack of a proper intra-anal retractor.

We use the same Sims position and Hill-Ferguson retractor described for the closed hemorrhoidectomy technique. Para-anal infiltration with lidocaine with epinephrine may be helpful but should not be used when cellulitis is present.

The common low anal fistula originating below the mucocutaneous junction usually can be palpated as a thin, firm tract leading to the anal canal from the external opening. The course of the tract may commonly correspond to "Goodsall's Rule." This generality, described in 1900, denotes the horizontal disposition of many low fistulae.[34] According to Goodsall, a fistula with an external opening in the anterior half of the perianum has a straight course to the anal canal. An external opening in the posterior half often denotes a fistula originating in the posterior midline of the anal canal. This is just a generality to which there are many exceptions, but it may assist in the search for the internal opening.

The site of the internal opening can be discovered in 85–90% of cases.[55, 68] If the internal opening is not readily apparent, pressure on the perianum with a stroking or milking action often causes fluid or frank pus to exude from and identify the aperture. This is the singly most useful and effective means of identifying an obscure internal opening. The same maneuver may produce "tugging" or dimpling at the internal opening. In any case, an appropriate probe then can be dropped into the opening and it can be opened from within outward to join the known external tract. If the internal opening is not found by the aforementioned means, the external opening may be opened as far as abnormal tissue is identifiable and then pressure in the depths of the external wound will extrude fluid, blood or pus from the internal opening under direct vision and a probe can be introduced. Impatience and heavy-handedness are the commonest causes of iatrogenic disasters. Probing of the external opening must be done gently to prevent creation of an abnormal tract or internal opening. Only simple, straight, or slightly curved tracts will accept a probe for the entire distance. We have not had much luck with the injection of dyes (too messy) or pastes (too thick) in fistula tracts to find the internal opening. If one wants to try an injection, ordinary milk is probably the best as it is fluid, opaque and white.

Upper extensions of anal fistulae are exceedingly rare and almost always iatrogenic. Palpation is the main diagnostic tool. A deep postanal fistula or abscess is best discerned by palpation with thumb and index finger. Palpable induration in the wall extending above the anorectal junction usually will delineate a high, intermuscular or submucosal tract which can be opened in its entirety transmucosally (intralumenally). An extrasphincteric fistula which embraces the sphincter ani muscles and the puborectalis muscle is so rare that one of us (J.A.F.) has seen only two in his professional career. One was iatrogenic and the other was secondary to sigmoid diverticular abscess.

Most fistulae are simply and effectively treated by fistulotomy of the entire tract. Recurrences develop usually because of inability to unroof the entire tract or early bridging of the site during healing. Total excision of the fistula, primary closure or skin grafting, add little to the results obtainable with a properly performed fistulotomy. Skin grafting of the fistulotomy wound is advocated by Hughes.[43] The fistula site is enlarged by excision of the overhanging edges so as to give a saucerlike shape to the wound. The primary graft is then applied. This was designed to reduce healing time of the large saucerlike wound. Although primary healing occurs, skin grafting is complicated, tedious and inappropriate for fistulae extending high in the ischioanal fossa.

We use minimal landscaping of the wound after fistulotomy. The width and depth of the wound are reduced by continuous suturing of the skin margin to the fistula base so as to "marsupialize" the area. This also provides effective hemostasis. The wide "cut-back" and saucerization of the wound practiced by many is avoided and healing time reduced.

Primary closure of a fistulotomy site was advocated by Starr[75] in 1949 under the cover of antibiotics. He claimed great success with the technique but Goligher[29] obtained primary healing in only 12 of 20 patients. The procedure is not generally in use. Its greatest applicability is for low, subcutaneous fistulae that are adequately treated by fistulotomy and marsupialization of the wound. Primary suture is useful with rectovaginal fistula or closure of high complicated fistula at the internal opening. The latter may require a colostomy or "medical colostomy" with intravenous hyperalimentation for successful primary healing.

Complete excision of the fistula tract rarely is of aid. Attempts at excision are frustrating, due to the wide area of surrounding fibrosis. A large wound and excision of a further portion of sphincter may result.

Parks[66] feels that surgical excision of the site of origin of the fistula at the anal crypt is important. While rational, for fistulae originating as intermuscular abscesses it has little practical application. The procedure involves surgical excision of a wedge of internal sphincter to include the internal opening and unroof the intersphincteric abscess. With the origin of the fistula exposed, it was hoped that further fistulotomy would be unnecessary and resolution of the remaining fistula would take place. For high, complicated fistulae or horseshoe fistulae, this has not proven to be the case. For low intermuscular or trans-sphincteric fistulae, we can see no advantage over simple fistulotomy.

Horseshoe fistulae seem to be a special problem. They presumably originate as high postanal abscesses which extend to one or both ischiorectal (ischioanal) fossae. This circumferential spread, in its classic form, resembles a horseshoe. There may be blind fistulae, multiple tracts or multiple external openings. Although horseshoe fistulae can develop between the internal and external sphincters or above the levator muscles, this is extremely rare.

Goligher[29] advocates complete unroofing of the horseshoe fistula. This results in a large, deep wound that is slow to heal. Hanley[37] advocates a method with which we have had excellent success. The essential aspect of the procedure is identification of the internal opening. The sphincters are incised posteriorly down to the postanal component as the fistula branches to either ischioanal fossa. This occurs high under the levator muscle and posterior to both sphincters. Tracts or abscesses to either side are opened at their anterior extension. The fistulae are curetted from the external opening to the postanal space. Such treatment usually results in spontaneous resolution of the ischioanal component if the posterior portion has been drained adequately. Unroofing of the ischioanal limb is avoided and healing time is lessened. In a ten-year study of this method, Hanley had no recurrences.

From a practical standpoint, most fistulae are treated adequately by fistulotomy. Fistula tracts originating at or below the mucocutaneous junction rarely result in significant incontinence. Any disability resulting from incising the sphincter often improves with healing of the wound. Care must be exercised for anal fistulae originating above the mucocutaneous junction. This is particularly true of anterior fistulae in women and patients with a prior history of diarrhea or incontinence. If there is any question of the amount of remaining muscle, a seton of nylon suture can be inserted along the fistula tract to encompass the muscle area in question. Goligher[29] advocates examination with the seton in place to determine if the puborectalis muscle can be palpated above the seton. Parks and Stitz[68] leave the seton in place for rare high fistulae encircling the puborectalis muscle. This presumably causes fibrosis and prevents wide separation of the muscle when subsequently incised several months later. Generally, setons are not necessary and we have not had occasion to use them.

High fistulae outside the external sphincter or puborectalis muscle usually are related to trauma (penetrating or factitial) or have a secondary cause in the pelvis such as inflammatory bowel disease or diverticulitis.[39] If no internal opening in the anal canal is evident and the probe passes in a cephalad direction to the upper reaches of the ischioanal fossa, then one should be suspicious of such a situation. High fistulae superficial to the puborectalis muscle (submucosal or intermuscular) are easily cured by fistulotomy and by marsupialization of the edges for hemostasis. We recently have seen three cases of such fistulae occurring anteriorly in women which were simply treated with no subsequent disability.

Results of Therapy

It is impossible to compare results of treatment of fistulae due to the vital importance of experience, surgical judgment and common sense of the operating surgeon. Recurrence rates vary in different patient populations. Inability to detect the internal opening, early bridging of the healing wound or undetected extension of a fistula causes most recurrences. Bennett and Goligher[7] could detect the internal opening in only 63% of cases yet reports recurrences or imperfections of healing in 10 of 108 patients seen in the previous six years. Parks and Stitz[68] analyzed 142 of 158 patients with high fistulae and had recurrences with slow healing in 16% of patients. Mazier[55] analyzed recurrence rates in a seven-year study of 1,000 patients. In 86% an internal opening was definitely found and the recurrence rate was 3.9%.

Disability from incontinence is subjective and not well reported. In the series of Bennett and Goligher,[7] 36% of patients with low anal fistulae and 55% of patients with high anal or horseshoe fistulae had some minor impairment or incontinence. In the series of Parks and Stitz[68] between 16 and 32% of patients had mild degrees of incontinence. Six of 139 patients (4.3%) had poor control of feces or flatus. Mazier's experience, in response to questionnaires, netted 79.2% good results, 14.7% good results with minor complaints and 6.1% unsatisfactory results.[55]

Anal fistulae rarely will be cured without delineation of the internal opening. Careful palpation usually will outline undetected sinuses or high extensions of fistulae. Most fistulae can be cured with minimal incontinence if a functionally intact puborectalis muscle is preserved. Anterior midline fistula tracts that do not encompass puborectalis fibers rarely embrace the entire external and internal sphincter muscle ring and preservation of a few fibers of internal sphincter muscle at the anorectal verge will ensure reasonable continence. In all cases preoperative documentation of the degree of continence obviously is imperative.

Summary

We have tried to present a comprehensive survey of present-day management of hemorrhoids, fistulae and fissures, be it in the office or in the hospital. There is great socioeconomic pressure lately for cost-containment, which is apt to effect better medical judgment in the selection of type and place of management. Minor operations can and should be done, as always, on an outpatient basis. General anesthesia is not a minor matter and hemorrhoidectomy is not a minor operation.

The major function of outpatient service in the management of anal disease is that of accurate and comprehensive diagnosis. Hundreds of patients come to us only because they fear cancer and it is not enough for us to hunt for and treat the vague little disorders of which they complain. The incidence of cancer of the colon and rectum in this country just recently has slightly surpassed that of lung cancer. Adjuvant treatments (e.g., chemotherapy, radiotherapy, immunotherapy and their combinations) are promising but still in the investigational stage. Early diagnosis is our finest weapon with subsequent surgical management.

The challenge and responsibility for early diagnosis of colorectal cancer is ours alone. We must first recognize it and then meet it firmly and squarely. We must feel for (digital rectal), look for (sigmoidoscopy), and search for (barium enema x-ray examination) colorectal cancer in all of our patients regardless of the insignificance of anal symptoms and anal findings. Our countrymen fear cancer. We have the devices to allay their fears or to cure their cancers if they are found early enough. We have a straightforward moral commitment and a national trust.

REFERENCES

1. Ackland, T. H.: The treatment of prolapsed, gangrenous hemorrhoids, Aust. N.Z. J. Surg. 30:201, 1961.
2. Alexander-Williams, J., and Crapp, A. R.: Conservative management of hemorrhoids: Part I, injection, freezing and ligation, Clin. Gastroenterol. 4:595, 1975.
3. Allgower, M.: Conservative management of hemorrhoids: Part III, partial internal sphincterotomy, Clin. Gastroenterol. 4:608, 1975.
4. Allingham, W.: *Fistula, Hemorrhoids, Painful Ulcer, Stricture, Prolapsus, and Other Diseases of the Rectum, their Diagnosis and Treatment* (London: J. and A. Churchill, Ltd., 1971), pp. 86–97.
5. Barron, J.: Office ligation of internal hemorrhoids, Am. J. Surg. 105:563, 1963.
6. Bekhit, F.: Hemorrhoidectomy: a new technic of extramucous excision, Int. Surg. 35:788, 1961.
7. Bennett, R. C.: A review of the results of orthodox treatment for anal fistulae, Proc. R. Soc. Med. 55:756, 1962.
8. Bennett, R. C., Friedman, M. H. W., and Goligher, J. C.: The late results of hemorrhoidectomy by ligation and excision, Br. Med. J. 2:216, 1963.
9. Bennett, R. C., and Goligher, J. C.: Results of internal sphincterotomy for anal fissures, Br. Med. J. 2:1500, 1962.
10. Blaisdell, P. C.: Prevention of massive hemorrhage secondary to hemorrhoidectomy, Surg. Gynecol. Obstet. 106:485, 1958.
11. Blaisdell, P. C.: Pathogenesis of anal fissure and implications as to treatment, Surg. Gynecol. Obstet. 65:672, 1937.
12. Buie, L. A.: *Practical Proctology* (Springfield, Illinois: Charles C Thomas, Publisher, 1960).
13. Burkitt, D. P., and Graham-Stewart, C. W.: Hemorrhoids—fistulated pathogenesis and proposed prevention, Postgrad. Med. J. 51:631, 1975.
14. Chiari, H.: Uber die Nalen Divertikel der Rectumschlienehaut und Thre Beziehung zu den Anal Fistelu, Wein Med. Press 19:1482, 1878.

15. Clark, C. G., Giles, G. R., and Goligher, J. C.: Results of conservative management of hemorrhoids, Br. Med. J. 2:12, 1967.
16. Corman, M. L., and Veidenheimer, M. C.: The new hemorrhoidectomy, Surg. Clin. North Am. 53:417, 1973.
17. Crapp, A. R., and Alexander-Williams, J.: Fissure in ano and anal stenosis, Part I: conservative management, Clin. Gastroenterol. 4:619, 1975.
18. Earle, S. T.: Diseases of the Anus, Rectum and Sigmoid (Philadelphia: J. B. Lippincott, 1911).
19. Eisenhammer, S.: Proper principles and practices in the surgical management of hemorrhoids, Dis. Colon Rectum 12:288, 1968.
20. Eisenhammer, S.: The internal anal sphincter: its surgical importance, S. Afr. Med. J. 27:266, 1953.
21. Eisenhammer, S.: The evaluation of the internal anal sphincterotomy operation with special reference to anal fissure, Surg. Gynecol. Obstet. 109: 583, 1959.
22. Eisenhammer, S.: A new approach to anorectal fistulous abscess on the high intramuscular lesion, Surg. Gynecol. Obstet. 106:595, 1958.
23. Fansler, M. A., and Anderson, J. K.: A plastic operation for certain types of hemorrhoids, JAMA 101:1064, 1933.
24. Ferguson, J. A., and Heaton, J. R.: Closed hemorrhoidectomy, Dis. Colon Rectum 2:176, 1959.
25. Ferguson, J. A., Mazier, W. P., Ganchrow, M. I., and Friend, W. G.: The closed technique of hemorrhoidectomy, Surgery 7:480, 1971.
26. Ferguson, J. A.: Fissure in ano and anal stenosis part II: radical surgical management, Clin. Gastroenterol. 4:629, 1975.
27. Gabriel, W. B.: Principles and Practice of Rectal Surgery, (4th ed; London: Lewis, 1948).
28. Ganchrow, M. I., Mazier, W. P., Friend, W. G., and Ferguson, J. A.: Hemorrhoidectomy revisited: a computer analysis of 2,038 cases, Dis. Colon Rectum 14:128, 1971.
29. Goligher, J. C.: Surgery of the Anus, Rectum and Colon (London: Cassel, 1961).
30. Goligher, J. C.: Cryosurgery for hemorrhoids, Dis. Colon Rectum 19:213, 1976.
31. Grace, R. H., and Creed, A.: Prolapsing thrombosed hemorrhoids: outcome of conservative management, Br. Med. J. 3:354, 1975.
32. Graham-Stewart, C. M.: Injection treatment of hemorrhoids, Br. Med. J. 1:213, 1962.
33. Graham-Stewart, C. W.: The etiology and treatment of fissure in ano, Int. Abst. Surg. 115:511 (in Surg. Gynecol. Obstet. 115:6, 1962).
34. Goodsall, D. H., and Miles, W. E.: Diseases of the Anus and Rectum (London: Longman's, 1900).
35. Hancock, B. D., and Williams, P.: The internal sphincter and hemorrhoids, Eur. Surg. Res. 2 (Suppl.):20, 1973.
36. Hardy, K. J., and Cutherbertson, A. M.: Lateral sphincterotomy: an appraisal with special reference to sequelae, Austr. N.Z. J. Surg. 39:91, 1969.
37. Hanley, P. H.: Conservative surgical correction of horseshoe abscess and fistula, Dis. Colon Rectum 8:364, 1968.

38. Hawley, P. R.: The treatment of chronic fissure-in-ano: a trial of methods, Br. J. Surg. 56:915, 1969.
39. Heaton, J. R., and Cohen, R. S.: Complicated para-anal fistulas of obscure etiology, Dis. Colon Rectum 8:437, 1965.
40. Hoffman, D. C., and Goligher, J. C.: Lateral subcutaneous internal sphincterotomy in treatment of anal fissure, Br. Med. J. 3:673, 1970.
41. Howard, P. M., and Pingree, J. H.: Immediate radical surgery for hemorrhoidal disease with acute extensive thrombosis, Am. J. Surg. 116:777, 1968.
42. Hughes, E. S. R.: Treatment of anal fissure, Br. Med. J. 2:803, 1953.
43. Hughes, E. S. R.: Primary skin grafting in proctological surgery, Br. J. Surg. 41:639, 1953.
44. Jones, C. B., and Schofield, P. F.: A Comparative study of methods of treatment for hemorrhoids, Proc. R. Soc. Med. 67:51, 1974.
45. Keighley, M. R. B., Arabi, Y., and Alexander-Williams, J.: Anal pressures in hemorrhoids and anal fissure, Br. J. Surg. 63:665, 1976.
46. Kline, J. R., Spencer, R. J., and Harrison, E. G., Jr.: Carcinoma associated with fistula-in-ano, Arch. Surg. 89:989, 1964.
47. Kratzer, G. L.: Outpatient anorectal surgery. Am. Fam. Physician 11:94, 1975.
48. Laurence, A. E., and Murray, A. J.: Histopathology of prolapsed and thrombosed hemorrhoids, Dis. Colon Rectum 5:56, 1962.
49. Lieberman, W.: The place of suppositories and ointments in proctological practice (a re-appraisal and new data), Am. J. Proctol. 17:371, 1966.
50. Lewis, M. I., De La Cruz, T., Gazzaniga, D. A., and Ball, T. L.: Cryosurgical hemorrhoidectomy: preliminary report, Dis. Colon Rectum 12:371, 1969.
51. Lord, P. H.: A new regime for the treatment of hemorrhoids, Proc. R. Soc. Med. 61:935, 1968.
52. Macintyre, I. M. C., and Balfour, T. W.: Results of the Lord nonoperative treatment of hemorrhoids, Lancet 1:1094, 1972.
53. Mazier, W. P.: Emergency hemorrhoidectomy: a worthwhile procedure, Dis. Colon Rectum 16:200, 1973.
54. Mazier, W. P.: An evaluation of the surgical treatment of anal fissures, Dis. Colon Rectum 15:222, 1972.
55. Mazier, W. P.: The treatment and care of anal fistulas: a study of 1,000 patients, Dis. Colon Rectum 14:134, 1971.
56. Miles, W. E.: Observations upon internal piles, Surg. Gynecol. Obstet. 29: 497, 1919.
57. Miles, W. E.: Rectal Surgery (London: Cassell, 1939).
58. Milligan, E. T. C., and Morgan, C. N.: Surgical anatomy of the anal canal, Lancet 2:1150, 1934.
59. Milligan, E. T. C., Morgan, C. N., Jones, L. J., and Officer, R.: Surgical anatomy of the anal canal and the operative treatment of hemorrhoids, Lancet 2:1119, 1937.
60. Mitchell, A. B.: A simple method of operating on piles, Br. Med. J. 1:482, 1903.
61. Nothmann, B. J., and Schuster, M. M.: Internal anal sphincter derangement with anal fissures, Gastroenterology 67:216, 1974.

62. Notaras, M. J.: Lateral subcutaneous sphincterotomy for anal fissure—a new technique, Proc. R. Soc. Med. 62:713, 1969.
63. Parks, A. G.: The surgical treatment of hemorrhoids, Br. J. Surg. 43:337, 1956.
64. Parks, A. G.: The management of fissure-in-ano, Hosp. Med. 1:737, 1967.
65. Parks, A. G.: Hemorrhoidectomy, Adv. Surg. 5:1, 1970.
66. Parks, A. G.: Pathogenesis and treatment of fistula-in-ano, Br. Med. J. 1: 463, 1961.
67. Parks, A. G., Gordon, P. H., and Hardcastle, J. D.: A classification of fistula in ano, Br. J. Surg. 63:1, 1976.
68. Parks, A. G., and Stitz, R. M.: The treatment of high fistula-in-ano, Dis. Colon Rectum 19:487, 1976.
69. Petit, J. L.: Traite des Maladies Chirurgicales et des Operations qui leur Conviennent, Paris 2:737, 1775.
70. Rankin, F. W., Bargen, J. A., and Buie, L. A.: *The Colon, Rectum and Anus* (Philadelphia: W. B. Saunders, 1932).
71. Rudd, W. W. H.: Hemorrhoidectomy in the office: methods and precautions, Dis. Colon Rectum 13:438, 1970.
72. Rudd, W. W. H.: Lateral subcutaneous internal sphincterotomy for Chronic anal fissure, an outpatient procedure, Dis. Colon Rectum 18:319, 1975.
73. Rowe, R. J., Benjamin, H. G., McGirney, J. Q., Nesselrod, J. P., Terrell, R., and Todd, I. P.: Symposium: management of hemorrhoidal disease, Dis. Colon Rectum 11:127, 1968.
74. Sampson, R. B., and Stewart, W. R. C.: Sliding skin grafts in treatment of anal fissures, Dis. Colon Rectum 13:372, 1970.
75. Starr, K. W.: Primary closure in proctology, Postgrad. Med. 14:365, 1953.
76. Steinberg, D. M., Leigois, H., and Alexander-Williams, J.: The longer-term evaluation of rubber-band ligation, Proc. R. Soc. Med. 67:24, 1974.
77. Stelzner, F.: Dtsch. Med. Wochenschr. 88:689, 1963.
78. Stelzner, R.: *Die Anorectalen Fistelu* (Berlin: Springer-Verlag, 1959).
79. Thomson, W. H. F.: The nature and cause of hemorrhoids, Proc. R. Soc. Med. 68:574, 1975.
80. Walls, A. D. F., and Rackley, C. V.: A five-year follow up of Lord's dilatation for hemorrhoids, Lancet 1:1212, 1976.
81. Watts, J. McK., Bennett, R. C., Duthie, H. L., and Goligher, J. C.: Healing and pain after hemorrhoidectomy, Br. J. Surg. 51:808, 1964.
82. Watts, J. McK., Bennett, R. C., and Goligher, J. C.: Stretching of anal sphincters in treatment of fissure-in-ano, Br. Med. J. 2:342, 1964.
83. Whitehead, W.: The surgical treatment of hemorrhoids, Br. Med. J. 1:148, 1882.

Development of Cancer in Transplantation Patients

ISRAEL PENN, M.D.

Department of Surgery, University of Colorado School of Medicine and Veterans Administration Hospital, Denver, Colorado

Many surgical procedures are destructive, leading to loss of portions of the body and alteration of normal physiology. The trend in modern surgery is more and more toward procedures that conserve tissue, or replace diseased structures with prosthetic materials or with the patient's own organs and tissues, or with those obtained from other individuals. The field of organ transplantation has been growing rapidly. Restoration of function and return to a satisfactory state of health have been achieved on a long-term basis in recipients of renal, hepatic, cardiac, pancreatic, bone marrow and other grafts. Unfortunately, the ideal of replacing diseased structures with healthy ones is marred by a variety of complications encompassing technical, immunologic, infectious and other problems. Among these is an increased incidence of cancer. Transplantation must now be added to the list of iatrogenic manipulations that may lead to malignancy.[1-10]

Some of the tumors encountered have been uncommon types, have unusual anatomic locations or have exhibited extraordinary behavior patterns. It is important to study these neo-

Supported in part by research grant 6985 from the Veterans Administration, by grants AI-AM-08898 and AM-07772 from the National Institutes of Health; and by grants RR-00051 and RR-00069 from the General Clinical Research Center Program of the Division of Research Resources, National Institutes of Health.

0065-3411/78/0012-0155$03.75

plasms, as they may shed some light on our understanding of the problem of malignancy.

This paper is based on material collected in an informal tumor registry maintained by the author since 1968. Physicians working in transplant centers all over the world have generously contributed data concerning their patients. Material collected up to December 1977 is included in this analysis. I shall consider three categories of neoplasia: (1) tumors present before transplantation; (2) malignancies inadvertently transmitted with the homograft; and (3) cancers which arise de novo after transplantation.

Organ Transplantation and Immunosuppressive Therapy

Before discussing the malignancies it is necessary to outline briefly the therapeutic manipulations involved in organ transplantation. Grafting organs between identical twins evokes no immunologic reaction and usually no immunosuppressive therapy is necessary. In transplantation between all other individuals histocompatibility differences exist. These stimulate a variable immune response by the host, which, if left untreated, usually will destroy the graft. Immunosuppressive therapy therefore, is given to prevent or treat this rejection reaction. Immunosuppression serves to dampen the activities of the lymphoreticular system. Ideally we would prefer to interfere only with the response to the foreign antigens in the transplanted organ. This is not possible in the present state of our knowledge. In consequence, we are forced to use blanket immunosuppressive therapy which depresses the host's response to a wide variety of antigens, including those of bacteria, viruses, protozoa and fungi. Infectious complications therefore are common in the immunologically compromised host.

Various pharmacologic agents are the cornerstone of immunosuppressive therapy. Most patients are given a combination of azathioprine (Imuran), a derivative of the cytotoxic compound 6-mercaptopurine, and one of the corticosteroids, usually prednisone or methylprednisolone. In some centers antilymphocyte or antithymocyte globulin (ALG or ATG, respectively) is also given during the first few weeks after transplantation. Cyclophosphamide (Cytoxan) sometimes is used as a substitute for azathioprine. Actinomycin C or D may be given for a very brief period in the treatment of episodes of threatened rejection and may be supplemented by small doses of radiotherapy to the homograft. The immunosuppressive drugs are given in large doses during the first few weeks or months after transplantation, when the problem of acute rejection is most likely to occur. Thereafter, dosage is reduced to maintenance levels which are continued indefinitely.

In addition to the pharmacologic agents other procedures occasionally are used to further blunt the host's immune response to the homograft. These include splenectomy, thymectomy, drainage of thoracic duct lymphocytes, intralymphatic infusion of colloidal radioisotopes, extracorporeal irradiation of peripheral whole blood or lymph, and total body irradiation.

Immunosuppressive therapy in bone marrow transplantation differs from that used in transplantation of solid organs such as the kidney, liver or heart. The aim is to obtain persistent immunologic tolerance of the donor marrow by the recipient. The patient is conditioned to receive the graft by massive immunosuppressive therapy given a short time before transplantation. Several regimens are in use: either total body irradiation, large doses of cyclophosphamide or a combination of various cancer chemotherapeutic agents. After grafting, no other immunosuppressive therapy is used except for intermittent doses of methotrexate during the first 100 days to prevent the dangerous complication of a graft-versus-host reaction. Should this occur, ATG may be given to treat it.

Besides immunosuppressive therapy, transplant patients may receive a number of other pharmacologic agents to prevent or treat various complications. Because of frequent infections, antibiotics often are used. Antihypertensive drugs, antacids to combat the gastric effects of the corticosteroids, and anticonvulsant drugs to control seizure disorders in patients with hypertensive encephalopathy also may be required.

Tumors Present before Transplantation

Some patients have cancers before transplantation. These frequently are removed before the procedure, sometimes during the operation and occasionally after transplantation. In some cases the surgeon has no choice, as in liver transplantation for hepatic malignancies, where he must remove the diseased liver and replace it with a healthy one during the same procedure. In contrast, primary renal malignancies may be removed and the patient treated with hemodialysis until such time that the surgeon feels that it is safe for the patient to undergo transplantation. There is controversy as to whether immunosuppressive therapy may interfere with the immune response to residual cancer cells, thus facilitating their growth and dissemination. Some surgeons[11] feel that the final outcome is not altered and are willing to perform renal transplantation simultaneously with, or soon after, removal of renal tumors. Others adopt a more cautious attitude,[8, 12-17] preferring to wait for an arbitrary period of time, usually a year or more after removal of the neoplasm. Transplantation thus is avoided in many patients who develop recurrences or metastases during this interval. We shall now consider the fate of patients who had a variety of pre-existing malignancies. There are two categories: those who underwent transplantation as part of the treatment of cancers of the liver, kidney, bone marrow or other organs, and those who had tumors that were incidental to renal transplantation.

HEPATIC NEOPLASMS

When conventional hepatic resections are not feasible, as with tumors involving the hepatic hilum or both lobes of the liver, the whole organ may be removed and replaced with a homograft, provided that there is no evidence of distant spread of the neoplasia. Transplants have been performed for hepatomas, cholangiocarcinomas and other primary hepatic malignancies,[18, 19] and, occasionally, in the treatment of tumors metastatic to the liver.[19] Although long-term tumor-free survival for 3½, 5 and nearly 8 years has been achieved in 3 patients, overall results have been disappointing. Thirty-two of 56 patients (57%) had evidence of recurrence or metastases. If we exclude those with a short follow-up of less than two months we are left with 44 recipients of whom 28 (64%) had recurrent or metastatic tumor. This figure may prove to be higher, as some of the survivors have been followed for only a short time.

The poor results are not surprising in view of the advanced

nature of most hepatic tumors that require transplantation. In many cases micrometastases presumably were present at the time of operation and became clinically overt several weeks or months later. Tumor growth in several instances occurred at a spectacular rate and the homograft itself became the seat of numerous metastases. On theoretical grounds the cancers that may have the best prognosis when treated with transplantation are those arising in the biliary system at the junction of the right and left with the common hepatic ducts. These neoplasms usually are small and frequently do not metastasize, but kill by obstructing the biliary system. The transplant experience accumulated thus far is too small to make any clear-cut statements about their prognosis.

RENAL AND URETERAL TUMORS

In view of the controversy surrounding the timing of renal transplantation we analyzed the results obtained in 79 patients in order to establish practical guidelines regarding the management of individuals with renal and ureteral tumors. Two groups may be identified,[8] recipients with asymptomatic renal carcinomas that were discovered incidentally, and those with symptomatic renal or ureteral tumors. The former category includes 18 patients in whom the neoplasm was discovered incidentally during the work-up of chronic renal failure, or following bilateral nephrectomy in preparation for transplantation. Sixteen were removed less than a year before transplantation and two, more than 12 months before transplantation. Six other patients were found to have incidental malignancies in their native kidneys 2–11 months after transplantation, when these were removed (usually for persistent hypertension) or examined at autopsy. These malignancies may well have been present before transplantation, but we cannot exclude the possibility that they may have arisen at some time after the procedure. With the exception of one patient whose tumor was an incidental finding at autopsy examination, the other 23 recipients had no evidence of recurrence or metastases in an average follow-up of 25 months (range, 2 days to 65 months).

Several factors may account for the favorable prognosis in this group. The diagnosis may have been erroneous in some cases;

pathologists have great difficulty in distinguishing between large renal adenomas and small, well-differentiated carcinomas.[12, 20] Often the distinction is made on size alone; those over 2 cm in diameter are considered malignant. A second possibility is that while malignant histologically, the tumors may be relatively benign biologically. The fortuitous discovery of the neoplasms at a very early stage also may contribute to the satisfactory outcome, since the size of renal carcinomas is related to their ability to metastasize. Bell[21] found only one instance of metastasis in 39 patients whose tumors were smaller than 3 cm in diameter, but metastases occurred in 66 of 84 patients whose tumors were larger than 5 cm. Despite these encouraging findings it is wise to adopt a cautious attitude toward these neoplasms, as this is only a small series and the average length of follow-up is short. It is well known that renal neoplasms may give rise to late metastases.

The patients with symptomatic malignancies may be divided into two groups: 36 who underwent transplantation 12 months or less after completion of treatment of their cancers, and 19 in whom the interval was greater than 12 months. The tumors in the two groups were renal cell carcinomas in 29 patients, Wilms' tumors in 17, transitional cell carcinomas in 3, carcinomas of the ureter in 2, squamous cell carcinoma of the renal pelvis in 1, leiomyosarcoma in 1, neuroblastoma invading the kidney in 1, and in 1 recipient the histologic type of malignancy was uncertain. Twenty-eight of the 55 patients (51%) had bilateral neoplasms. The distribution of the tumors was similar in the two groups. However, the outcome was very different. Of the 36 patients with a waiting interval of less than 12 months, 19 (53%) developed recurrences or metastases in a follow-up ranging from 1 week to 102 months (average time, 25 months). In contrast, none of the 19 recipients whose tumors were removed from 15 to 185 (average, 50) months before transplantation had recurrence or metastases. The length of follow-up ranged from 1 to 134 (average, 28) months. These results indicate that whenever possible, transplantation should be delayed for a minimum period of one year after completion of cancer therapy. This recommendation is supported by numerous reports, received by the author, of patients who underwent nephrectomy for renal cancers but who did not receive transplants because they died of metastases during the 12-month waiting period.[8] This policy avoids needless waste of precious kidneys on patients with a poor prognosis. Occasionally, however, the surgeon may be forced to forego the waiting period, for example, in very young children with Wilms' tumors, who may be very difficult to treat with hemodialysis for prolonged periods.[8]

ACUTE LEUKEMIA TREATED BY BONE MARROW TRANSPLANTATION

Bone marrow transplantation is used in patients with acute leukemia who cannot be controlled adequately with chemotherapy. As described, total body irradiation or intensive chemotherapy is used to destroy as many of the leukemia cells as possible. Marrow transplantation then is performed in the hope that the graft will obliterate any residual tumor, and also to restore depleted blood cells. Most successes have been obtained with grafts from identical twins or HL-A-identical siblings. Of 100 patients with acute myelogenous or acute lymphoblastic leukemia treated with marrow grafts from HL-A-identical siblings, 13 currently are alive, without recurrent leukemia 1 – 4½ years after transplantation.[22, 23] Relapse of leukemia occurred in 31 recipients. A remarkable finding was the development of leukemia in the transplanted donor cells in two recipients.[24]

LARYNGEAL TUMORS AND SMALL BOWEL NEOPLASMS

One patient had a laryngeal carcinoma resected with immediate replacement by a laryngeal homograft. He died of recurrent cancer 10 months later.[25]

Another patient had a recurrent desmoid tumor involving the jejunum, ileum and right colon, all of which were resected. Sixteen months later she received a partial small bowel transplant from an HL-A-identical sibling. The recipient died of septic complications 2½ months after transplantation. No residual tumor was present at autopsy examination.

SPLENIC TRANSPLANTATION FOR ADVANCED MALIGNANCIES

Patients with advanced cancers often have marked depression of immunity.[26] It has been hoped that provision of a continuous source of immunocompetent cells by splenic transplantation might induce a graft-versus-host tumor reaction. This procedure was attempted in five patients, but no worthwhile long-term results were obtained.[27]

CANCERS INCIDENTAL TO RENAL TRANSPLANTATION

Fifty-four patients who underwent renal replacement had pre-existing tumors in various organs treated within 5 years of transplantation. Follow-up ranged from a minimum of 2 months up to 102 months. Twenty-nine recipients had malignancies of various internal organs and 25 had skin cancers (Table 1). As was done for renal tumors, the results were analyzed according to whether the neoplasms were removed less or more than a year before transplantation. In patients with neoplasms of the internal organs, the only recurrences occurred in 3 of 13 patients (23%) who were treated less than a year before transplantation. The tumors were a persistent myeloma, a bladder carcinoma and a carcinoma of the thyroid gland with lymph node

TABLE 1.—MALIGNANCIES INCIDENTAL
TO RENAL TRANSPLANTATION

TYPE OF MALIGNANCY	NO. OF PATIENTS
Cancers of internal organs	
Carcinoma of the urinary bladder	4
Carcinoma of the thyroid gland	4
Carcinoma of the breast	4
Carcinoma of the cervix of uterus	3
(in situ, 2; invasive, 1)	
Carcinoma of the body of uterus	2
Seminoma of testis	2
Carcinoma of bronchus	2
Carcinoma of colon	2
Sarcomas of small bowel (lymphosarcoma;	2
omental recurrence of leiomyosarcoma)	
Multiple myeloma causing renal failure	2
Carcinoma of the parathyroid gland	1
Chronic lymphocytic leukemia in remission	1
Total	29
Skin cancers	
Basal cell carcinomas	10
Squamous cell carcinomas	9
Basal and squamous cell carcinomas	1
Type of tumor not specified	3
Malignant melanoma	2
Total	25

metastases. We had no data on how long the individual with chronic lymphocytic leukemia had been in remission. The other 15 patients were treated from 20–60 (average, 34) months before transplantation and had no recurrences. Therefore, it appears that a waiting period of at least a year also is of value in patients with this group of tumors. However, the waiting time can be shortened considerably in recipients having neoplasms with a good prognosis, such as in situ carcinomas of the uterine cervix.

Recurrent skin cancers occurred in 13 of the 25 patients (52%), including both individuals with malignant melanoma (see Table 1). The incidence of recurrence could not be related to the length of the pretransplant waiting period. Therefore, renal transplantation can be undertaken at any time after treatment of most skin cancers, with the possible exception of the malignant melanomas where a substantial waiting period may be a wise precaution. Paradoxically, the two patients with melanoma developed metastases despite waiting periods of 21 and 48 months, respectively, an indication of the capricious natural history of these malignancies.

Conclusions Regarding Patients with Pre-existing Tumors

Study of the various groups described suggests that if a neoplasm has been eradicated thoroughly before transplantation, the patient will not have further problems with that particular tumor. However, he is as prone as other transplant recipients to develop unrelated de novo malignancies, as shall be seen in a later section dealing with these cancers. The patient who is left with residual cancer cells at the time of transplantation inevitably will develop local recurrences or distant metastases. Whether or not immunosuppressive therapy enhances their growth is not certain. However, the spectacular growth rate of metastases in several patients with hepatoma[18, 28] suggests that it may do so in the case of certain neoplasms.

Transplanted Malignancies

Tumor transplantation in animals is an important area of cancer research. Inbred strains frequently are used to avoid histocompatibility differences between the donor of the cancer cells and the recipient, as these will cause rejection of the grafts. Where incompatibility exists it is necessary to use a modified recipient animal, either a congenitally immunodeficient one such as the "nude" mouse which will even accept human cancer cells, or one that has been made immunodeficient by immunosuppressive therapy.

Transplantation of cancer cells between humans has been studied extensively by Southam.[29] This is unsuccessful except in recipients who have advanced malignancies and who demonstrate marked impairment of immune reactivity.[26] Transplantation of neoplasia into healthy humans is, fortunately, extremely rare; otherwise, the surgeon who accidentally pricks a finger in the course of doing a cancer operation would be at great risk. A unique case has been reported of transplantation of malignant melanoma from a daughter to her healthy mother, who eventually died of the tumor.[30] Presumably there was a close histocompatibility match which permitted the growth and dissemination of the malignancy in the recipient. In organ transplantation, where significant histocompatibility differences usually are present, immunosuppressive therapy may permit the survival of cancer cells inadvertently transplanted with the homograft obtained from a donor with cancer. The cells may multiply, invade surrounding structures and even disseminate widely.[2, 3, 5, 6, 9, 10, 31, 32]

We have data on 65 patients[2, 3, 5, 6, 9, 10, 31-44] who received organs from donors with cancer, excluding those with primary malignancies confined to the brain, which seldom spread outside the central nervous system.[45, 46] They were mostly kidney transplant recipients, with the exception of one who received a cardiac homograft. Fifty-two organs were obtained from cadaver donors and 13 were obtained from living volunteers.

CADAVER DONORS

All homografts obtained from cadavers appeared grossly normal and free of cancer. One donor had been treated five years previously for carcinoma of the colon and had no tumor at autopsy examination. After transplantation, primary renal carcinomas developed in two recipients, but we cannot determine whether these had been present in the donors or had developed de novo at a later period. At the time that the kidneys were harvested, all the other donors had cancers, many of which were widely disseminated. The most frequent were carcinomas of the bronchus,[19] kidney,[7] colon or rectum[5] or malignant melanoma.[5] A donor with a renal carcinoma of one kidney was the father of a recipient. The contralateral kidney was transplanted and the patient has had no evidence of neoplasia in a follow-up of more than six years.

Living Donors

Living donors had been treated for cancer within 5 years before nephrectomy or were found to have neoplasia at the time of donation, or developed evidence of it within 18 months after the procedure. The most common type of malignancy, found in six patients, was carcinoma of the kidney. One was in a "free" kidney, removed from a patient as treatment for a hypernephroma. The organ was deliberately transplanted into a patient dying of uremia, during the early years of transplantation when very few cadaver donors were available. The patient died 15 weeks after transplantation and at autopsy the cancer was found to have invaded adjacent structures. In four instances a malignant nodule was found in the donor kidney at the time of nephrectomy. This was excised promptly with a wide margin of healthy tissue in two cases and the kidneys were then transplanted. A third kidney was removed after 48 hours when the final biopsy report indicated that the suspicious nodule was, indeed, malignant. In the case of the fourth kidney the initial biopsy report was equivocal. Re-exploration of the homograft three months after transplantation showed an increase in size of the nodule; a partial nephrectomy was performed and the diagnosis of carcinoma was confirmed. None of these four patients has had further evidence of malignancy when followed up to 5 1/2 years.

Several months after transplantation a donor developed an anaplastic carcinoma in the nephrectomy site. The recipient manifested an identical tumor in the homograft and died of widespread metastases ten months after transplantation.

Malignancy in Recipients

In an extensive autopsy study Muiznieks et al.[42] found that patients with head and neck carcinomas had a 5% incidence of renal metastases, while those with bone, uterine, visceral and soft tissue sarcomas had a 10% incidence. In the present series of 65 patients, 24 (37%) had evidence of malignancy that involved the homograft. The actual incidence is higher if we exclude some donors who had neoplasms that were most unlikely to spread to the organs used for transplantation. One had had an in situ carcinoma of the cervix removed 2 years previously. One had a large basal cell carcinoma of the neck and 2 had had successful excisions of carcinomas of the colon and tongue, respectively, 5 years previously. In the case of the recipients who did not show evidence of malignancy we presume that the homografts were free of cancer or that transmitted malignant cells failed to survive after transplantation.

The 24 recipients who developed malignancies are listed in Table 2. The tumors were histologically identical to those in the

TABLE 2. – TRANSPLANTED MALIGNANCIES*

| PRIMARY MALIGNANCY IN DONOR | DONOR | MALIGNANCY IN RECIPIENT | | |
		HOMOGRAFT ONLY	HOMOGRAFT AND LOCAL STRUCTURES	DISTANT SPREAD
Lung	Cadaver			+
Lung	Cadaver			+
Lung	Cadaver		+	
Lung	Cadaver			+
Lung	Cadaver			+
Lung	Cadaver			+
Lung	Cadaver			+
Kidney	Cadaver			+
Kidney	Cadaver			+
Kidney	Cadaver			+
Kidney	Cadaver	+		
Kidney	Cadaver	+		
Kidney	Living	+		
Kidney	Living	+		
Kidney	Living		+	
Kidney	Living			+
Malignant melanoma	Cadaver			+
Malignant melanoma	Cadaver			+
Breast	Cadaver	+		
Breast	Cadaver	+		
Thyroid	Cadaver	+		
Hepatoma	Cadaver			+
Pyriform sinus	Cadaver			+
Choriocarcinoma	Cadaver			+

*Excludes two kidneys from living donors as the tumors were removed before transplantation.

original donors. Twenty patients received organs from cadaver donors and 4 received organs from living volunteers. In 7 patients the malignancy was confined to the homograft. Two were in kidneys obtained from living donors and have been described above. The other 5 were discovered at the time of nephrectomy or at autopsy performed during the first few weeks after transplantation. Two patients had local spread of the neoplasms, one being the patient into whom a hypernephroma had been deliberately transplanted.

Fifteen patients had widespread metastases. Only one received a homograft from a living donor. Cadaver donors with primary carcinomas of the lung or kidney, or with malignant melanoma, were the major source of the organs that transmitted the tumors. One patient who received a kidney from a donor with widespread choriocarcinoma had cancer cells in the kidney but no histologic proof of dissemination, the diagnosis of which was based on high levels of human chorionic gonadotropin (hCG).

Most of the recipients with metastases died of neoplasia. However, two patients demonstrated regression and, ultimately, complete disappearance of malignancy following reduction of the tumor burden by nephrectomy and cessation of immunosuppressive therapy.[31, 44] Presumably their depressed immune systems were able to recover and to reject the cancers. There is suggestive evidence that a similarly satisfactory outcome occurred in two other patients.[34, 37] One was the recipient with choriocarcinoma, whose elevated hCG levels fell slowly over a period of 8 weeks following nephrectomy and discontinuation of immunosuppression. No evidence of tumor was found at autopsy examination 7 months after transplantation. A fifth recipient with an anaplastic adenocarcinoma of a renal homograft with metastases did not respond to these measures and died 2 months after diagnosis of the neoplasm.[41] Presumably the extensive cancer had overwhelmed his immune defenses.

PREVENTION OF TUMOR TRANSPLANTATION

Most of the experience with transmitted malignancies was accumulated in the early years of transplantation, when the hazards of grafting organs from donors with malignancy into immunosuppressed recipients were not appreciated. Today such hazards rarely occur because the transplant surgeon has learned some valuable lessons. The most important is that one should not use donors with neoplasms, except those with low-grade skin cancers or with primary tumors confined to the central nervous system, as these rarely spread to other parts of the body.[45, 46] Even in the latter group great caution is necessary, because an occult primary tumor, usually of the bronchus, may spread to the brain and mimic a primary cerebral malignancy. Only through obtaining a tissue diagnosis of all brain tumors will we be able to avoid this pitfall.

What should the surgeon do when he finds a suspicious nodule in a kidney that is being harvested for transplantation? He should perform a biopsy of the lesion and obtain a frozen section diagnosis.[4] If the report indicates malignancy, the kidney should not be used.[47] Sometimes the initial report may be negative for cancer; but several days after transplantation, study of the definitive paraffin sections may indicate that the original diagnosis was in error. The surgeon must now reoperate and either remove the homograft[4] or perform a wide excision of the affected area.[48] As mentioned above, two patients underwent the latter procedure. After 6 weeks one lost his homograft because of rejection, but is free of cancer nearly 5 years later. The second patient remains well 5½ years after partial nephrectomy.

Tumors Arising De Novo after Transplantation

We have data on 585 patients with neoplasms appearing after transplantation. Of these, 574 were recipients of renal homografts, 9 of cardiac homografts and 2 of hepatic homografts.

INCIDENCE, AGE AND SEX

Examination of two large series of kidney transplant patients gives us an idea of the incidence of the complication. In the first 678 recipients in the University of Colorado Medical Center and the Denver Veterans Administration Hospital series, 40 patients (5.9%) developed these malignancies. The Australasian series of 1,884 patients found 126 patients (7%) affected.[49] The incidence is approximately 100 times greater than in individuals in the general population in the same age range.[2]

The patients were mostly young with an average age at the

time of transplantation of 39.9 (range 5–70) years. Forty-eight percent of the recipients were under 40 years of age.

Males were affected in 64% and females in 36% of instances. This does not signify a male predilection for cancer, but merely that males make up 62% and females 38% of renal transplant recipients[50] who comprise the bulk of patients in this study.

Interval between Transplantation and Malignancy

The average time between transplantation and the diagnosis of neoplasia was 37 (range 1–158) months. This period was shorter in recipients who developed lymphomas (26 months), than in those with nonlymphomatous tumors (40 months). The short time interval for the development of neoplasia is in contrast with the long latent period of 5–15 years or more that has been observed between exposure to an oncogenic stimulus such as ionizing radiation or tobacco, and the development of malignancy.

The incidence of cancer increases with the length of time following transplantation.[49, 51] Thus, in the Australasian series the frequency in those who survived beyond 1 year and 5 years was 11 and 24%, respectively.[49] All transplant patients therefore should be followed indefinitely. It will be of great interest to see what the incidence of cancer will be in a large group followed for 15 years or more.

Recipients with Previous Malignancies

Twelve of the 585 patients had previous malignancies treated at intervals ranging from 17 years to several weeks before transplantation, or at the time of this procedure. In 9 recipients the neoplasms that appeared after transplantation had no relationship to the previous tumors. However, there may have been a morphologic or etiologic connection between the two types of cancer in 3 other patients. Basal cell carcinomas were treated before transplantation in one patient who subsequently developed a malignant melanoma of the skin. The second recipient had been treated successfully for multiple myeloma and subsequently developed a pulmonary infiltrate that was diagnosed histologically as an "immunoblastoma." However, we cannot

exclude the possibility that it might have been a poorly differentiated plasmacytoma. The third patient had received radiotherapy for a gastric lymphosarcoma 17 years previously and after
transplantation presented with a gastric adenocarcinoma.

Apart from the 12 recipients described above it is possible that
some of the others may have had tumors that were present at
the time of transplantation, but which were clinically silent.
Thirty-four of the 585 patients (5.8%) manifested malignancies
within the first four months after transplantation.

Cancer in the Organ Donors

The homografts were obtained from 690 donors, of whom 235
were living related volunteers, 7 unrelated living donors and
448 were cadavers. One cadaver donor had had a carcinoma of
the colon removed five years previously and was free of tumor at
autopsy examination. The recipient subsequently developed a
reticulum cell sarcoma of the brain. Six other donors had cancers including medulloblastoma (3 patients), intracranial neu-
roepithelioma, carcinoma of the bronchus and metastatic cylindroma of salivary gland origin. The neoplasms that developed in
the recipients had no known relationship to these tumors. They
consisted of reticulum cell sarcoma, gastric leiomyosarcoma,
carcinoma of the breast, squamous cell carcinoma of the skin,
carcinoma of the endometrium and carcinoma of the rectum.

Types of De Novo Malignancy

The types of cancers encountered in the 585 patients are listed
in Table 3. Nonlymphomatous tumors occurred in 462 patients,
solid lymphomas in 118 and both a nonlymphomatous neoplasm
and a solid lymphoma in each of 5 recipients. Twenty-four patients had two different types of neoplasia, so that there was a
total of 609 tumor varieties.

Most surveys of cancer statistics omit consideration of nonmel-
anoma skin cancers and carcinoma in situ of the uterine cervix.
In order to compare the distribution of tumors in transplant recipients with that for the general population we shall, for the
moment, exclude recipients with these neoplasms, leaving us
with 374 patients. A most unusual feature in this series is a dis-

TABLE 3.—DE NOVO TUMORS IN ORGAN
HOMOGRAFT RECIPIENTS

TYPE OF CANCER	NO. OF PATIENTS*
Cancers of skin and lips	238
Solid lymphomas	124
Carcinomas of uterus	47
Cervix (43); body (4)	
Carcinomas of the lung	31
Head and neck carcinomas (excluding skin and lip)	21
Thyroid (7); tongue (3); parotid (3);	
floor of mouth (2); other (6)	
Carcinomas of colon and rectum	18
Leukemias	17
Metastatic carcinomas (primary site unknown)	17
Carcinomas of breast	13
Carcinomas of urinary bladder	13
Carcinomas of the kidney	10
Host kidney (7); homograft kidney (3)	
Carcinomas of liver and bile ducts	9
Testicular carcinomas	8
Soft tissue sarcomas	6
Ovarian cancers	5
Cancers of stomach (1 carcinoid tumor)	4
Brain tumors	4
Carcinomas of prostate gland	4
Carcinomas of the pancreas	4
Miscellaneous cancers	16
Total	609

*Twenty-four patients had more than one type of neoplasm.

proportionately high incidence of lymphomas present in 123 patients (33%), compared to an incidence of only 3–4% in the general population.[52] The common types of malignancy in the population at large infrequently are observed in transplant patients—carcinoma of the colon and rectum (14% versus 4.8%), carcinoma of the prostate (17% versus <2%), carcinoma of the female breast (26% versus 9%), invasive carcinoma of the uterine cervix (14% versus 7%) and carcinoma of the lung in males (22% versus 7%). The incidence of lung cancer in women (10%) was slightly higher than in the general population (6%), but this may be artifact because of the small number of patients involved. The relatively young age of the transplant recipients may account for the infrequent occurrence among them of common types of malignancy that usually are encountered in older people in the general population.

TABLE 4. – MALIGNANCIES OF
THE SKIN AND LIPS

TYPE OF CANCER	NO. OF PATIENTS
Squamous cell carcinomas	135
Basal cell carcinomas	63
Squamous and basal cell carcinomas	26
Malignant melanoma	10*
Unclassified	4
Total	238

*One patient also had a squamous cell carcinoma, and another had multiple basal cell carcinomas.

Malignancies of the Skin and Lips

The most common malignancies were those of the skin and lower lip, which were found in 238 of the 585 patients (41%). Skin only was involved in 188 recipients, the lip only in 27 and the skin and the lip in 23. Table 4 indicates the types of lesions that were encountered. The tumors differed in several respects from those in the general population. Whereas basal cell carcinomas outnumber the squamous cell lesions in the public at large,[53] the opposite was found to be the case in transplant patients (see Table 4). In renal transplant recipients squamous cell carcinomas were 36 times more frequent than in the general population, whereas skin cancers as a group were 7 times more common.[54] On the average, recipients were 30 years younger than persons with similar lesions in the general population.[55] Multiple tumors were more common in transplant patients (39%) compared with a 16%[56] to 22%[53] incidence in the public at large. Therefore, repeated follow-up examinations of transplant recipients with skin cancer are most important.

Nearly all the neoplasms occurred on areas exposed to sunlight, emphasizing the importance of this agent as an etiologic factor.[57, 58] In addition, most of the patients with these tumors lived in areas exposed to prolonged sunshine, mostly in Australasia and the southwest portion of the United States.

Most of the skin cancers were of low-grade malignancy, but 16 patients had dangerous lesions. Regional lymph node metastases occurred in 12 – 10 with squamous cell carcinomas and 2 with melanomas. Six of these recipients died of metastases (Fig 1), as did another 4 who had no lymph node involvement. Half of

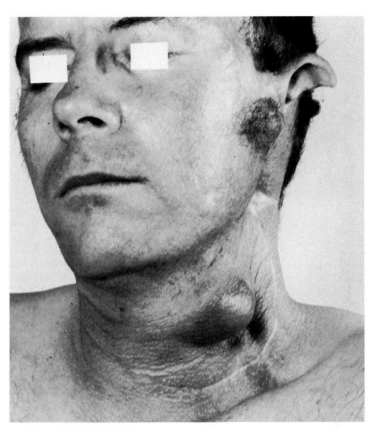

Fig 1.—Male, 30 years old at time of transplantation, developed multiple squamous cell carcinomas of face, neck and left hand 36 months later. These were excised or treated with topical 5-fluorouracil. Three years later he developed carcinoma of the left ear with an enlarged cervical lymph node, requiring excision of a major portion of the ear and a radical neck dissection. Six months later recurrent tumor appeared in the lower neck with metastases in the lumbar spine, liver and brain, causing death 7½ years after transplantation.

the deaths occurred in patients with malignant melanoma and half occurred in patients with squamous cell carcinoma.

Hyperkeratoses and warts frequently are observed on sun-exposed skin areas in transplant recipients.[57] The former lesions appear to undergo malignant transformation more readily than in the general population.[59] A spectrum of abnormalities ranging from hyperkeratoses and keratoacanthomas to frank carcinomas may be present.[51] At times it may be very difficult to dis-

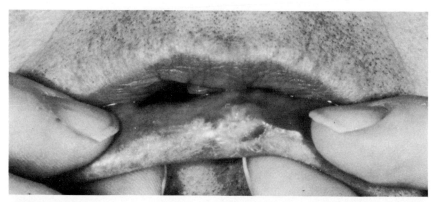

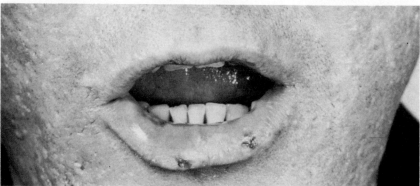

Fig 2 (top).—Male, 39 years old at time of transplantation, developed a classical squamous cell carcinoma of the lip three years later. Excision with clear margins was followed by a recurrence three years later, which again was excised with satisfactory margins. This recurred 2½ years later and was treated with radiotherapy. The patient remains well 11½ years after transplantation. (Reprinted with permission from Penn, I.: Immunosuppression and cancer: importance in head and neck surgery, Arch. Otolaryngol. 101:667, 1975. Copyright 1975 by the American Medical Association.)

Fig 3 (bottom).—Man, 21 years old at time of transplantation, developed multiple warts, hyperkeratoses and squamous cell carcinomas of the upper extremities, face and right knee 78 months later. These were treated by excision or with 5-fluorouracil cream. Thirty months later biopsy of two persistent superficial ulcers of the lower lip demonstrated squamous cell carcinomas which were widely excised. No recurrences of the lip lesions have appeared but the patient had further skin cancers. He currently is alive more than 13½ years after transplantation. He has been on dialysis and off immunosuppressive therapy for approximately two years. (Reprinted with permission from Penn, I.: Immunosuppression and cancer: importance in head and neck surgery, Arch. Otolaryngol. 101:667, 1975. Copyright 1975 by the American Medical Association.)

tinguish the various lesions from one another; whenever there is any hint of malignancy, a biopsy should be taken.

Lip cancers also may present diagnostic problems, as they may have atypical features. Although some carcinomas present with a classical rolled everted edge and indurated base (Fig 2), many lack these features and present as one or more superficial ulcers (Fig 3). A wise policy is to perform biopsy for all lip lesions that persist for more than a month.

Patients who live in areas with plentiful sunlight should be cautioned against prolonged exposure. If the recipients' occupations or hobbies do not permit this, it is advisable to apply an aminobenzoic acid sunscreen lotion twice daily.[57]

Malignant melanomas are treated by surgical excision, whereas squamous or basal cell carcinomas respond well to excision, radiotherapy or cryotherapy. Patients with multiple superficial skin cancers often can be managed satisfactorily with repeated applications of topical chemotherapeutic agents such as 5-fluorouracil cream. In most recipients with skin cancer it is not necessary to decrease or discontinue immunosuppressive therapy as is sometimes practiced in patients with high grade malignancies.

Solid Lymphomas

Since the classification of the lymphomas is controversial[60, 61] and as some of the newer terminology is not yet widely accepted, the older nomenclature will be used in this paper (Table 5). The broad term "lymphoma" is used in cases where the pathologist was not willing to make a more specific diagnosis. Reticulum

TABLE 5.—SOLID LYMPHOMAS IN ORGAN TRANSPLANT RECIPIENTS

Reticulum cell sarcomas	81*
Kaposi's sarcomas	16*
Lymphomas	12
Lymphosarcomas	6
Hodgkin's disease	3
Plasma cell lymphomas	3
Lymphoreticular tumors	2
Histiocytic reticulosis	1
Total	124

*One patient had Kaposi's sarcoma and a reticulum cell sarcoma.

cell sarcoma includes cases diagnosed as "reticulosarcoma," histiocytic lymphoma," "cerebral microglioma" and "immunoblastic sarcoma." There is much debate about the identity of the primary cell of Kaposi's sarcoma. We have included this tumor among the lymphomas because some physicians regard it as belonging to this group.[62-64]

Fig 4.—Nine months after transplantation a man, 55 years old at time of transplantation, developed extensive areas of Kaposi's sarcoma of the anterior abdominal wall, left thorax (shown) and the right leg. The immunosuppressive therapy was reduced and three months later the lesions appeared to be regressing. (Courtesy of Dr. Margaret C. Douglass, Dr. Nathan Levine and Dr. C. Cruz, Henry Ford Hospital, Detroit.)

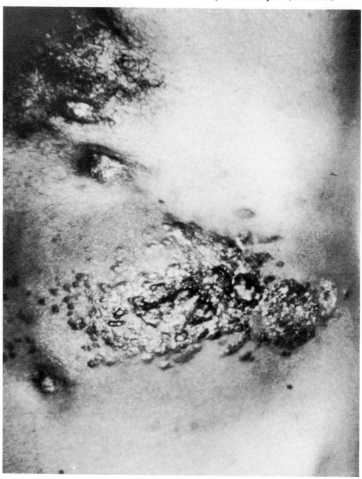

In the general population Hodgkin's disease comprises 34% of the lymphomas[52] and is the most common lymphoid tumor in all age groups.[65] In striking contrast, the incidence in transplant recipients was found to be very low (see Table 5), comprising only 3 of 124 lymphomas (2%). The predominant type of lymphoma was the reticulum cell sarcoma (65%), which was 350 times more common in renal transplant recipients than in the general population.[66] Most reticulum cell sarcomas probably belong to the class of "immunoblastic sarcomas"[60] as they have all the morphologic features of antigen-stimulated lymphocytes. These tumors may represent an abnormal immune response to the foreign histocompatibility antigens of the homograft or to the antigens of various infectious agents that frequently attack immunosuppressed patients.

In the general community Kaposi's sarcoma is a rare entity, but it occurred in 16 of the 585 transplant recipients (3%). Eleven had involvement of the skin of one or more extremities. Additional lesions affected the skin of the thorax and abdomen in 1 patient (Fig 4); the skin of the abdomen (1 patient); the skin of the penis (1 patient); the tonsil (1 patient); and the mucosa of the mouth and nose (1 patient). Visceral Kaposi's sarcoma occurred in 5 patients. Most of the lesions occurred in the alimentary tract and lungs.

The 108 recipients with other lymphomas (see Table 5) may be divided into two groups: those with widespread lesions and those with disease localized to a single viscus.[7] There were 50 recipients in the former group, in which the distribution of the neoplasms was similar to that in the general population. They involved mainly the liver, spleen, lymph nodes, bone marrow and lungs (Fig 5).

The organs affected by the localized lymphomas are listed in Table 6. It is important to emphasize the frequency of CNS involvement (Fig 6). Apart from the 40 patients with lesions limited to this area, there were another 8 who had tumors involving the brain and other organs.* Thus 48 of the 108 recipients (44%) with non-Kaposi's sarcoma had CNS lesions. This is in sharp contrast with a less than 2% incidence in the general population.[67, 68] The brain lymphomas frequently had a multicentric distribution (see Fig 6). The high frequency of CNS involvement

---

*Excluding two patients with widespread tumor in whom the only CNS involvement was the pituitary gland in one and the pia mater in the other.

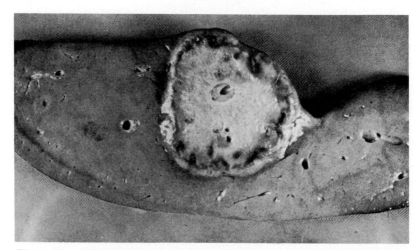

Fig 5.—Man, 23 years old at time of transplantation, underwent emergency partial gastrectomy for severe bleeding 30 months later. The source was multiple ulcers of the stomach, each of which was the site of reticulum cell sarcoma. At autopsy examination several days later, tumor also was found in the liver (shown), thyroid gland, lungs, pituitary gland, skin and the psoas muscle. (Reproduced with permission from Penn, I., Hammond, W., Brettschneider, L., and Starzl, T. E. Malignant lymphomas in transplantation patients, Transplant. Proc. 1:106, 1969. Courtesy of the editor.)

may be related to the poor immunologic reactions of this area. A lymphoma that has arisen in CNS itself or that has been transmitted there from other organs, is much more likely to grow in this relatively immunologically privileged site than in other organs.[69]

TABLE 6.—ORGANS AFFECTED BY LOCALIZED LYMPHOMAS

ORGAN	NO. OF PATIENTS
Brain	39
Spinal cord	1
Liver	5
Small bowel	3
Lung	3
Esophagus	1
Colon	1
Vagina	1
Stomach	1
Submandibular nodes	1
Kidney homograft	1
Vertebral bone marrow	1
Total	58

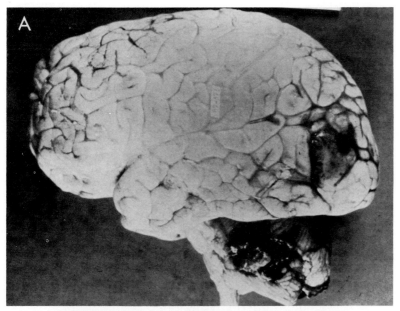

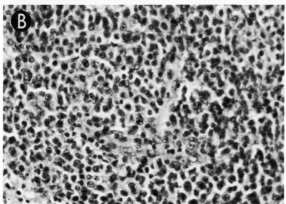

Fig 6.—Boy, 14 years old, developed neurologic symptoms 5½ months after transplantation. Craniotomy and biopsy revealed a cerebellar reticulum cell sarcoma. **A,** the patient died within a few weeks and was found to have four discrete areas of tumor in the brain, two of which are seen in the left occipital lobe and cerebellum. There was no tumor elsewhere in the body. **B,** the large uniform cells with indistinct cytoplasm and round to oval nuclei are characteristic of reticulum cell sarcoma (×350). (Reproduced with permission from Penn, I., Hammond, W., Brettschneider, L., and Starzl, T. E. Malignant lymphomas in transplantation patients, Transplant. Proc. 1:106, 1969. Courtesy of the editor.)

The occurrence of neurologic symptoms in a transplant recipient must always arouse suspicion of complications such as hypertensive encephalopathy, meningitis, brain abscess or intracranial bleeding. To this list we must add CNS lymphomas. A prompt work-up is indicated. This may include examination of the cerebrospinal fluid, electroencephalography, brain scan, computerized cerebral tomography and cerebral angiography.

Experiments in animals indicate that lymphomas may be of donor or host origin, usually the latter.[70] The question arises as to whether some of the tumors in man may be of donor origin, in view of the fact that the homograft inevitably contains numerous lymphocytes. Thus far the source of these cells has been studied in only three patients. In each instance they arose from the recipient's lymphocytes.[5, 71, 72]

The lymphoid tissues in transplant patients are exposed to and may react to numerous antigens, including those of the homograft, a large number of infectious agents, ALG or ATG, and a variety of other medications. The surgeon and the pathologist must beware of several lymphoproliferative processes that may, on occasion, mimic the lymphomas. Lymphoid hyperplasia may be induced by ALG therapy.[73] A few cases have been described of lymphoid hyperplasia that was histologically identical to reticulum cell sarcoma, which completely regressed following cessation of ATG therapy.[74] Diphenylhydantoin (Dilantin), which is used to prevent and control convulsions in chronic hemodialysis and renal transplant patients, may cause pseudolymphomas (which may regress following cessation of this therapy) and even lymphomas.[75, 76] Other conditions that may cause confusion are immunoblastic lymphadenopathy,[77, 78] lymphomatoid granulomatosis[79] and toxoplasmosis.[80, 81] Some workers report that atypical lymphoproliferative reactions to the Epstein-Barr virus also may simulate lymphomas.[82]

Carcinoma of the Uterus

Dysplasia of the uterine cervical epithelium occurs after treatment with a number of immunosuppressive agents including azathioprine.[83-86] It is possible that these changes may progress to malignancy. Carcinoma of the cervix frequently has been encountered (see Table 3). Of 209 female patients, 43(21%) had this problem. Thirty-three recipients (77%) had carcinoma in situ, 6(14%) had invasive cancer and in 4(9%) the stage of the disease was not reported. The incidence of in situ carcinoma is approximately 14 times greater than in the general community.[85] The fact that 1 of 5 females is likely to develop a cervical carcinoma emphasizes the need for all postadolescent patients to have pelvic examinations and cervical smears performed before transplantation and at regular intervals thereafter. These neoplasms respond well to conventional therapy either with simple hysterectomy, cone excision of the cervix or cryosurgery.

In contrast to the cervical lesions, carcinoma of the body of the uterus was uncommon (see Table 3). Perhaps this is a reflection of the youth of most transplant recipients; carcinoma of the uterine body usually is seen in postmenopausal women.

Leukemia

Leukemia occurred in 17 patients. Chronic myelogenous leukemia (CML) occurred in 7 patients, acute myeloblastic leukemia in 3 and a variety of other types, in 7. The incidence of CML in transplant recipients was estimated to be approximately five times greater than that in the general population.[87] The preponderance of CML is surprising as the leukemias that have developed after cancer chemotherapy have been overwhelmingly of the acute myeloblastic or acute myelomonoblastic varieties.[88]

Metastases of Undetermined Source

Of 45,728 patients with cancer listed in the tumor registry of Charity Hospital in New Orleans there were 56 with unknown primary neoplasms at the time of diagnosis in whom the primary site was later found. There were an additional 1,512 patients (3%) in whom the primary site was never found.[89] An identical incidence was found in 17 of the 585 patients in the present series.

Multiple Neoplasms

The risk of developing a new independent primary malignancy is 1.29 times greater in individuals who already have a cancer than in those who never have had neoplasia.[90] In the general population more than half of the cases of multiple cancers in-

volve the same organ or bilaterally paired organs.[91] Organ
transplant patients have a similar incidence of multiple malignancies. We have already alluded to the frequency of multiple
skin cancers and the multicentricity of cerebral lymphomas. In
addition, two recipients each had several carcinoids of the small
bowel; another patient had a squamous cell carcinoma and an
adenocarcinoma of the uterine cervix. The incidence of multiple
primary malignancies of different organs or tissues ranges from
2.8%[91] to 8.1%[92] in the general population. Twenty-four transplant recipients (4.1%) had such neoplasms.

Relationship to Immunosuppressive Therapy

Table 7 summarizes the immunosuppressive measures that
were used. The development of cancer cannot be related to any
particular immunosuppressive measure, but appears to be an
effect of immunosuppression in general. The treatment given to
patients with lymphomas differed little from that given to recipients with other tumors, other than that a higher percentage
(37% versus 25%) were treated with ALG or ATG.

Treatment of Tumors

Besides treatment of the malignancy per se, the question arises as to whether it is necessary to reduce or discontinue immu-

TABLE 7. – IMMUNOSUPPRESSIVE
MEASURES USED*

AGENT	NO. OF PATIENTS
Prednisone	579
Azathioprine	583
Local irradiation of the homograft	179
ALG	163†
Splenectomy	132
Actinomycin	91
Cyclophosphamide	35
Thoracic duct fistula	13
Thymectomy	11

*Other treatments included endolymphatic irradiation
(3 patients); total body irradiation (3); thymic irradiation
(2); 5-fluorouracil (2); 6-mercaptopurine (2); extracorporeal
irradiation of the peripheral blood (1); methotrexate (1);
and azaserine (1).
†Two patients received ALG after the appearance of
the tumors.

nosuppressive therapy to permit the recipient's depressed immune system to recover in the hope that it may play a role in eliminating the cancer. We have already mentioned several patients with transplanted malignancies who had a satisfactory outcome following cessation of immunosuppressive therapy. Such drastic treatment is unnecessary in the management of low-grade cancers of the skin, lip and uterine cervix. As regards the more highly malignant neoplasms there is a difference of opinion. Some surgeons do not modify immunosuppressive therapy, while others – including the author – prefer to reduce or completely discontinue it. Thus far only a small number of patients have been treated in this manner and several have done well. An example is one of our patients who had a cerebral lymphoma and who is well more than nine years after the tumor was diagnosed.

In patients with widespread cancers requiring chemotherapy it is important to remember that such treatment has profound effects on bone marrow. It is therefore wise to discontinue immunosuppressive therapy with azathioprine or cyclophosphamide, which also cause marked depression of marrow activity. Despite this, satisfactory homograft function may continue, as many of the cancer therapeutic agents have immunosuppressive side effects. Should rejection of a renal homograft occur, it may be removed and the patient treated with hemodialysis. Unlike in kidney transplantation there are no satisfactory artifical supports for patients with failing liver or cardiac homografts. The surgeon must bear this in mind before making a decision to discontinue immunosuppression in hepatic or cardiac transplant recipients who develop cancer.

PROGNOSIS

Of the patients followed, 309 (53%) currently are alive. Of recipients with lymphomas, 19% are still living, as are 62% of those with other neoplasms. These figures paint an unduly gloomy picture. Although we readily admit that a substantial number of patients with high-grade malignancies die of cancer, many of the deaths are from other causes, especially infections caused by immunosuppressive therapy, homograft failure caused by rejection, and cardiovascular complications. In some recipients the tumors were incidental findings at autopsy examination.

An accurate outlook for these patients may be obtained from a study of the first 678 renal transplant patients treated at the University of Colorado Medical Center and the Denver Veterans Administration Hospital. Almost 6% developed cancer but less than 1% died from this cause. Confirmation of these favorable figures is obtained from the Australasian Renal Transplant survey,[93] in which there were 2,302 recipients of whom 907 died, with only 30 deaths (3%) from de novo malignancies.

ETIOLOGY OF DE NOVO NEOPLASMS

The cause of the increased incidence of malignancies of organ homograft recipients is unclear, but a complex interplay of multiple factors probably is responsible. These are considered in detail in other publications.[2, 7, 10] Among the factors that deserve consideration are alterations in immunity, activation of oncogenic viruses, oncogenic or co-oncogenic effects of the immunosuppressive agents or occasionally of other drugs (such as diphenylhydantoin or isoniazide), and genetic factors. Transplant patients with and without malignancies require intensive study to enable us to learn more about factors that lead to oncogenesis in man.

Implications for the Future Use of Immunosuppressive Agents

Does the development of cancer serve as a deterrent to future endeavors in the field of organ transplantation? The answer is an emphatic "no!". Though the incidence of malignancies is increased, we have shown that many are of low grade and are readily treatable by conventional techniques. Even if the high-grade neoplasms and other serious complications of immunosuppressive therapy are taken into consideration, organ transplantation still is a worthwhile undertaking. It is the only satisfactory treatment for many patients with end-stage disease of the kidney, liver, heart and other organs. Nevertheless, we should not be satisfied with the status quo. We must find a substitute for current immunosuppressive therapy with its broad, nonspecific depression of the immune system. This must be some form of immune unresponsiveness directed only at the antigens of the homograft.

This study has implications far beyond the field of organ

transplantation. Immunosuppressive therapy currently is being used to treat a variety of disorders including chronic renal disease, rheumatoid arthritis, systemic lupus erythematosus, hepatitis, Wegener's granulomatosis and other diseases of obscure etiology.[3, 6, 9] In addition, many of the cancer chemotherapeutic agents have immunosuppressive and other side effects and, paradoxically, may even cause malignancies to develop.[3, 6, 9, 88, 94] There are no accurate statistics on the incidence of malignancy in nontransplant patients with nonmalignant diseases treated with immunosuppressive agents. These will be obtainable only through prospective controlled trials of large numbers of patients treated for prolonged periods. Thus far we have collected data on 80 patients who developed 83 malignancies, of which 25% were lymphomas and 18% were leukemias.[9] These findings suggest that the long-term use of immunosuppressive agents should be restricted to those for whom all other forms of therapy have failed to control their illnesses.

There has been an increased incidence of malignancy in cancer patients who receive chemotherapy.[3, 6, 9, 94] Several thousand patients treated for Hodgkin's disease, multiple myeloma or ovarian cancer have had a significantly increased frequency of acute leukemia.[88, 95] In patients with these types of advanced cancers the risk of development of additional neoplasms must be accepted, as it is far outweighed by the months or years of control of the original tumors. We are more concerned about the late effects of chemotherapy in patients with minimal disease or those receiving treatment after resection of all clinically evident disease (adjuvant chemotherapy). Conflicting results have been obtained following treatment of various malignancies. A decreased relapse rate in premenopausal women with breast cancer has been reported in two studies[96, 97] evaluating mastectomy and adjuvant chemotherapy. The median follow-up period was about a year and no patient had a second cancer during this time. Obviously a much longer period of follow-up is necessary to assess the risk of possible second cancers. In contrast with these encouraging early results Jamieson and Ludbrook[98] quote reports indicating that adjuvant chemotherapy in colorectal cancer has proved unrewarding. This treatment apparently has enhanced neoplastic recurrence in patients with lung cancer as well as in those with breast cancer in a small clinical trial.[98] In addition, Lerner[99] described the development of acute myeloblastic leukemia in 3 of 13 women who received the alkylating agent chlorambucil as adjuvant treatment for breast cancer. It is obvious that great caution is necessary with adjuvant chemotherapy, particularly in patients at low risk for relapse, as in those with negative regional nodes. Similar caution is advisable with regimens in which chemotherapy is given with radiation therapy, a combination that is likely to enhance the risk of carcinogenesis.[100]

Acknowledgment

The author is grateful to numerous colleagues working in transplant centers throughout the world for their generous contribution of data concerning their patients.

REFERENCES

1. Penn, I., Hammond, W., Brettschneider, L., and Starzl, T. E.: Malignant lymphomas in transplantation patients, Transplant. Proc. 1:106, 1969.
2. Penn, I.: *Malignant Tumors in Organ Transplant Recipients* (New York: Springer-Verlag, 1970).
3. Penn, I., and Starzl, T. E.: The effect of immunosuppression on cancer, in *Seventh National Cancer Conference Proceedings* (Philadelphia: J. B. Lippincott Co. 1973), pp. 425–436.
4. Penn, I.: Transplantation of kidneys containing primary malignant tumors, Transplantation 16:674, 1973.
5. Penn, I.: Malignancies in recipients of organ transplants, in Beers, R. F., Jr., Tilghman, R. C., and Bassett, E. G., (eds.): *The Role of Immunological Factors in Viral and Oncogenic Processes, Johns Hopkins Med. J.* (suppl. 3): 211–221, 1974.
6. Penn, I.: Chemical immunosuppression and human cancer, Cancer 34: 1474, 1974.
7. Penn, I.: Immunosuppression and malignant disease, in Good, R. A., and Twomey, J. J. (eds.): *The Immunopathology of the Lymphomas* (New York: Plenum Press) (in press).
8. Penn, I.: Transplantation in patients with primary renal malignancies, Transplantation 24:424, 1977.
9. Penn, I.: Malignancies associated with immunosuppressive or cytotoxic therapy, Surgery 83:492, 1978.
10. Penn, I.: Tumors arising in organ transplant recipients, in Klein, G., and Weinhouse, S. (eds.): *Advances in Cancer Research*, Vol. 28 New York: Academic Press (in press).
11. Belzer, F. O., Schweizer, R. T., Kountz, S. L., and Delorimer, A. A.: Malignancy and immunosuppression. Renal homotransplantation in patients with primary renal neoplasms, Transplantation 13:164, 1972.
12. Cronin, R. E., Kaehny, W. D., Miller, P. D., Stables, D. P., Gabow, P. A.,

Ostroy, P. R., and Schrier, R. W.: Renal cell carcinoma: Unusual systemic manifestations, Medicine 55:291, 1976.
13. Editorial: Renal cell carcinoma, Lancet 2:887, 1976.
14. Ehrlich, R. M., Goldman, R., and Kaufman, J. J.: Surgery of bilateral Wilms' tumors: The role of renal transplantation, J. Urol. 111:277, 1974.
15. Fetner, C. D., Barilla, D. E., Scott, T., Ballard, J., and Peters, P.: Bilateral renal cell carcinoma in von Hippel-Lindau syndrome: Treatment with staged bilateral nephrectomy and hemodialysis, J. Urol. 117:534, 1977.
16. Matas, A. J., Simmons, R. L., Buselmeier, R. J., Kjellstrand, C. M., and Najarian, J. S.: Successful renal transplantation in patients with prior history of malignancy, Am. J. Med. 59:791, 1975.
17. Parker, R. M., Timothy, R. P., and Harrison, J. H.: Neoplasia of the solitary kidney, J. Urol. 101:283, 1969.
18. Starzl, T. E.: *Experience in Hepatic Transplantation* (Philadelphia: W. B. Saunders Co., 1969), pp. 350–367.
19. Williams, R., Smith, M., Shilkin, K. B., Herbertson, B., Joysey, V., and Calne, R. Y.: Liver transplantation in man: The frequency of rejection, biliary tract complications, and recurrence of malignancy based on an analysis of 26 cases, Gastroenterology 64:1026, 1973.
20. Bennington, J. L.: Cancer of the kidney—etiology, epidemiology and pathology, Cancer 32:1017, 1973.
21. Bell, E. T.: *Renal Diseases* (Philadelphia: Lea and Febiger, 1950), p. 428.
22. Thomas, E. D., Fefer, A., Buckner, C. D., and Storb, R.: Current status of bone marrow transplantation for aplastic anemia and acute leukemia, Blood 49:671, 1977.
23. Thomas, E. D., Buckner, C. D., Banaji, M., Clift, R. A., Fefer, A., Flournoy, N., Goodell, B. W., Hickman, R. O., Lerner, K. G., Neiman, P. E., Sale, G. E., Sanders, J. E., Singer, J., Stevens, M., Storb, R., and Weiden, P. L.: One hundred patients with acute leukemia treated by chemotherapy, total body irradiation, and allogeneic marrow transplantation, Blood 49:511, 1977.
24. Thomas, E. D., Bryant, J. I., Buckner, C. D., Clift, R. A., Fefer, A., Johnson, F. L., Neiman, P., Ramberg, R. E., and Storb, R.: Leukaemic transformation of engrafted human marrow cells in vivo, Lancet 1:1310, 1972.
25. Kluyskens, P., and Ringoir, S.: Follow up of a human larynx transplantation, Laryngoscope 80:1244, 1970.
26. Eilber, F. R., and Morton, D. L.: Impaired immunologic reactivity and recurrence following cancer surgery, Cancer 25:362, 1970.
27. Marchioro, T. L., Rowlands, D. R., Jr., Rifkind, D., Waddell, W., and Starzl, T. E.: Splenic homotransplantation. Ann. N.Y.Acad. Sci. 120:626, 1964.
28. Penn, I., Corman, J., Gustafsson, A., Halgrimson, C. G., Putnam, C. W., Schroter, G. T., Groth, C. G., and Starzl, T. E.: Experience in orthotopic liver transplantation: Indications, results and future prospects, in Lie, R. S., and Gutgemann, A. (eds.): *Liver Transplantation* (Baden-Baden, West Germany: Gerhard-Witzstrock Co., Ltd., 1974), pp. 27–38.
29. Southam, C. M.: Host defense mechanisms and human cancer, Ann. Inst. Pasteur 107:585, 1964.

30. Scanlon, E. F., Hawkins, R. A., Fox, W. W., and Smith, W. S.: Fatal homo-transplanted melanoma. A case report, Cancer 18:782, 1965.
31. Wilson, R. E., Hager, E. B., Hampers, C. L., Corson, J. M., Merrill, J. P., and Murray, J. E.: Immunologic rejection of human cancer transplanted with a renal allograft, N. Engl. J. Med. 278:479, 1968.
32. Wilson, R. E., and Penn, I.: Fate of tumors transplanted with a renal allo-graft, Transplant. Proc. 7:327, 1975.
33. Cerilli, G. J., Nelsen, C., and Dorfmann, L.: Renal homotransplantation in infants and children with the hemolytic uremic syndrome, Surgery 71: 66, 1972.
34. Gokal, J. M., Rjosk, H. K., Meister, P., Stelter, W-J., and Witte, J.: Meta-static choriocarcinoma transplanted with cadaver kidney. A case report, Cancer 39:1317, 1977.
35. Jeremy, D., Farnsworth, R. H., Robertson, M. R., Annetts, D. L., and Murgnaghan, G. F.: Transplantation of malignant melanoma with ca-daver kidney, Transplantation 3:619, 1972.
36. Kuss, R., Legrain, M., Mathé, G., Nedey, R., and Camey, M.: Homologous human kidney transplantation. Experience with six patients, Postgrad. Med. J. 38:528, 1962.
37. Lanari, A., Rodo, J. E., Barcat, J. A., Mollins, M., Morando, G. G., Ague-ro, M. T., and Blanco, O. L.: Cuatro casos de desarrollo de un cancer del dado en el rinon injertado, Medicina 32:79, 1972.
38. Maclean, L. D., Dossetor, J. B., Gault, M. H., Oliver, J. A., Inglis, F. G., and Mackinnon, K. J.: Renal transplantation using cadaver donors, Arch. Surg. 91:288, 1965.
39. Martin, D. C., Rubini, M., and Rosen, V. J.: Cadaveric renal homotrans-plantation with inadvertent transplantation of carcinoma, JAMA 192:82, 1965.
40. McPhaul, J. J., Jr., and McIntosh, D. A.: Tissue transplantation still vex-es, N. Engl. J. Med. 272:105, 1965.
41. Mocelin, A. J., and Brandina, L.: Inadvertent transplant of a malignancy, Transplantation 19:430, 1975, (Letter to the Editor).
42. Muiznieks, H. W., Berg, J. W., Lawrence, W., Jr., and Randall, H. T.: Suitability of donor kidneys from patients with cancer, Surgery 64:871, 1968.
43. Tunner, W. S., Goldsmith, E. I., and Whitsell, J. C.: Human homotrans-plantation of normal and neoplastic tissue from the same organ, J. Urol. 105:18, 1971.
44. Zukoski, C. F., Killen, D. A., Ginn, E., Matter, B., Lucas, D. O., and Seig-ler, H.F.: Transplanted carcinoma in an immunosuppressed patient, Transplantation 9:71, 1970.
45. Rubinstein, L. J.: Extracranial metastases in cerebellar medulloblasto-ma, J. Pathol. 78:187, 1959.
46. Willis, R. A.: The Spread of Tumours in the Human Body. (St. Louis: C. V. Mosby, Co., 1952).
47. Fox, M.: Renal carcinoma in a living kidney graft donor, Transplantation 15:523, 1973.
48. Baird, R. N., White, H. J. O., and Tribe, C. R.: Renal carcinoma in a ca-daver kidney graft donor, Br. Med. J., 2:371, 1975.

49. Sheil, A. G. R.: Cancer in renal allograft recipients in Australia and New Zealand, Transplant. Proc. 9:1133, 1977.
50. Advisory Committee to the Renal Transplant Registry: The 13th report of the human renal transplant registry, Transplant. Proc. 9:9, 1977.
51. Marshall, V.: Pre-malignant and malignant skin tumours in immunosuppressed patients, Transplantation 17:272, 1974.
52. Silverberg, E.: Cancer statistics 1977, Cancer 27:26, 1977.
53. Bergstresser, P. R., and Halprin, K. M.: Multiple sequential skin cancers. The risk of skin cancer in patients with previous skin cancer, Arch. Dermatol. 111:995, 1975.
54. Hoxtell, E. O., Mandel, J. S., Murray, S. S., Schuman, L. M. and Goltz, R. W.: Incidence of skin carcinoma after renal transplantation, Arch. Dermatol. 113:436, 1977.
55. Mullen, D. L., Silverberg, S. G., Penn, I., and Hammond, W. S.: Squamous cell carcinoma of the skin and lip in renal homograft recipients, Cancer 37:729, 1976.
56. Phillips, C.: Multiple skin cancer; statistical and pathologic study, South. Med. J. 35:583, 1942.
57. Koranda, F. C., Dehmel, E. M., Kahn, G., and Penn, I.: Cutaneous complications in immunosuppressed renal homograft recipients, JAMA 229:419, 1974.
58. Koranda, F. C., Loeffler, R. T., Koranda, D. M., and Penn, I.: Accelerated induction of skin cancers by ultraviolet radiation in hairless mice treated with immunosuppressive agents, Surg. Forum 26:145, 1975.
59. Walder, B. K., Robertson, M. R., and Jeremy, D.: Skin cancer and immunosuppression, Lancet 2:1282, 1971.
60. Lukes, R. J., and Collins, R. D.: Immunologic characterization of human malignant lymphomas, Cancer 34:1488, 1974.
61. Case Records of the Massachusetts General Hospital. Case 30-1977. N. Engl. J. Med. 297:206, 1977.
62. Moertel, C. G., and Hagedorn, A. B.: Leukemia or lymphoma and coexistent primary malignant lesions: A review of the literature and a study of 120 cases, Blood 12:788, 1957.
63. Ormsby, O. S., and Montgomery, H.: *Diseases of the Skin* (8th ed.; Philadelphia, Pa.: Lea and Febiger, 1954), p. 1503.
64. Warner, T. F. C. S., and O'Loughlin, S.: Kaposi's sarcoma: a byproduct of tumor rejection, Lancet 2:687, 1975.
65. Levin, D. L., Devesa, S. S., Godwin, J. D., II., and Silverman, D. T.: *Cancer Rates and Statistics* (2d ed.; U.S. Department of Health, Education and Welfare, 1974).
66. Hoover, R., and Fraumeni, J. F., Jr.: Risk of cancer in renal transplant recipients, Lancet 2:55, 1973.
67. Richmond, J., Sherman, R. S., Diamond, H. D., and Craver, L. F.: Renal lesions associated with malignant lymphomas, Am. J. Med. 32:184, 1962.
68. Rosenberg, S. A., Diamond, H. D., Jaslowitz, B., and Craver, L. F.: Lymphosarcoma: A review of 1269 cases, Medicine (Baltimore) 40:31, 1961.
69. Schneck, S. A., and Penn, I.: De novo cerebral neoplasms in renal transplant recipients, Lancet 1:983, 1971.
70. Gleichmann, E., Gleichmann, H., Schwartz, R. S., Weinblatt, A. and

Armstrong, M. Y. K.: Immunologic induction of malignant lymphoma: Identification of donor and host tumors in the graft-versus-host model, J. Natl. Cancer Inst. 54:107, 1975.

71. Brown, R. S., Schiff, M. and Mitchell, M. S.: Reticulum cell sarcoma of host origin arising in a transplanted kidney, Ann. Intern. Med. 80:459, 1974.

72. Portmann, B., Schindler, A-M., Murray-Lyon, I. M. and Williams, R.: Histological sexing of a reticulum cell sarcoma arising after liver transplantation, Gastroenterology 70:82, 1976.

73. Iwasaki, Y., Porter, K. A., Amend, J. R., Marchioro, T. L., Zühlke, V., and Starzl, T. E.: The preparation and testing of horse antidog and antihuman antilymphoid plasma or serum and its protein fractions, Surg. Gynecol. Obstet. 124:1, 1967.

74. Iwatsuki, S., Geis, W. P., Molnar, Z., Giacchino, J. L., Ing, T. S., and Hano, J. E.: Systemic lymphoblastic response to antithymocyte globulin in renal allograft recipients: An initial report, J. Surg. Research (in press).

75. Editorial. Is phenytoin carcinogenic? Lancet 2:1071, 1971.

76. Li, F. P., Willard, D. R., Goodman, R., and Vawter, G.: Malignant lymphoma after diphenylhydantoin (dilantin) therapy, Cancer 36:1359, 1975.

77. Lukes, R. J., and Tindle, B. H.: Immunoblastic lymphadenopathy: A hyperimmune entity resembling Hodgkin's disease, N. Engl. J. Med. 292:1, 1975.

78. Spector, J. I., and Miller, S.: Immunoblastic lymphadenopathy. A report of two cases, JAMA 238:1263, 1977.

79. Hammar, S., and Mennemeyer, R.: Lymphomatoid granulomatosis in a renal transplant recipient, Hum. Pathol. 7:111, 1976.

80. Kayhoe, D. E., Jacobs, L., Beye, H. K., and McCullough, N. B.: Acquired toxoplasmosis; observations on two parasitologically proved cases treated with pyrimethamine and triple sulfonamides, N. Engl. J. Med. 257:1247, 1957.

81. Kayhoe, D. E.: Discussion of Pirofsky, B., Beaulieu, R., and Bardana, E. J. (Jr.): Antithymocyte antisera therapy in the presence of human lymphoid neoplasia, Behring Institute Mitteilungen 51:212, 1972.

82. Hertel, B. F., Matas, A. J., Dehner, L. P., Rosai, J., Simmons, R. L., and Najarian, J. S.: Lymphoproliferative disorders in organ transplant recipients (abstract), Proceedings of the Third Annual Meeting of the American Society of Transplant Surgeons, Chicago, June 2–4, 1977.

83. Gupta, P. K., Pinn, V. M., and Taft, P. D.: Cervical dysplasia associated with azathioprine (Imuran) therapy, Acta Cytol. (Baltimore) 13:373, 1969.

84. Kay, S., Frable, W. J., and Hume, D. M.: Cervical dysplasia and cancer developing in women on immunosuppression therapy for renal homotransplantation, Cancer 26:1048, 1970.

85. Porreco, R., Penn, I., Droegemueller, W., Greer, B., and Makowski, E.: Gynecologic malignancies in immunosuppressed organ homograft recipients, Obstet. Gynecol. 45:359, 1975.

86. Schramm, G.: Development of severe cervical dysplasia under treatment with azathioprine (Imuran), Acta Cytol. (Baltimore) 14:507, 1970.
87. Adler, K. R., Lempert, N. and Scharfman, W. B.: Chronic granulocytic leukemia following successful renal transplantation, Cancer (in press).
88. Sieber, S. M.: Cancer chemotherapeutic agents and carcinogenesis, Cancer Chemother. Rep. 59:915, 1975.
89. Krementz, E. T., Cerise, E. J., Ciavarella, J. M., Jr., and Morgan, L. R.: Metastases of undetermined source, Cancer 27:289, 1977.
90. Schoenberg, B. S.: Multiple primary neoplasms in Fraumeni, J. F., Jr. (ed.): *Persons at High Risk of Cancer. An Approach to Cancer Etiology and Control* (New York: Academic Press, 1975), pp. 103–119.
91. Moertel, C. G., Dockerty, M. B., and Baggenstoss, A. H.: Multiple primary malignant neoplasms. I. Introduction and presentation of data, Cancer 14:221, 1961.
92. Schottenfeld, D.: The epidemiology of multiple primary cancers, Cancer 27:233, 1977.
93. Sheil, A. G. R.: The Australasian Renal Transplant Survey (personal communication, 1977).
94. Penn, I.: Second malignant neoplasms associated with immunosuppressive medications, Cancer 37:1024, 1976.
95. Reimer, R. R., Hoover, R., Fraumeni, J. F., Jr., and Young, R. C.: Acute leukemia after alkylating-agent therapy of ovarian cancer, N. Engl. J. Med. 297:177, 1977.
96. Bonadonna, G., Brusamolino, E., Valagussa, P., Rossi, A., Brugnatelli, L., Brambilla, C., De Lena, M., Tancini, G., Bajetta, E., Musumeci, R., and Veronesi, U.: Combination chemotherapy as an adjunctive treatment in operable breast cancer, N. Engl. J. Med. 294:405, 1976.
97. Fisher, B., Carbone, P., Economou, S. G., Frelick, R., Glass, A., Lerner, H., Redmond, C., Zelen, M., Band, P., Katrych, D. L., Wolmark, N., and Fisher, E. R.: L-Phenylalanine mustard (L-PAM) in the management of primary breast cancer: A report of early findings, N. Engl. J. Med. 292: 117, 1975.
98. Jamieson, G. G., and Ludbrook, J.: Adjuvant chemotherapy for cancer, Arch. Surg. 112:119, 1977.
99. Lerner, H.: Second malignancies diagnosed in breast cancer patients while receiving adjuvant chemotherapy at the Pennsylvania Hospital, Proc. Am. Assoc. Cancer Res. 18:340, 1977.
100. Chabner, B. A.: Second neoplasm—a complication of cancer chemotherapy, N. Engl. J. Med. 297:213, 1977.

Metabolism during the Hypermetabolic Phase of Thermal Injury

DOUGLAS W. WILMORE, M.D.; L. HOWARD
AULICK, Ph.D.; and BASIL A. PRUITT, Jr., M.D.

United States Army Institute of Surgical Research
Brooke Army Medical Center, Fort Sam Houston, Texas

The hypermetabolic response to thermal injury is the most exaggerated catabolic response associated with any disease process. Increased oxygen consumption begins within the first 48 hours of injury, varies with the extent of the burn and may reach levels two times higher than normal in more extensively injured patients. The increased rate of heat production reaches a peak during the first to second week postinjury, gradually returning to normal with coverage of the burn wound. This report summarizes our knowledge to date about burn metabolism during the hypermetabolic phase of illness. Although marked physiologic changes occur in many organ systems during this time period, we will specifically limit our discussion to posttraumatic metabolic changes and will refer to thermoregulatory and circulatory alterations only as they relate to the regulation of energy flux and distribution of blood flow for heat transfer and metabolic purposes. The metabolic changes that occur during burn shock will be mentioned in order to establish the time course for

---

The opinions and assertions contained herein are the private views of the authors and are not to be construed as official or as reflecting the views of the Department of the Army or the Department of Defense.

the events as they occur following injury. Many burn patients sustain the life-threatening complications of septicemia, but a discussion of the impact of invasive infection on burn metabolism is outside the scope of this review.

This paper, then, will discuss the metabolic alterations that occur in febrile, hyperdynamic, hypermetabolic burn patients who break down body tissue at accelerated rates during a time when the wound is healing. The changes to be measured are of such magnitude that a study of metabolism in burn patients having no other disease processes allows a specific description and quantification of the body's metabolic and hormonal response to extensive injury. Application of this knowledge is possible not only in the treatment of burn patients, but also in other critically ill individuals who have sustained injury, infection and multiorgan system failure.

Mediators of the Metabolic Response to Burn Injury

After injury or infection, afferent stimuli signal the brain that tissue damage and/or microbiologic invasion has occurred. These signals set into motion an integrated neurohormonal response that results in metabolic alterations programmed to aid host defense and facilitate tissue repair. The magnitude of these signals depends primarily on the extent of stress (in burn patients, this response is related initially to the mass of tissue damage as quantitated by burn size), although the tissue response to these signals may be modulated by the age and sex of the patient, physiologic reserve (i.e., stress capacity), nutritional status and underlying disease processes. The causative factors and afferent signals that evoke the injury response are related to the time course of the posttraumatic response. Cuthbertson and Tilstone[1] described the first part of the response to injury as the "ebb" phase, which occurs immediately after injury and is characterized by a general depression of the body's physiologic function. Following successful resuscitation and restoration of blood volume, cardiopulmonary function increases, heat production and body temperature rise and substrate is mobilized from body tissues. This generalized elevation in physiologic activity characterizes the "flow" phase of injury which describes metabolic and hemodynamic alterations associated with tissue repair and patient recovery.

During the ebb phase, three general types of stimuli cause recognition of the injury and/or initiate homeostatic adjustment by the organism after burn injury.

FLUID LOSS. — Fluid loss from the vascular compartment occurs immediately after burn injury and results in stimulation of volume and pressure receptors, initiating a series of CNS-mediated homeostatic adjustments. With progressive fluid loss into the area of the burn, cardiac output drops markedly and hypoperfusion occurs, resulting in a reduction in tissue oxygenation and disturbances in the acid-base equilibrium. Chemoreceptor stimulation thus serves as additional afferent input. Because loss of fluid volume following thermal trauma is related closely to the extent of tissue damage, these specific mechanisms allow an initial quantitative physiologic response to occur after burn injury in man (i.e., the response is directly proportional to the size of the burn).

Early postburn hypovolemia and a decrease in cardiac output reach their nadir during the first 24 hours postburn and mimic those circulatory alterations occurring during hemorrhagic shock. The initial fall in oxygen consumption at this time reflects a decrease in the perfusion of the total body mass. Studies by Asch et al.[2] examined changes in organ blood flow and cardiac output following a 40%, histologically confirmed full-thickness scald burn in an animal model. When these animals were not resuscitated, the cardiac index decreased from a control level of 5.77 L/minute·m² to 3.78 L/minute·m² by the end of one hour after injury. At this time, studies with microspheres revealed that blood flow was reduced to the kidneys by 41%, to the liver by 34%, to the small intestines by 60% and to the carcass by 43%, while flow to the brain, heart, stomach, duodenum, large intestine, spleen and pancreas remained unchanged. Perfusion was restored to normal following fluid resuscitation. Alterations in organ system function have been described by Stoner[3] during the ebb phase of injury and normal function returns with restoration of blood volume.

AFFERENT SENSORY NERVE FIBERS. — Afferent sensory nerve fibers provide the most direct and quickest route for signals to arrive at the CNS following stress. It frequently has been suggested that pain may serve as the initial afferent signal after injury, and a variety of studies suggest that such neurogenic signals originating in the burn area are essential for the initial excitation of the pituitary-adrenal axis. The adrenocortical response to a burn injury placed on a dog's hind leg was not observed in animals after section of the peripheral nerves to the area of injury, transection of the spinal cord above the injury, or section through the medulla oblongata.[4] A similar pattern of response to denervation before injury has been described in man.[5, 6] In addition, a number of factors that accompany the "stress" of critical illness — restraint, immobilization and environmental disturbances — are most likely perceived by nervous afferent impulses.

CIRCULATING FACTORS. — Circulating factors may directly or indirectly stimulate the CNS and set the injury response into motion. Exogenous factors such as bacterial exotoxins or endotoxins are potent stimuli that cause major metabolic adjustments. Alterations in serum electrolytes, release of cell breakdown products, changes in the amino acid pattern and release of endogenous pyrogen may all be considered to be possible intrinsic chemical mediators of the initial injury response.

In patients who survive the acute injury, the ebb phase evolves into the flow phase response, which is characterized by hypermetabolism and the increased loss of nitrogen and other intracellular constituents from the body. During the flow phase, the initial increase in vascular permeability resolves and blood volume and other fluid compartments return to normal. At this point, hypovolemia or abnormalities in acid-base composition of the blood are corrected and are no longer considered responsible for flow phase responses. However, the close relationship between the metabolic responses and the size of the body surface burn suggests that in some manner, signals from the wound reach the CNS and determine the magnitude of the generalized or systemic response.

To determine the role of afferent nervous signals from the area of burn injury during the flow phase response, a variety of studies have been conducted in thermally injured patients.[7] First, a patient with traumatic spinal cord transection with burns of the lower extremities has been studied: hypermetabolism and the associated metabolic responses occurred despite central sensory afferent interruption from a major portion of the wound. In three patients, a topical anesthetic was applied to the burn wound to achieve total anesthesia. No alteration in metabolic rate or core temperature occurred after the initial application or maintenance of the topical anesthetic for up to six hours, although most patients were rendered pain-free and slept throughout the study. Finally, a spinal anesthetic was administered and maintained for four hours in a patient with multiple long bone fractures and 33% total body surface burns over the lower extremities. Once again, no significant effect on metabolic rate or core temperature was detected following interruption of sensory signals from the injured area.

At one time it was thought that the increased evaporative heat loss from the burn wound stimulated cold receptors and provided afferent signals to the brain; the resultant hypermetabolism was considered the thermoregulatory response to restore body temperature. As will be discussed in further detail, the hypermetabolism following thermal injury is temperature sensitive but is not temperature dependent. Although heat production can be minimized by treating burn patients in a warm ambient environment, the marked elevation in metabolic rate does not return to normal with external heating.

Although nervous afferent excitation may not be essential for the flow phase response, pain after treatment and patient manipulation will increase metabolism even further during the flow phase of injury. However, when burn patients were studied in ambient comfort conditions and allowed to sleep with or without analgesics, the hypermetabolic response was minimized to only 50–80% above normal but was not abated. Patient care should be oriented to minimize all painful stimuli: judicious use of analgesics and tranquilizers may be necessary in the treatment of critically ill patients.

Because of the inability to identify specific nervous afferent stimuli as initiators and propagators of the flow phase injury response, a search has begun for a circulating factor or factors that serve as the afferent signal to the brain following injury. In one study, heparinized blood was collected from burn patients and normal controls in pyrogen-free syringes.[8] A microaliquot of each sample was injected through indwelling chronic cannulae in rabbits, placed by standard stereotactic technique so that the distal tip lay in the preoptic area of the hypothalamus. Injection of normal serum in the rabbits resulted in no more than a 0.1 C rise in rectal temperature in samples from the 6 control subjects. Serum from 9 of the 13 patients elicited a febrile response (0.6–0.9 C over two hours) following hypothalamic injection.

Limulus lysate assay for endotoxin was negative in all these samples. After heat treatment of the serum, the febrile response was attenuated, suggesting that endogenous pyrogens (the product of the body's cells participating in the inflammatory reaction) mediated this febrile response.

Prostaglandins are known to affect hypothalamic function. Increased concentrations of these substances are found in lymph-draining areas of injury and in exudate from burn wounds.[9] To evaluate these substances as possible "wound hormones," arterial and venous concentrations of PGA, E, and F were determined using specific antibody assay techniques.[8] Twenty-one patients were studied and blood was drawn from the femoral vein in 15 of these subjects to determine the contribution of injured tissue to the prostaglandin level. However, arterial and venous concentrations of these prostaglandins were similar to those observed in normal subjects: patients with and without leg burns showed similar concentrations of these substances in the femoral vein when studied between the 3d to 31st day postinjury.

In contrast, prostaglandins have been shown to play a role in the hypermetabolic response in a small animal model.[10] The 30% increase in metabolic rates of these animals was attenuated by intraperitoneal injections of indomethacin, R02-5720 (Hoffman-LaRoche), and meclofenamate, drugs that interfere with prostaglandin activity. With this method of administration, however, one remains uncertain as to the peripheral or central actions of these agents on prostaglandin activity. Therefore, while prostaglandin metabolism may play a role in the hypermetabolic activity of small animals, the lack of peripheral release from burned limbs and the failure to blunt the metabolic response in man by high levels of salicylates[7] indicate that they probably do not act as circulating afferent signals for the hypermetabolism in burn patients. This does not eliminate, however, the possibility that central alterations in thermoregulatory reset process may involve prostaglandin synthesis and release within the hypothalamus.

Considered together, these studies suggest that circulating (rather than neurogenic) signals arising from the wound mediate the injury response during the flow phase. The endogenous pyrogens studied are products of leukocytes and other phagocytic cells that participate in the inflammatory response and wound healing. Whether the endogenous pyrogen is the single mediator of the metabolic response to injury, or whether it is just one of a number of circulating factors that mediate posttraumatic events, is not known.

CNS Adjustments after Burn Injury

The brain receives peripheral signals and integrates this afferent input. The CNS is an essential element of the hypermetabolic response to injury: patients with "brain death" and associated extensive thermal injury fail to mount a "flow" phase response. Similarly, morphine anesthesia, which markedly reduces hypothalamic function, has been shown to result in a prompt decrease in hypermetabolism, rectal temperature and cardiac output in severely burned patients.[11] Evidence to date suggests that a variety of adjustments occur within the hypothalamus and pituitary gland and that these alterations in neurohumoral control appear to dictate the compensatory adjustments to stress. These alterations in CNS control alter thermoregulatory mechanisms, increase heat production and regulate substrate mobilization and intraorgan energy transfer.

Marked adjustments in thermoregulation occur during the flow phase in injured patients. At this time, burn patients are febrile and at ambient temperatures studied (19–33 C) maintain core and mean skin temperatures 1–2 C above normal.[12] When allowed to adjust ambient temperature, burn patients selected a warmer environment to achieve comfort than did normal subjects, in spite of the fact that the patients had elevated core and mean skin temperatures.[13] The selected ambient temperature generally was related to burn size. This suggests that thermal injury results in an elevation of the central reference temperature and that body temperature is controlled by an upward "reset" in the hypothalamic thermostat. Administration of a variety of pharmacologic agents known to affect actual temperature setpoint in man (aspirin, L-Dopa, and calcium) has not reduced the hypermetabolism and hyperpyrexia that occur after injury.[11] As previously noted, the injury response in a rat burn model was consistently reduced by the administration of prostaglandin-blocking agents, possibly through their direct effects on the thermoregulatory center.

Other alterations in hypothalamic function also occur during

TABLE 1.—hGH RESPONSE AFTER PROVOCATIVE STIMULATION IN THERMALLY INJURED PATIENTS (mean ± SEM, nG/ml)

	NORMAL SUBJECTS (NO.=5)		ACUTE BURN PATIENTS (NO.=9)		RECOVERED BURN PATIENTS (NO.=7)	
	BASAL*	PEAK RESPONSE	BASAL	PEAK RESPONSE†	BASAL	PEAK RESPONSE
Insulin hypoglycemia	0.8±0.1	32.6±7.6	1.7±0.2	12.6±2.8	1.7±0.4	27.8±12.0
Arginine infusion	1.0±0.1	10.1±1.4	1.8±0.3	3.9±0.9	1.8±0.5	9.3± 5.1

*Basal level of normal individuals different from acute and recovered patients, $p<0.001$.
†Mean peak response of acute burn patients different from normal individuals and recovered patients, $p<0.01$.

the flow phase. Pituitary function has been assessed by examining specific hormone responses to various provocative stimuli. Human growth hormone response to insulin hypoglycemia and arginine infusion was measured in 9 burn patients and 5 normal controls.[13] Initial studies were carried out between the 3d and 24th days postburn and were repeated in the surviving patients after wound closure. The provocative tests for human growth hormone release were performed on consecutive days in the early morning. On the first day, 0.3 unit/kg body weight insulin was administered to burn patients and 0.15 unit/kg body weight to recovered patients and normal individuals. Serial blood samples were obtained for estimation of blood glucose concentration and hGH. On the subsequent morning, 30 gm of a 10% solution of arginine hydrochloride was infused intravenously over 30 minutes and blood was serially assayed for glucose, blood urea nitrogen, hGH and insulin.

Fasting hGH was significantly elevated above normal in the burned patients during the hypermetabolic phase of injury and during recovery, and elevated hGH levels occurred during the period of acute injury despite the associated fasting hyperglycemia. The hGH response to hypoglycemia was more rapid, but the peak response was diminished in the burned patient when compared with recovery and with controls. An attenuated response also was observed after arginine infusion (Table 1).

In a second study, serum concentrations of thyroid hormones were determined sequentially for the first two weeks after injury.[14] Thyrotoxin (T_4) and triiodothyronine (T_3) concentrations were significantly reduced and reversed T_3 (rT_3) concentrations

TABLE 2.–THYROID STUDIES IN BURN PATIENTS
(mean N = 5)

POSTBURN DAY	T_4 (μG%)	FREE THYROID INDEX	T_3 (nG%)	RT_3 (nG%)	TSH (μ IU/ML)
3	2.5	3.8	52	94	4.1
6	2.5	3.0	26	104	2.2
8	3.7	6.1	36	76	4.2
10	5.1	6.2	31	85	3.2
13	3.8	5.0	16	56	3.7
15	5.0	6.3	44	66	4.7
Normal range	4.5–11.5	3.8–13.4	80–180	36–84	<10

TABLE 3.—TSH (μIU/ML) RESPONSE OF 12 BURN PATIENTS TO TRH (400 μU IV, MEAN $\pm$ SEM)

| PATIENT GROUP | NO. | TIME IN MIN FOLLOWING TRH | | | | | | PEAK RESPONSE | Δ RESPONSE | INTEGRATED RESPONSE ABOVE BASAL (μIU-MIN/ML) |
		0	15	30	45	60	90			
Without complications	5	3.6±1.0	10.3± 1.8	12.1±1.9	12.3±1.9	12.9±2.1	9.3±1.6	13.8±2.0	10.2±1.5	593±90
Bacteremia	3	6.2±1.4	28.7±13.5	21.3±5.2	30.5±5.8	25.0±6.1	23.8±3.2	42.2±6.9*	36.0±8.2*	1618±102†
Bacteremia (dopamine infusion)	4	2.0±0.2	2.4±0.4	3.0±0.5	3.1±0.4	2.5±0.3	3.1±0.6	1.6±0.4*	1.6±0.4*	66±25†

*$P<0.01$ when compared to patients without complications.
†$P<0.001$ when compared to patients without complications.

TABLE 4.—CHARACTERISTICS OF PATIENTS (MEAN ± SEM OR RANGE)

PATIENT GROUP	NO.	AGE (YEARS)	TOTAL BODY SURFACE BURN (%)	POSTBURN DAY STUDIED	RECTAL TEMPERATURE (C)	POSITIVE BLOOD CULTURES AT TIME OF STUDY	BASAL HORMONE CONCENTRATIONS			
							T_4 (µG/DL)	T_3 (µG/DL)	rT_3 (nG/DL)	CORTISOL (µG/DL)
Without complications	5	32 (18–26)	58.5 (38–73)	13 (3–31)	38.6±0.2	0/5	3.2±1.0	100±32	129±10	31±5
Bacteremia (stable)	3	22 (19–28)	62.5 (45–94)	11 (5–16)	37.2±0.4*	3/3	3.2±0.5	41±30	319±63*	52±5*
Bacteremia (dopamine infusion)	4	39 (15–61)	66.0 (45–79.5)	7 (4–14)	37.8±0.4	3/4	3.4±0.5	72±29	423±85*	53±7*

*$P<0.05$ when compared to patients without complications.

became elevated, findings consistent with observations in other disease processes (Table 2). These alterations in thyroid hormone levels occurred while TSH remained normal. To assess the pituitary responsiveness of TSH, 12 additional thermally injured patients with a mean burn size of 62% (range 38–94%) were studied.[15] Thyrotropin-releasing hormone, the hypothalamic hormone which stimulates TSH release, was given as a 400 μg intravenous bolus and serial TSH levels were monitored. In four critically ill patients requiring dopamine infusions for cardiocirculatory support, the TSH response to TRH was attenuated, a finding consistent with the pituitary suppression known to occur with dopaminergic stimulation of the pituitary gland (Table 3). Five burn patients without complications demonstrated a normal rise of TSH after administration of TRH. In contrast, three patients with bacteremia and hypothermia demonstrated an exaggerated TSH response. These persons demonstrated significantly higher cortisol and rT_3 concentrations when compared with the patients without complications (Table 4). However, these bacteremic patients were relatively hypothermic, a stress that is known to increase pituitary release of ACTH and TSH. Because the hyperresponsive patients demonstrated lower body temperatures at the time of testing, this study suggests that the inability to maintain core temperature provided physiologic stimulation of the pituitary gland, resulting in a concomitant release of ACTH (reflected by the elevated cortisol response) and an augmented TSH response. Thus, the pituitary TSH response to TRH was appropriate and normal in the patients without complications; TSH release was suppressed with dopamine and accentuated by cold exposure. Alterations in peripheral thyroid hormone concentrations (low T_4 and T_3, high rT_3) could not be explained by alterations in TSH or changes in the pituitary control of the thyroid gland. The appearance of rT_3 in patients with complicated illnesses suggests that it is associated with the catabolic process and, like its precursor amino acids, tyrosine and phenylalanine,[16] serves as a metabolic marker of body catabolism.

These studies suggest that specific compensatory adjustments occur within the hypothalamus and pituitary gland of thermally injured patients. Specific areas in the hypothalamus play a central role in many visceral regulatory mechanisms. They act to maintain homeostasis via the integration of numerous afferent signals and subsequent modulation of spinal preganglionic autonomic neurons. Hypothalamic control of body temperature, appetite and glucose metabolism are of particular importance to the burn patient. "Setpoint" readjustments in temperature and metabolic control within the brain are expressed by an increase in both sympathetic and parasympathetic activity following stress, but evidence suggests that the sympathetic nervous system effect dominates. The sympathetic response is modulated by the concurrent actions of pituitary and adrenal hormones.

Flow Phase Metabolism — The Hypermetabolic Response

Burn hypermetabolism, the result of increased sympathetic outflow, is associated with the elaboration of high quantities of catecholamines.[12, 17] Catecholamines are elevated after thermal injury and adrenergic activity has been related to the extent of the burn and to the oxygen consumption of the patient. Carefully controlled adrenergic blockade in patients with large surface area burns has demonstrated a consistent decrease in metabolic rate with combined α- and β- or β-adrenergic blockade alone.[12] This evidence suggests that catecholamines (increased adrenergic activity) are the major calorigenic mediators responsible for the hypermetabolic response following injury. Limited increases in calorigenesis also have been noted, however, with growth hormone administration and infusion of glucagon.[18] The physiologic significance of these effects is yet to be determined, but these hormonal mediators may act to augment or potentiate the catecholamine-directed heat production in the injured patient.

The ability to respond to a stimulus requiring catecholamine calorigenesis depends on the availability of catecholamine reserves and the ability of tissues to respond to increased catechol stimuli. Reports evaluating catecholamine stores in patients who die after injury and stress demonstrate depletion of these neurotransmitter reserves in adrenal medulla, sympathetic nerve endings, sympathetic ganglia and heart.[19] Dopamine turnover in burn patients is increased markedly, possibly reflecting substrate limitation.[20] Patients with injuries of more than 40% of body surface appear to maintain maximal or near-maximal rates of catecholamine synthesis and utilization. Exposing these patients to a cool environment (21C) results in a mild cold stress and stimulates catecholamine elaboration. Patients who eventually survive respond by increasing heat production as a result of greater elaboration of catecholamines.[12] In contrast, patients who lack catecholamine reserves or tissue responsiveness to these mediators fail to generate additional heat to maintain heat balance in the 21C environment and become hypothermic. All of the nonresponding patients in the study described above subsequently died from complications of their injuries. This suggests that these patients did not have the autonomic reserve to respond to the additional challenges of body cooling, infection and hemorrhage.

In the normal individual, approximately two-thirds of resting metabolic heat production takes place in the head and trunk. Splanchnic oxygen consumption in a limited number of burn patients has been reported to increase 50-60% above normal resting levels.[22] Peripheral oxygen consumption has been determined in burned and unburned legs of patients by measuring limb blood flow and femoral arteriovenous oxygen differences. Leg oxygen consumption was unaffected by the local presence of a burn wound but remained a relatively constant proportion of total body oxygen consumption (5-6%) in the legs of both hypermetabolic burn patients and normal controls.[23] This relationship between limb and total body aerobic metabolism is in good agreement with Stolwijk's estimate of 5.9%.[24] Since splanchnic oxygen consumption increases following thermal injury and peripheral oxygen uptake remains a fixed portion of total aerobic metabolism in the patient, burn hypermetabolism appears to be a generalized or systemic response involving the entire body. Consequently, the general increase in body heat production appears to be distributed in a relatively normal fashion—two-thirds of the heat being produced in the visceral tissues and the other one-third taking place in the extremities (Table 5).

In the normal individual, limited amounts of evaporative heat loss occur continuously from normal, nonsweating skin as water diffuses through the epidermis and vaporizes, a process called "insensible perspiration." This form of passive heat loss through the total skin surface amounts to about 10 kcal/hour, or roughly 12-15% of basal metabolic heat production. Vaporization of water from the respiratory passages increases the level of

TABLE 5.—ESTIMATED CHANGES IN OXYGEN
CONSUMPTION AND BLOOD FLOW FOLLOWING
50% TOTAL BODY SURFACE BURN*

	OXYGEN CONSUMPTION (ML/MIN)	BLOOD FLOW (ML/MIN)
TOTAL BODY		
Controls	220–260	4,500–5,500
Burn	440–480	12,000–14,000
Change (%)	90	160
SPLANCHNIC		
Controls	52–55	1,200–1,300
Burns	83	1,500–1,750
Change (%)	55	33
LEG		
Controls	10–14	240–310
No leg burn	19–24	270–330
Leg burn (60%)	19–24	700–900
Change (%)	90	10–200
SKIN		
Controls	8–24	200–500
Burns	4–12	1,700
Change (%)	−50	+400

*70-kg man; 1.73 m² surface area.

obligatory wet heat loss to about 17 kcal/hour or 20–25% of basal heat production.

Thermal injury involving the middle third of the epidermis essentially eliminates the normal water diffusion barrier and greatly accelerates the rate of evaporative heat loss from the wound.[25] For example, a patient with a 50% total body surface burn will lose about 60–80 kcal/hour through vaporization of water from the wound. This increased rate of wet heat loss occurs when the patient is resting quietly in an ambient temperature of 25C, and represents about 45% of the total heat production.[26] Increasing the room temperature to 33C, a more comfortable thermal environment for this patient, will raise surface heat energy and accelerate evaporative heat loss to account for about 70–75% of metabolic heat production. In this warm environment, normal patients will also lose most of their metabolic heat load via evaporation, but, unlike the burn patient whose evaporative water loss occurs via passive diffusion through the wound, the normal individual must actively sweat; under clinical conditions, it is rare that the burn patient sweats.

When skin temperature exceeds that of the environment, heat is lost from the body surface by radiation, convection and conduction. The predominant factor affecting these forms of "dry" heat loss is the temperature difference between the skin and the environment. To minimize these particular avenues of surface heat transfer, the individual must lower skin temperatures by cutaneous vasoconstriction. The ability to reflexly vasoconstrict the wound and limit core to surface heat flow is severely impaired in the thermally injured patient.

To fully appreciate alterations in surface blood flow following thermal injury, one must first be aware of the general circulatory adjustments to this form of stress. Total body blood flow rises above normal resting levels as soon as plasma volume is restored after injury.[27] This increase in cardiac output generally is related to the extent of injury and may reach levels three to four times higher than normal in the more severely injured patient with adequate cardiovascular reserve. Much of this extra blood flow is directed to peripheral tissues, since splanchnic perfusion in burn patients increases slightly but represents a smaller portion of the cardiac output (14–17%) than it does in normal persons (23%) or patients with postoperative infection (22%).[22] The relationship between burn size and cardiac output suggests that the wound has some influence on these hemodynamic changes but does not establish that the extra blood flow is directed specifically to the wound, since increased peripheral vasodilation may occur in normal muscle and uninjured skin as well.

The rate of heat transfer from the body core to the skin,* a commonly used index of superficial blood flow, is twice normal in burn patients over a wide range of thermal environments, indicating that much of the increased peripheral circulation is directed to the skin.[26] This high rate of deep to superficial heat flux is considered responsible for the elevated skin temperatures of burn patients, which occur despite increased rates of evaporative cooling of the wound. While these data do suggest that burn patients are unable to appropriately vasoconstrict the surface, it remains unclear whether this elevated surface flow was confined to the wound or also involved normal skin.

---

*The coefficient of core-to-skin heat transfer or "thermal conductivity" of the body is determined by:

$$\text{thermal conductivity in kcal/hr} \cdot \text{m}^2 \cdot \text{C} = \frac{\text{rate of metabolic heat production (kcal/hr} \cdot \text{m}^2}{T_{core} - T_{skin}(C)}$$

In order to partition superficial blood flow into wound and normal skin components, total limb blood flow has been measured in burned and unburned legs by venous occlusion plethysmography.[28] Limb blood flow is essentially normal in the uninjured legs of burn patients but rises in a curvilinear fashion with the size of the leg surface burn. This suggests that most of the extraperipheral blood flow is directed to the superficial wound: a conclusion which was later supported by muscle blood flow studies demonstrating that skeletal muscle perfusion was the same in burned and unburned legs as it was in the limbs of normal controls.[29]

The estimated cardiac index of a "typical" patient with a 50% total body surface burn would exceed 7.0 L/minute · m². Based on actual measurements of splanchnic,[22] limb,[28] muscle[29] and renal (unpublished data) blood flow, and assuming no change in brain circulation and a rise in coronary perfusion proportional to changes in total flow, one may partition the cardiac index of this hyperdynamic patient during the flow phase of injury (Fig 1). This illustrates the general shift in the distribution of total body circulation toward the periphery, with the major portion of the extra flow going to the wound. This increase in superficial flow, however, is well within maximum levels of cutaneous flow observed in resting patients under severe heat stress.[30]

Leg blood flow in uninjured legs of burn patients is normal despite elevated rectal temperatures. A comparable degree of hyperthermia in a resting normal individual would result in a four- to fivefold increase in leg blood flow.[30] Control levels of blood flow to the uninjured limbs suggest that these febrile patients vasoconstrict the normal skin. Since cutaneous vasoconstriction is an appropriate heat conservation response during fever, why does the wound remain dilated? The selected elevation in wound blood flow cannot be explained by a complete loss of intrinsic vascular smooth muscle tone.[28] This was demonstrated by the capacity of severely burned legs with high basal flows to vasodilate further when limb surface temperature was increased. The burn wound appears to be "functionally" denervated, however, since it fails to vasodilate when its temperature is held constant and the patient's core temperature is elevated 0.4 – 0.5C by external heating.[31] This loss of neurogenic vasomotor control of the burn wound is most likely the combined result of (1) actual physical disruption of sympathetic vasomotor

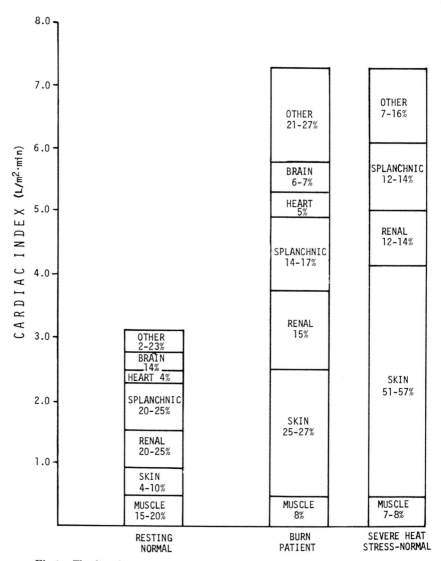

Fig 1.—The distribution of cardiac index in resting normals and burn patients.

nerves at the time of injury; and/or (2) presence of local inflammatory and metabolic factors that interfere with neuromuscular transmission in vessels that retain their innervation. Possible chemical vasodilators identified in the burn wound include such inflammatory products as histamine, kinins and various prostaglandins.[9, 32, 33] Increased rates of lactate production may contribute to local vasodilation and interfere with extrinsic vasomotor influences.[34] Actual physical denervation of wound microvasculature is most apparent after inflammation subsides and the wound is completely healed. Although local chemistry should approach that of normal skin with wound closure, reflex vasomotor control to the healed wound still is reduced markedly. The most likely explanation for this lag in reinnervation of the burn wound is the evidence that regeneration of sympathetic nerves in granulation tissue is slow and vascular reinnervation often is incomplete, particularly if split-thickness skin grafts are used.[35, 36]

The high obligatory levels of wound perfusion act to promote healing but severely compromise the heat conservation efforts of these febrile burned patients. The increased wound flow raises surface temperature — thus not only accelerating dry heat loss, but also supplying additional heat energy to the granulating wound and increasing heat loss by evaporation. This inability to effectively vasoconstrict the burn wound creates an insulative deficit for the burn patient which (1) increases in proportion to the size of the surface injury; (2) raises the requirements for metabolic heat production in a cool room; and (3) increases the susceptibility to hypothermia in cooler environments.

Accelerated rates of peripheral vascular heat loss combined with increased visceral heat production and storage greatly exaggerate normal differences between body core and central intravenous blood temperatures (Fig 2). As blood entered the lower inferior vena cava, for example, it averaged 0.8C below rectal temperature in a group of burned patients as compared to only 0.2C in a group of afebrile controls studied earlier by Eichna et al.[37] Increased heat content of the viscera of the burn patients, however, rapidly reduced the difference between venous blood and rectal temperature until the normal relationship observed in afebrile patients was established as the blood entered the pulmonary circulation. Considering the marked alterations in body heat fluxes between febrile, hyperdynamic, hypermetabolic burn patients and normal subjects, it is surprising that the basic relationship between central intravenous blood temperature and rectal temperature was essentially the same in both groups.

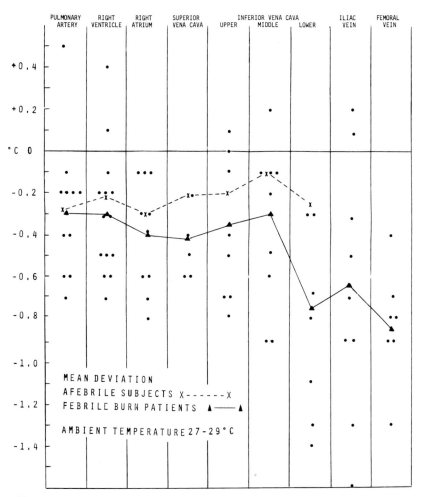

Fig 2.—Multiple intravascular temperatures were measured in 11 burn patients and the difference between each intravascular temperature and rectal temperature of each patient plotted. Individual temperature differences are shown by the closed circles and the mean of the burn group is represented by the triangles. The temperature relationships are similar to those observed in afebrile individuals (x), when relating central vascular measurements with core temperatures.[37] However, blood returning from the legs of burn patients is relatively much cooler than that observed in normals, but is rapidly warmed by the increased heat produced in the viscera.

The Hyperpyrexia of Burn Injury: A Consequence of Burn Hypermetabolism

A number of factors support the thesis that an upward shift in the body's thermostat occurs in thermally injured persons. They include:

1. The maintenance of elevated body temperatures (core, intravascular and skin) over a wide range of thermal environments.[12, 23, 26]
2. The preference for above-normal ambient temperatures to achieve thermal comfort despite elevated body temperatures.[13]
3. Vasoconstriction of the unburned skin to maintain the febrile state.[28, 31]

Can the increased rate of heat production and elevated body temperatures be explained solely by a rise in thermoregulatory setpoint? In other words, do patients produce heat to remain febrile or are they febrile because they are hypermetabolic?

Although still controversial,[38] there is a great deal of experimental evidence to suggest that increased metabolic heat production in the burn patient is not solely to satisfy a thermoregulatory reset. It was thought initially that hypermetabolism was related to the increased evaporative cooling of the burn wound through cold receptor stimulation. This conclusion was based on studies that demonstrated a reduction in the metabolic rates of small animals upon blocking their superficial heat loss.[39, 40] Other studies demonstrated that burn patients reduced their metabolic rates when ambient temperature was increased from 21 – 32C.[41] The significance of evaporative cooling as a metabolic stimulus was challenged by Zawacki et al.[42] These investigators were unable to demonstrate any consistent change in the metabolic activity of burn patients after blocking their evaporative water loss by wrapping the wound in a water-impermeable membrane. More recently, seven patients were placed in a 30C environment and heated by a series of radiant lamps.[43] Despite an average 0.8C increase in rectal temperature for the group, again there was no consistent change in resting metabolic rate (Table 6). Many of these subjects sweated from unburned skin and a few stated that they "felt hot," indicating this external

TABLE 6.–THE EFFECTS OF HEATING
SEVEN PATIENTS SLEEPING IN A
30C ENVIRONMENT

Mean burn size (% body surface)	65% (40.5–86)
Postburn day studied	11 (8–15)
Rectal temperature (C)	
Before	38.6 ± 0.3
After	39.4 ± 0.2
Metabolic rate (kcal/m²/hr)	
Before	76.5 ± 3.7
After	73.9 ± 3.6

heat load had exceeded their central reference temperature (thermostat) without reducing metabolic heat production. Additional studies in our institute[44] and elsewhere[45] have demonstrated that increasing room temperature may reduce the accelerated rate of heat production but does not return it to normal resting levels. This concept has been confirmed recently in an animal model.[46] These studies suggest that although there may be thermoregulatory influences on burn hypermetabolism, the increased rate of heat production is determined primarily by a metabolic reset; that is, burn hypermetabolism is temperature-sensitive but not temperature-dependent.

Interorgan Transfer of Substrate and Energy

To support the increased energy demands of the burn patient, stored energy or exogenous substrate is oxidized at accelerated rates. In addition, substrate is transferred from body stores to provide the energy or synthetic requirements essential to host defense mechanisms or to facilitate wound healing. This intraorgan transfer involves alterations in the metabolism of carbohydrate, protein, and fat: hyperglycemia commonly occurs after injury and infection, and the elevation of fasting blood glucose above normal is generally related to the severity of the stress. Oral or intravenous glucose intolerance tests obtained from patients following hemorrhage or burn shock (ebb phase) usually show a diabeticlike curve with prolonged disappearance of glucose from the blood stream and a persistent elevation of fasting glucose. However, the tendency toward hyperglycemia and prolonged glucose disappearance has resulted in terms such as "traumatic diabetes" and "diabetes of injury," which generally suggest an insulin-deficient state, although hormonal responses and glucose dynamics have not been assessed. Moreover, the concept of insulin deficiency is appealing, for it explains in part the increased protein catabolism that occurs in critically ill patients. In contrast, Long and associates[47] have demonstrated increased glucose flow through the extracellular fluid compartment in critically ill patients. Other hepatic catheterization studies suggest that insulin inhibition of hepatic gluconeogenesis is not dampened after injury.[48]

In studies of burn patients,[49, 50] the rate of glucose disappearance and the mass flow of glucose through the glucose space (extracellular fluid compartment) were calculated using the model of Hlad, Elrick and Witten.[51] During the initial period of burn shock, serum glucose and body glucose (serum glucose × body glucose space) were elevated and mass flow of glucose through the expanded glucose space (extracellular fluid compartment) was only slightly greater than normal (Table 7). During the period of burn shock, the elevated body glucose appeared to be a function of a decrease in the rate of glucose disappearance, which reflected a reduction in peripheral uptake during resuscitation, a finding previously reported by Allison, Hinton and Chamberlain.[52] As the integrity of the extracellular fluid compartment was re-established and normal circulation was achieved after resuscitation, patients moved from the ebb phase of injury to the flow phase. At this point (6 – 16 days postinjury), the rate of glucose disappearance returned to normal in spite of a persistent hyperglycemia which was observed in the burn patients. Glucose flow was elevated significantly in the burn patients compared to that in normal persons, suggesting that the increase in blood glucose observed in these individuals was a consequence of increased hepatic production of glucose rather than altered peripheral disappearance. Glucose flow was related to the extent of injury and returned to normal with closure of the burn wound.

To determine which peripheral tissues use this large quantity of glucose produced by the liver, substrate flux was measured across injured and uninjured extremities of severely burned patients, matched for age, weight and extent of the total body surface burn.[23] Both groups of patients demonstrated similar systemic responses to injury, as reflected by cardiac index, oxygen consumption and body temperature (Table 8). Net glucose flux

TABLE 7.—GLUCOSE DYNAMICS AFTER INJURY

	NO.	FASTING SERUM GLUCOSE (MG/100 ML)	GLUCOSE SPACE (L/KG)	BODY GLUCOSE (MG/KG)	K (100 MIN^{-1})	GLUCOSE FLOW (MG/KG/MIN)	BASAL INSULIN (μU/ML)	INSULINOGENIC INDEX
Controls	12	70 ± 2	0.152 ± 0.010	106 ± 5	4.01 ± 0.56	3.29 ± 0.32	22 ± 3	0.48 ± 0.10
Burn shock resuscitation	4	140 ± 11	0.349 ± 0.010	483 ± 22	1.21 ± 0.12	5.81 ± 0.44	20 ± 6	0.21 ± 0.07
Burns (6–16 days)	17	113 ± 5	0.117 ± 0.010	200 ± 11	5.27 ± 0.51	10.12 ± 0.95	22 ± 2	0.52 ± 0.07

TABLE 8.–COMPARISON OF PATIENTS WITH SMALL AND
LARGE LEG BURNS (MEAN AND RANGE OF SEM)

	SMALL LEG BURNS	LARGE LEG BURNS
Patient characteristics		
No. of subjects	8	7
No. of studies	9	7
Age (yr)	28	27
	(17–50)	(18–50)
Weight (kg)	73.2	70.1
	(57.5–89.4)	(58.6–83.7)
Body surface area (m²)	1.89	1.88
	(1.63–2.10)	(1.70–2.07)
% total body surface burn	40.5	42
	(12–57.5)	(12–61.5)
% total leg burn	9.5	58.0
	(0–17.5)	(37.5–82.5)
Postburn day studied	12	14
	(8–19)	(7–22)
Systemic responses		
Cardiac index (L/m²·min)	7.82 ± 0.70	7.46 ± 0.81
Oxygen consumption (ml/m²·min)	204 ± 12	241 ± 22
Rectal temperature (C)	38.5 ± 0.3	38.3 ± 0.3
Mean skin temperature (C)	36.1 ± 0.2	36.1 ± 0.2
Peripheral responses		
Mean leg skin temperature (C)	35.2 ± 0.3	35.5 ± 0.3
Leg blood flow (ml/100 ml leg·min)	4.22 ± 0.43	8.02 ± 0.51‡
Arterial oxygen concentration (ml/100 ml)	15.08 ± 0.40	15.29 ± 0.72
A-FV§ oxygen difference (ml/100 ml)	4.40 ± 0.87	3.08 ± 0.26
Leg oxygen consumption (ml/100 ml leg·min)	0.187 ± 0.037	0.240 ± 0.010
Arterial glucose concentration (mg/100 ml)	89 ± 10	81 ± 4
A-FV glucose difference (mg/100 ml)	1 ± 1	4 ± 1*
Leg glucose uptake (mg/100 ml leg·min)	0.037 ± 0.033	0.336 ± 0.077†
Arterial lactate concentration (mg/100 ml)	17.2 ± 3.4	17.6 ± 3.6
A-FV lactate difference (mg/100 ml)	−1.4 ± 1.4	−3.6 ± 0.9
Leg lactate release (mg/100 ml leg·min)	0.060 ± 0.055	0.299 ± 0.075*

*p < 0.05.
†p < 0.01.
‡p < 0.001.
§Arterial-femoral vein.

across the uninjured extremities was low, suggesting that fat, not glucose, was the primary fuel for skeletal muscle, a finding similar to that observed in normal individuals. However, increased glucose uptake occurred in extensively injured extremities. While oxygen uptake by the extensively injured extremity is sufficient to account for complete oxidation of glucose in the burned extremity, a large quantity of lactate is produced in these limbs. Calculated on a weight basis, the lactate produced accounts for a major portion of the glucose consumed by the extensively injured limb, suggesting that little or no oxygen is used for glucose metabolism in the extensively injured limbs. Presumably, the oxygen consumed in the peripheral tissues must be utilized to oxidize fat, which occurs primarily in skeletal muscle.

Glucose consumption and lactate production by the burn wound are compatible with our knowledge of the biochemistry of granulation tissue. Fibroblasts, leukocytes and new epithelial cells are glycolytic and demonstrate a major capacity for anaerobic metabolism.[53, 54] The increased hepatic glucose that is produced serves as a primary fuel for the healing wound and is not used by the uninjured limb. The lactate that is produced by glycolysis in the wound is recycled by the liver to new glucose; what glucose is oxidized is replaced by amino acids that arise from skeletal muscle and are transported to the liver to serve as additional gluconeogenic precursors (Fig 3). This rate of alanine release from the extremity generally is related to total body burn size,[55] and the nitrogen residue is processed in the liver to urea, which is excreted in the urine. Thus, the rate of gluconeogenesis is related closely to the rate of ureagenesis. The energy required to support hepatic gluconeogenesis is derived from fat. That fat is the major oxidized fuel for the body is confirmed by the respira-

Fig 3. — The flow of six- and three-carbon units after injury.

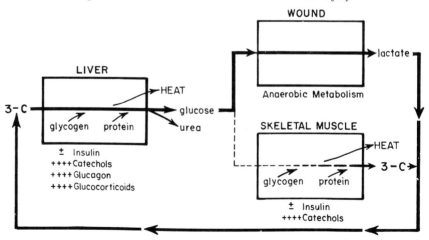

tory exchange ratio (RQ), which ranges between 0.70–0.76 in these and other injured patients.

The mechanism and mediators of the increased glucose flow and accelerated nitrogen loss following injury have been clarified only recently. Cahill and associates[56] studied proteolysis and gluconeogenesis in a starvation study and found that amino acids (primarily alanine) are released from the muscle bed, transported to the liver and converted to new glucose. This provides a constant flow of a readily available fuel to maintain function of essential glucose-dependent tissue. Because glycogen stores are limited and fatty acids cannot be converted to new glucose, this flow of alanine provides an ongoing supply of glucose at the expense of body protein. Increased gluconeogenesis and ureagenesis thus reflect the body's protein catabolic response to injury. This same sequence of metabolic events occurs with infection, prolonged exercise and cold exposure, i.e., any physiologic stress.

After thermal injury, hormones that stimulate mobilization of body fuels are increased relative to insulin, the hormone that regulates storage of body fuels. As previously noted, catecholamines are elevated.[12] This increased sympathetic nervous system activity stimulates increased elaboration of glucagon.[57] Cortisol level is elevated, especially in the early phase of injury, but may return to normal in the stable patient without complications.[58] These hormones all promote hepatic gluconeogenesis and ureagenesis when they are increased relative to insulin (Fig 4). During burn shock resuscitation, insulin levels are low, but in the uncomplicated fed patient, they return to normal levels. During the flow phase, pancreatic β cell response is normal following a standard provocative stimulus.[50]

In addition to the interacting effects these hormones exert on hepatic metabolism, they also stimulate mobilization of body fuel from peripheral tissues.[7] Insulin appears central to the regulation of skeletal muscle protein metabolism and relative changes of plasma insulin levels are associated with muscle amino acid uptake or release. Glucagon does not appear to have a peripheral effect on amino acid release, but acts centrally on the liver. Catecholamines stimulate an outpouring of lactic acid from muscle, which is followed by an efflux of three-carbon amino acid fragments which serve as carbon intermediates for hepatic conversion to new glucose. Cortisol augments transloca-

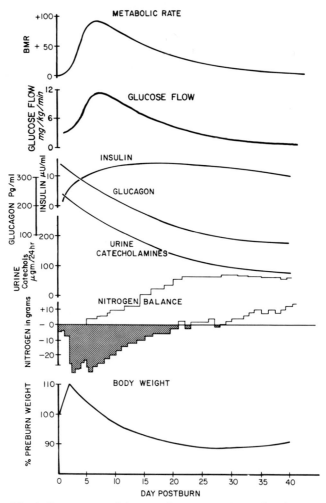

Fig 4.—Metabolic events and hormonal concentrations after burn injury until closure of the burn wound is achieved.

tion of skeletal muscle amino acids from the periphery to the viscera. Catecholamines also stimulate release of fat from peripheral stores to provide the primary oxidized body fuel.

Although all of these interacting hormonal systems are important in mediating the posttraumatic response, the primary regulatory substances that determine mobilization or storage of body fuels after thermal injury appear to be catecholamines (increased sympathetic activity) and insulin. Adrenal ablation studies in experimental animals reveal that the increase in postburn catabolism is not diminished in adrenalectomized animals receiving maintenance corticosteroids.[10] However, a diminished response occurs with administration of adrenergic blocking agents. Moreover, the importance of the hormonal interaction between insulin and catecholamines has been demonstrated in a series of studies which document the ability of insulin, insulin and carbohydrate,[59] carbohydrate through stimulation of insulin, or carbohydrate substituted isocalorically for fat[60] to spare nitrogen in markedly catabolic stressed patients. Glucose and insulin administration do not alter the increased oxygen consumption that occurs following injury, but exerts a major effect on substrate flow, diminishing nitrogen loss and preserving lean body mass in these critically ill patients.

The Metabolic Support of Burn Patients

Although the integrated care and treatment of burn patients is thoroughly detailed in the literature,[61, 62] and is beyond the scope of this review, several aspects of care are intimately related to metabolic events in burn patients and are applicable in the treatment of other critical illnesses:

1. Minimize external stimuli: minimize pain associated with treatment and treat patients in a warm environment.
2. Vigorously feed the patient: energy and protein requirements for equilibrium are markedly increased. Severe erosion of body mass occurs if a vigorous feeding program is not initiated.[63]
3. Maintain an active muscle mass: deposition and incorporation of amino acids into skeletal protein is facilitated by use of the muscle cell. Burn patients have marked limitation of their activity and require a planned exercise program to maintain an active and functional skeletal mass.
4. Prevent and treat infection: sepsis exaggerates the metabolic response to injury and may disrupt the physiologic responses.
5. Close the burn wound: the metabolic response to thermal injury occurs because of a large, open cutaneous wound. With closure, the hypercatabolic phase abates and, with adequate nutritional support, weight gain and a rebuilding of body mass are achieved.

REFERENCES

1. Cuthbertson, D., and Tilstone, W. J.: Metabolism during the postinjury period, Adv. Clin. Chem. 12:1, 1969.
2. Asch, M. J., Meserol, P. M., Mason, A. D., Jr., and Pruitt, B. A., Jr.: Regional blood flow in the burned unanesthetized dog, Surg. Forum 22:55, 1971.
3. Stoner, H. B.: Changes in the central nervous system and their role in the metabolic response to injury, in Wilkinson, A. W. and Cuthbertson, D. (eds.): *Metabolism and the Response to Injury* (Kent: Pitman Publishing Corp, 1977), p. 179.
4. Hume, D. M., and Egdahl, R. H.: The importance of the brain in the endocrine response to injury, Ann. Surg. 150:697, 1959.
5. Newsome, H. H., and Rose, J. C.: The response of human adrenocorticotrophic hormone and growth hormone to surgical stress, J. Clin. Endocrol. Metab. 33:481, 1971.
6. Hume, D. M.: The endocrine and metabolic response to injury, in Schwartz, S. E. (ed.): *Principles of Surgery* (New York: McGraw-Hill, 1969), p. 2.
7. Wilmore, D. W.: Hormonal responses and their effect on metabolism, Surg. Clin. North Am. 56:999, 1976.
8. Wilmore, D. W.: Studies of the Effect of Variations of Temperature and Humidity on Energy Demands of the Burned Soldier in a Controlled Metabolic Room. US Army Institute of Surgical Research Annual Progress Report, 1 July 1975 – 30 June 1976.
9. Arturson, G.: Prostaglandins in human burn wound secretion, Burns 3: 112, 1977.
10. Herndon, D., Wilmore, D. W., Mason, A. D., Jr., and Pruitt, B. A., Jr.: Humoral mediators of non-temperature dependent hypermetabolism in 50% burned adult rats, Surg. Forum 28:37, 1977.
11. Taylor, J. W., Hander, E. W., Skreen, R., and Wilmore, D. W.: Effect of CNS narcosis on the sympathetic response to stress, J. Surg. Res. 20:313, 1976.
12. Wilmore, D. W., Long, J. M., Mason, A. D., Jr., et al: Catecholamines: mediator of the hypermetabolic response to thermal injury, Ann. Surg. 180: 653, 1974.
13. Wilmore, D. W., Orcutt, T. W., Mason, A. D., Jr., and Pruitt, B. A., Jr.: Alterations in hypothalamic function following thermal injury, J. Trauma 15:697, 1975.
14. Becker, R., Johnson, D. W., Woeber, K. A., and Wilmore, D. W.: Depressed serum triiodothyronine (T_3) levels following thermal injury, Fed. Proc. 35: 316, 1976.
15. Becker, R. A., Wilmore, D. W., Johnson, D. W., Wurtofsky, L., Burman, K. D., and Woeber, K. A.: Alterations in thyroid economy and pituitary responsiveness following thermal injury (in press).
16. Herndon, D., Wilmore, D. W., Mason, A. D., Jr., and Pruitt, B. A., Jr.: Abnormalities of phenylalanine and tyrosine kinetics: Significance in septic and nonseptic burned patients, Arch. Surg. 113:133, 1978.
17. Harrison, T. S., Seaton, J. F., and Feller, L.: Relationship of increased oxy-

gen consumption to catecholamine excretion in thermal burns, Ann. Surg. 165:169, 1967.

18. Aulick, L. H., Wilmore, D. W., and Mason, A. D., Jr.: Mechanism of glucagon calorigenesis, Fed. Proc. 35:401, 1976.

19. Goodall, McC., and Moncrief, J. A.: Sympathetic nerve depletion in severe thermal injury, Ann. Surg. 162:893, 1965.

20. Goodall, McC., and Alton, H.: Dopamine (3-hydroxytyramine) replacement and metabolism in sympathetic nerve and adrenal medullary depletions after prolonged thermal injury, J. Clin. Invest. 48:1761, 1969.

21. Cannon, W. B.: The Wisdom of the Body (New York, W. W. Norton Co., 1967).

22. Gump, F. E., Price, J. B., Jr., and Kinney, J. M.: Blood flow and oxygen consumption in patients with severe burns, Surg. Gynecol. Obstet. 130:23, 1970.

23. Wilmore, D. W., Aulick, L. H., Mason, A. D., Jr., and Pruitt, B. A., Jr.: Influence of the burn wound on local and systemic responses to injury, Ann. Surg. 186:444, 1977.

24. Stolwijk, J. A. J.: Mathematical model of thermoregulation, in Hardy, J. D., and Gagge, A. P. (eds.): Physiological and Behavioral Temperature Regulation (Springfield: Charles C Thomas Co., 1970), pp. 703–721.

25. Harrison, H., Moncrief, J. A., Duckett, J. W., and Mason, A. D., Jr.: The relationship between energy metabolism and water loss from vaporization in severely burned patients, Surgery 56:203, 1964.

26. Wilmore, D. W., Mason, A. D., Jr., Johnson, D. W., and Pruitt, B. A., Jr.: Effect of ambient temperature on heat production and heat loss in burn patients, J. Appl. Physiol. 38:593, 1975.

27. Unger, A., and Haynes, B. W., Jr.: Hemodynamic studies in severely burned patients, Surg. Forum 10:356, 1959.

28. Aulick, L. H., Wilmore, D. W., Mason, A. D., Jr., and Pruitt, B. A., Jr.: Influence of the burn wound on peripheral circulation in thermally injured patients, Am. J. Physiol. 233(4):H520, 1977.

29. Aulick, L. H., Wilmore, D. W., and Mason, A. D., Jr.: Muscle blood flow in burned patients, Physiologist 20(4):3, 1977.

30. Wyss, C. R., Brengelmann, G. L., Johnson, J. M., Rowell, L. B., and Niederberger, M.: Control of skin blood flow, sweating and heart rate: role of skin vs. core temperature, J. Appl. Physiol. 36:726, 1974.

31. Aulick, L. H., Wilmore, D. W., Mason, A. D., Jr., and Pruitt, B. A., Jr.: Peripheral blood flow in thermally injured patients, Fed. Proc. 36:417, 1977.

32. Anggard, E., and Johnson, D. -E.: Efflux of prostaglandin in lymph from scalded tissue, Acta Physiol. Scand. 81:440, 1971.

33. Edery, H., and Lewis, G. P.: Kinin-forming activity and histamine in lymph after tissue injury, J. Physiol. (Lond) 169:568, 1963.

34. Remensnyder, J. P., and Majno, G.: Oxygen gradients in healing wounds, Am. J. Pathol. 52:301, 1968.

35. Clark, E. R., Clark, E. L., and Williams, R. G.: Microscopic observations in the living rabbit of the new growth of nerves and establishment of nerve-controlled contractions of newly formed arterioles, Am. J. Anat. 55:47, 1934.

36. Fitzgerald, M. J. T., Martin, F., and Paletta, F. X.: Innervation of skin grafts, Surg. Gynecol. Obstet. 124:808, 1967.
37. Eichna, L. W., Berger, A. R., Rader, B., and Becker, W. H.: Comparison of intracardiac and intravascular temperatures with rectal temperatures in man, J. Clin. Invest. 30:353, 1951.
38. Arturson, M. G. S.: Transport and demand of oxygen in severe burns, J. Trauma 17:179, 1977.
39. Caldwell, F. T., Jr.: Metabolic response to thermal trauma: II. Nutritional studies with rats at two environmental temperatures, Ann. Surg. 155:119, 1962.
40. Lieberman, Z. H., and Lansche, J. M.: Effects of thermal injury on metabolic rate and insensible water loss in the rat, Surg. Forum 7:83, 1956.
41. Barr, P., -O., Birke, G., Liljedahl, S. -O, and Plantin, L. -O.: Oxygen consumption and water loss during treatment of burns with warm dry air, Lancet 1:164, 1968.
42. Zawacki, B. E., Spitzer, K. W., Mason, A. D., Jr., and Jones, L. A.: Does increased evaporative water loss cause hypermetabolism in burn patients? Ann. Surg. 171:236, 1970.
43. Wilmore, D. W., Aulick, L. H., Mason, A. D., Jr., and Pruitt, B. A., Jr.: Will Increasing Body Temperature Reduce Burn Hypermetabolism? A Negative Answer. Paper presented at the Ninth Annual Meeting of the American Burn Association, Anaheim, California, April, 1977.
44. Aulick, L. H., and Wilmore, D. W.: Unpublished data.
45. Davies, J. W. L., Lamke, L. -O., and Liljedahl, S. -O: Treatment of severe burns, Acta Chir. Scand. (suppl. 468), 1977.
46. Herndon, D. N., Wilmore, D. W., and Mason, A. D., Jr.: Development and analysis of a small animal model simulating the human postburn hypermetabolic response (in press).
47. Long, C. L., Spencer, J. L., Kinney, J. M., and Geiger, J. W.: Carbohydrate metabolism in man: effect of elective operations and major injury, J. Appl. Physiol. 31:110, 1971.
48. Gump, F. E., Long, C., Killian, P., and Kinney, J. M.: Studies of glucose intolerance in septic injured patients, J. Trauma 14:378, 1974.
49. Wilmore, D. W., Mason, A. D., Jr., and Pruitt, B. A., Jr.: Alterations in glucose kinetics following thermal injury, Surg. Forum 26:81, 1975.
50. Wilmore, D. W.: Carbohydrate metabolism in trauma, in Alberti, K. G. M. M. (ed.): Clinics in Endocrinology and Metabolism, Vol. V (London: W. B. Saunders Publishing Co., 1976), p. 731.
51. Hlad, C. J., Jr., Elrick, H., and Witten, T. A.: Studies on the kinetics of glucose utilization, J. Clin. Invest. 35:1139, 1956.
52. Allison, S. P., Hinton, P., and Chamberlain, M. J.: Intravenous glucose-tolerance, insulin, and free-fatty acid levels in burn patients, Lancet 2: 1113, 1968.
53. Im, M. J. C., and Hoopes, J. E.: Enzyme activities in the repairing epithelium during wound healing, J. Surg. Res. 10:173, 1970.
54. Im, M. J. C., and Hoopes, J. E.: Energy metabolism in healing skin wounds, J. Surg. Res. 10:459, 1970.
55. Aulick, L. H., and Wilmore, D. W.: Leg amino acid turnover in burn patients, Fed. Proc. 37:536, 1978.

56. Cahill, G. F., Jr., Herrera, M. G., Morgan, A. P., Soeldner, J. S., Steinke, J., Levy, P. L., Reichard, G. A., and Kipnis, D. M.: Hormone-fuel interrelationships during fasting, J. Clin. Invest. 45:1751, 1966.

57. Wilmore, D. W., Lindsey, C. A., Moylan, J. A., et al: Hyperglucagonemia after burns, Lancet 1:73, 1974.

58. Batstone, G. F., Alberti, K. G. M. M. et al.: Metabolic studies in subjects following thermal injury: intermediate metabolites, hormones, and tissue oxygenation, Burns 2:207, 1976.

59. Hinton, P., Allison, S. P., Littlejohn, S., and Lloyd, J.: Insulin and glucose to reduce catabolic response to injury in burn patients, Lancet 1:767, 1971.

60. Long, J. M., III, Wilmore, D. W., Mason, A. D., Jr., and Pruitt, B. A., Jr: The effect of carbohydrate and fat intake on nitrogen excretion during total intravenous feedings, Ann. Surg. 185:417, 1977.

61. Artz, C. P., and Moncrief, J. A.: *The Treatment of Burns* (2d ed.; Philadelphia: W. B. Saunders Publishing Co., 1969).

62. Wilmore, D. W.: *The Metabolic Care of the Critically Ill* (New York: Plenum Publishing Co., 1977).

63. Wilmore, D. W.: Nutrition and metabolism following thermal injury, in Moncrief, J. A. (ed.): *Clinics in Plastic Surgery* (Philadelphia: W. B. Saunders Publishing Co., 1974), p. 603.

Renovascular Hypertension

CORNELIUS OLCOTT IV, M.D. AND EDWIN J. WYLIE, M.D.

Department of Surgery, University of California Medical Center, San Francisco, California

Interest in the relationship between the kidney and hypertension dates back to 1898, when Tigerstedt and Berman discovered that saline extracts of kidney tissue contained a pressor substance which they named renin.[1] This finding was confirmed subsequently by other investigators. In 1940, Page and Helmer demonstrated that renin was an enzyme that acted on a plasma substrate to produce an active pressor substance called angiotensin.[2]

The correlation between hypertension and renal ischemia first was demonstrated by Goldblatt, Lynch and Hanzal[3] in 1934 when they discovered that hypertension could be produced by impaired renal circulation.[3] In 1937 Butler reported curing a 7-year-old boy of hypertension by nephrectomy.[4] This report led to an initial wave of enthusiasm for nephrectomy in the treatment of hypertension.[5-10] A subsequent review by Smith in 1956 reported an 81% failure rate in 242 patients who underwent nephrectomy for treatment of hypertension thought to be due to unilateral renal disease.[11] Most of the patients in this report had unilateral pyelonephritis rather than extraparenchymal vascular disease. Nevertheless, this review led to a more critical look at the relationship between the kidney and hypertension.

The past two decades have seen the emergence of renovascular hypertension as a recognized remedial clinical entity.[12-14] The development of selective angiography, radioisotope scanning and renal vein assays has provided a more sophisticated

0065-3411/78...0012-0227$03.75

diagnostic approach to the patient with possible renovascular hypertension. Surgical techniques have advanced to the point that revascularization can be performed with an acceptably low morbidity and mortality and with a high degree of success.

There is no consensus as to the incidence of hypertension in the United States, although all physicians agree that it is an important entity not only in its own right but also as a risk factor for atherosclerosis. Edwards estimates that approximately 5 million people in the United States have hypertension.[15] Wilber and Barrow estimate that 10–15% of the adult population has elevated blood pressure and believe it to be the most common chronic condition seen in office practice.[16] What percentage of this patient population has hypertension on the basis of renovascular disease? In a report of a one-year experience at the University of Michigan, Correa and colleagues noted renal artery lesions in 6% of hypertensive patients studied angiographically.[17] Recently it has been stated that this figure may now approach 15%.[18] Other authors have reported an incidence as high as 28–37%.[19, 20] Obviously patient selection and referral practices will bias any such estimate, but certainly the number of hypertensive patients with renovascular disease is substantial.

Patient Assessment and Selection

Proper management of the patient with renovascular hypertension requires proper patient selection so that satisfactory results of surgical treatment may be anticipated. Investigative efforts have proceeded along two pathways. The first has been directed toward the development of screening tests to identify, in the pool of hypertensive patients, those whose hypertension probably is caused by renovascular disease. The second investigative effort has been to develop a method for predicting that an arteriographically demonstrated renal artery lesion is, in fact, the cause of hypertension. Although the results from these efforts have been promising, there has been a disappointingly large percentage of false-negatives. In our own clinic, arteriography remains the most accurate method for identifying a renovascular source of hypertension. In addition, the correlation of a demonstrated lesion and relief of hypertension by removal of the lesion remains higher than the index of predictability of success from various studies that have been developed. The bedside diagnosis of renovascular hypertension is virtually impossible, as there is no set clinical picture to aid in the diagnosis. Probably most important is a high index of suspicion on the part of the physician. Factors known to be associated with an increased incidence of renovascular disease are: (1) an upper abdominal or flank bruit; (2) abrupt onset or acceleration of hypertension; (3) hypertension occurring in a middle-aged female or a child less than 15 years of age; (4) hypertension occurring in a patient, particularly male, with associated atherosclerosis; and (5) history or suspicion of renal trauma or embolism.

A number of diagnostic tests have been used to select patients with renovascular hypertension and to attempt to predict who from that group will benefit from surgical therapy. As noted, these tests can be divided into two groups: screening tests for renovascular pathology and tests that attempt to differentiate significant from insignificant renal artery lesions. The former group includes intravenous pyelography, radioisotope renograms and renal arteriography. The latter includes split function studies, renin assays and angiotensin II suppression tests. It is in this group where the frequency of false-negative findings is high. Although this diagnostic work-up is extremely complex, a recent review has attempted to organize it into a workable algorithm.[21]

The intravenous pyelogram (IVP) remains a frequently used screening test. The Cooperative Study of Renovascular Hypertension reviewed the urograms of 1,128 patients, noting certain radiographic features that correlated well with the ultimate diagnosis of renovascular disease.[22] These included: (1) disparity in the caliceal appearance times; (2) disparity in kidney length (right kidney 2 cm shorter than the left or left kidney 1.5 cm shorter than the right); (3) contrast concentration within the collecting system of the ischemic kidney on late films; (4) ureteral notching from collateral vessels; and (5) parenchymal atrophy. However, there is a significantly high false negative return. Extensive collateral formation and the presence of bilateral disease greatly influence accuracy and account for most of the false negative results. Stanley and Fry reviewed urograms of patients with proven renovascular hypertension judged on the basis of postoperative results and noted abnormal studies in only 24% of pediatric patients, 47% of adults with fibromuscular dysplasia and 73% of patients with atherosclerosis.[23]

Hippuran, labeled with ^{131}I, also has been used as a screening test for renovascular hypertension.[12, 13] This is a relatively simple noninvasive test that provides a good index of renal vascularity and function. Although it is effective in detecting disparity in function between two kidneys, it cannot differentiate renal artery stenosis from renal parenchymal disease; and, like the IVP, it is subject to error in cases of extensive collateral supply or bilateral disease. Duston reviewed the results of this test and found a 14% false negative rate in patients with renal artery stenosis.[24] We, too, have used radioisotope scanning but have found it useful primarily in the immediate postoperative period to document patency of the reconstructed arteries. Newer techniques presently are being developed that will allow assessment of relative renal blood flow. These promise to be useful in comparing relative renal blood flow when bilateral lesions are present.

Arteriography remains the most reliable technique for selecting from the pool of hypertensive patients those with renal artery pathology. Originally, arteriograms were performed by the translumbar technique developed by Dos Santos.[25] Most centers now use the Seldinger technique,[26] a method that allows proper visualization of the orifices of the renal arteries and also allows selective renal artery visualization with definition of the branch vessels as well. One point to be stressed is the necessity of obtaining views in multiple projections.[27] The renal arteries frequently arise from the aorta slightly posterior to the midline. Standard anterior-posterior views without oblique views may fail to visualize properly the artery orifice, thereby missing a diagnosis of renal artery stenosis particularly when the lesion is atherosclerotic. Also, branch vessel lesions may require selective visualization in multiple projections to display properly the pathologic condition. A new technique for the angiographic evaluation of renal artery lesions is pharmacoangiography.[28] Recent evidence suggests that this may be useful in evaluating the hemodynamic significance of a renal artery lesion.

We use the Seldinger technique for arteriography. Patients are prepared with overnight hydration and the total dye dose is minimized, particularly in patients with abnormal renal function, to decrease the chance of transient renal failure as a reaction to the contrast medium. A flush aortogram should be performed first to display all renal arteries. Selective renal artery arteriograms then may be performed to display each artery more optimally. Special attention should be paid to visualizing collateral vessels.

Patients with atherosclerosis and significant aortoiliac disease should have simultaneous aortofemoral arteriography, as it may be appropriate to perform an aortofemoral reconstruction concomitant with the renal vascular procedure. Likewise, patients with fibromuscular dysplasia, particularly those with a carotid bruit, should have carotid arteriograms performed to evaluate the presence or extent of fibromuscular disease in the internal carotid arteries or intracranial berry aneurysms (both being frequent associated findings).

Although arteriography is accurate in detecting lesions of renal arteries, it does not always determine the significance of the lesion. One of the first tests to be used to aid in determining significance was the split-function test, which was described by Howard and Connor[29] and subsequently modified by Stamey et al.[30] These tests were based on the finding that the ischemic kidney will demonstrate decreased urine volume, decreased sodium concentration, increased creatinine concentration and increased concentration of para-aminohippuric acid. Bilateral ureteral catheterization is required, however, which is not well tolerated by some patients and has a predictable, albeit small, morbidity. Also, it has a definite false negative rate, estimated by Russell to be about 18%.[12] Dean and Foster[31] reported a 32% false negative rate using the classic Howard criteria and a 58% false negative rate with the classic Stamey criteria.[31] Because of the morbidity and the high false negative return, we no longer use this test.

At the present time the most frequent use of the split-function test is in conjunction with renal vein renin assays. Dean and Foster have used this combination and found that renal vein renin assays are more accurate than either the Howard or Stamey tests.[31] However, if only one of the tests had been used to determine operability, 8–10% of surgically cured patients would not have been selected for surgical therapy. Therefore, these authors recommend using split-function tests in conjunction with renal vein renin assays; it is their policy to recommend surgical treatment if either of these is positive.

The renal vein renin assay currently is the most widely used test to determine the hemodynamic significance of a renal artery lesion.[32-37] Renin, a proteolytic enzyme, is synthesized and secreted mainly by the kidney. Reninlike enzymes have been extracted from extrarenal sources; however, there is no evidence that any of these have a role in blood pressure regulation.[32] Renin cleaves its substrate, an α_2-globulin synthesized by the liver, to produce a decapeptide, angiotensin I. This is converted, primarily at the time of passage through the lung, to the octapeptide angiotensin II, which is a potent vasoconstrictor and stimulator of aldosterone production. Although the precise cellular mechanisms controlling renin release remain speculative, both changes in renal perfusion pressure and either concentration or amount of sodium in the distal tubule clearly have a regulatory effect.[32] Hence, renin hypersecretion is believed to furnish objective evidence of a significant renal artery lesion. Renin levels may be determined from a peripheral sample or from selective renal vein samples. The latter is the most frequently used, the accepted criteria for a positive result being a ratio of 1.5 or greater of renin activity from the involved kidney to the uninvolved kidney. This test also has been associated with a significant number of false negative results. Analysis by Dean and Foster revealed that using the 1.5 ratio, only 79% of patients cured by surgery were detected.[31] These investigators noted that if the renin vein ratio were liberalized to 1.3, then 90% of cured patients would be detected. This significant incidence of false negative results has been confirmed by other investigators as well.

The existence of inconsistencies in the current literature regarding the usefulness of renin assays has several explanations. First, there is great variability in the performance of the test. Some investigators measure basal renin, while others determine levels after stimulation of the renin-angiotensin system by reducing sodium intake, administering a natriuretic drug and/or withdrawing specimens from patients in the upright position. Second, patients frequently are taking medications known to suppress renin, e.g., reserpine, propranolol, and aldomet. Third, collateral development may alter renin secretion, as experimentally determined by Ernst, Daugherty and Kotchen.[35] Fourth, superselective sampling may be necessary to prevent dilutional errors where renal ischemia is segmental. Schambelan and colleagues have demonstrated that selective renal vein sampling can identify specifically a localized source of renin that may be overlooked by main renal vein sampling.[36]

Stanley, Gewertz and Fry have recommended using renal-systemic renin indices as a method of determining curability in patients with renovascular hypertension.[37] Renal-systemic renin indices (RSRI) are defined as individual renin activity minus systemic renin activity, divided by systemic renin activity. These investigators found that these indices reflected hypersecretion by the involved kidney in both cured and improved patients and were more reliable than the use of standard renal vein renin ratios only.

One of the principal problems with these tests is evaluation in the presence of bilateral renal artery involvement. Stanley believes that a beneficial response is most likely when renin hypersecretion, as determined by the RSRI, is associated with suppression of renin release from the contralateral kidney.[18, 23, 37] When cured and improved patients were compared, the RSRI did not differ significantly between the two groups, nor was there difference in the degree of renin secretion. However, nearly complete suppression of renin production by the contralateral kidney occurred in the cured group, whereas improved but not cured patients demonstrated some renin secretion from the contralateral kidney. The presence of a significant lesion in the artery of the contralateral kidney was associated with renin production and the second kidney frequently became a renin hypersecreter after reconstruction of the original renal artery.

Recently, further insight into the detection of renin-mediated hypertension has been gained through the use of saralasin, a competitive inhibitor of angiotensin II. Baer and colleagues found that 11 of 12 patients with a depressor response to angiotensin II blockade had renovascular hypertension.[39] Only 1 of 8 patients without a depressor response had evidence of renovascular disease. Thus it would appear that angiotensin blockade can be used for detecting renin-dependent forms of hypertension, unfortunately including those few cases of hyper-reninemic essential hypertension.

Marks, Maxwell and Kaufman have modified the saralasin

test so that testing is carried out after mild sodium depletion.[40] Ninety-four percent of their patients with renovascular hypertension responded to the saralasin test. Of 5 patients with documented renovascular disease who did not have lateralizing renin assays, 4 had a positive saralasin test. These authors also conclude that saralasin testing, particularly in the presence of modest sodium depletion, is an accurate means of detecting renin-mediated hypertension.

After a review of the above-described test modalities, one still wonders how to evaluate most efficiently the patient with suspected renovascular hypertension. At the present time, renal arteriography continues to be our principal diagnostic tool. All of the other diagnostic modalities, including renin assays, have too high a false negative rate for the decision regarding surgery to be based on their results alone. We do not hesitate to proceed directly to arteriography in any patient in whom routine screening has ruled out other common forms of hypertension. This is particularly true in those patients who are likely to have a vascular etiology for their hypertension, e.g., middle-aged women, children and patients with known atherosclerosis. We have been impressed that a significant arterial lesion demonstrated angiographically, especially in the presence of collateral vessels, will be associated with a good result in most patients following a technically adequate surgical procedure. We consider patients to be good candidates for operation if they (1) are less than 60 years old; (2) have moderate-to-severe hypertension not readily controlled by medical regimen; (3) have hypertension of short duration, preferably less than five years; and (4) have few, if any, other complications of atherosclerosis.

Pathology of Renovascular Hypertension

Any vascular lesion that impairs renal blood flow and initiates the renin-angiotensin-aldosterone system may produce renovascular hypertension. The most common pathologic lesions seen in most centers are atherosclerosis and fibromuscular dysplasia. At the University of California during the past ten years these two lesions have been seen with about equal frequency. Other pathologic entities we have found to be associated with renovascular hypertension include trauma, arteritis, aneurysms, congenital hypoplasia, neurofibromatosis, extrinsic com-

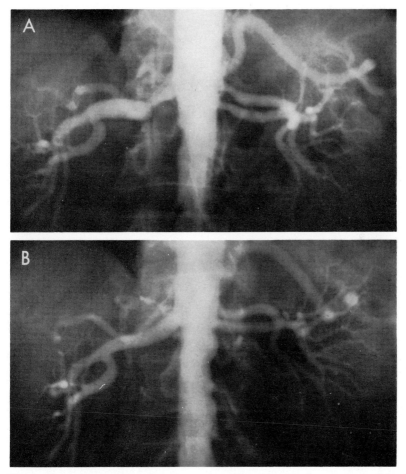

Fig 1.—Preoperative (A) and postoperative (B) aortograms in a patient with advanced stenosis in a single right renal artery and lesser lesions in paired left renal arteries. A normal lumen was restored in all three arteries by transaortic endarterectomy. The patient has remained normotensive for nine years.

pression, emboli, aortic dissections, arteriovenous malformations and homotransplant renal artery stenosis.

Atherosclerotic renal artery lesions generally are confined to the proximal portion of the artery (Fig 1). The endpoint between diseased intima and the distal normal intima is abrupt. The aortic intima at the level of the renal arteries and distal to them is grossly thickened.

The common anatomic pattern is one renal artery to each kidney. Stenosis often appears arteriographically to involve only one of the two renal arteries. Preoperative studies may indicate that the kidney on this side is the one responsible for hypertension. In other patients, a small but hemodynamically insignificant lesion may be present in the opposite renal artery. It is important to recognize that in the natural history of atherosclerosis in this area, the disease eventually becomes bilateral, and that unilateral operations for the treatment of hypertension in the two circumstances cited are subject to late failure once the contralateral lesions advance to the point of obstructing blood flow.

In many patients, one or more accessory renal arteries to one or both kidneys are present. These may vary in size from 1 to 4 mm. If there is stenosis in the main renal arteries, these usually will have some degree of stenosis at their origins as well. Since there are few, if any, collateral arterial connections within the renal parenchyma, failure to deal with these lesions may result in persistence of hypertension even after the lesions in the larger arteries are removed or bypassed.

Aortography may demonstrate stenosis of one main renal artery and total occlusion of the opposite main renal artery. When occlusion is the result of the progression of an atherosclerotic lesion, the development of capsular or periureteral collaterals may be adequate to sustain renal viability and even limited function. Although the kidney will be small, the urographic demonstration of opacification in the collecting system or the renal parenchyma identifies a kidney that may respond to a revascularization operation. Preservation of a smaller kidney distal to an occluded renal artery does not necessarily lessen the antihypertensive effect of the operation once the primary arterial lesion is removed.

One variation in the type of atherosclerosis in the aorta in the area of the renal arteries may have a profound effect on the choice of or indication for operation in patients with renovascular hypertension. This is characterized by necrotic degeneration of the perirenal aortic intima. Its luminal surface is fragmented, mushy and virtually can be removed with a spoon. These changes may be suspected in patients with frank aneurysms in the infrarenal aorta or preaneurysmal degeneration, as shown by aortography or operative inspection of the exterior of the aorta, or both. The application of occluding clamps on this type of aorta adjacent to the renal orifices may squeeze masses of necrotic intimal debris into the renal arteries and produce distal embolization unless appropriate precautions are taken. The added risk of operation in this type of patient must be balanced carefully against the need for surgical rather than merely medical management of hypertension.

Fibromuscular dysplasia is the second most common cause of renovascular hypertension, characteristically occurring in middle-aged women. This process involves the middle and distal thirds of the main renal artery and may extend into the branch vessels. The angiographic appearance is a string of beads (Fig 2). Extrarenal fibromuscular disease has been reported in 11% of patients with renal artery involvement.[41] Harrison and McCormack have classified these lesions based on the arterial layer involved:[42]

1. Intimal lesions: Intimal fibroplasia characterized by a circumferential or eccentric accumulation of loose, moderately cellular fibrous tissue with any lipid or inflammatory component. Secondary intimal fibroplasia may be found in a number of renal parenchymal diseases.

Fig 2.—Aortogram showing typical lesions of fibromuscular dysplasia with apparently more advanced lesions in the right renal artery. At operation both renal arteries were equally diseased, indicating the need for selective arteriography and multiple projections to demonstrate accurately the degree of stenosis created by the diaphragm-like irregularities characteristic of this disease.

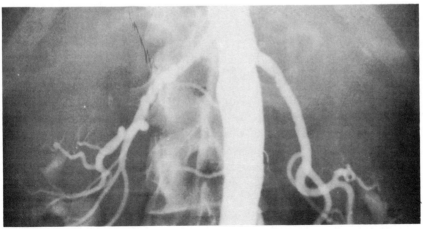

2. Medial dysplasia: This includes several subgroups.
   a. Medial fibroplasia with mural aneurysm occurs most frequently, comprising 60–70% of all stenoses. This is the lesion responsible for the string-of-beads lesion on arteriograms and comprises areas of stenosis alternating with areas of aneurysmal change.
   b. Medial hyperplasia is less common (5–15%) and is characterized by stenosis produced by hyperplasia of the arterial smooth muscle without aneurysm formation.
   c. Perimedial fibroplasia (15–25%) is characterized by a dense fibroplasia of the outer half of the media.
   d. Medial dissection (5–10%) is characterized by formation of a new channel in the outer third of the media. The media has zones of fibroplasia.
3. Adventitial lesions: Periarterial fibroplasia is the least common of all these lesions. Fibroplasia encompasses the adventitia and extends into the surrounding periarterial fibrofatty tissues.

Both atherosclerosis and fibromuscular dysplasia have been reported to be progressive lesions,[43] a finding we, too, have noted. Like atherosclerosis, the etiology of fibromuscular lesions remains an enigma. However, recent work from the University of Michigan suggests that impaired vasa vasoral blood flow may play a significant role in its etiology.[44]

Surgical Management and Results

For purposes of this review, surgical management and results have been broken down into four groups: pediatric patients, adults with fibromuscular dysplasia, adults with atherosclerosis and patients requiring ex vivo reconstructions. Results traditionally are reported as "cured," "improved" or "failures." In our own series we have defined cured patients as normotensive – off all antihypertensive medications – and improved patients as normotensive – on drug therapy or having diastolic pressures between 90–100 mm Hg, which are 15% lower than preoperative levels.

In preparing this report the authors have considered a major objective to be a comparison of the various surgical methods currently used in the treatment of renovascular hypertension, with respect to both the degree and duration of blood pressure response and the durability of the operative method. For a variety of reasons there are a number of obstacles to accomplishing this objective. These include:

1. Variations in the definition of "cured" and "improved";
2. Variations in time interval between operation and the assessment and reporting of the result;
3. Reporting on the basis of the result of a secondary operation (i.e., nephrectomy) when the primary operation has failed;
4. Inconstancy of obtaining serial or even single postoperative arteriograms in all patients;
5. Failure to use the life-table assessment technique when late results are reported in terms of percentages; and
6. Variations in the criteria used as indications for operation.

These factors should be weighed in the evaluation of data appearing in subsequent tables. Although these data represent general trends, the reader is urged to consult the referenced original reports.

Renovascular hypertension in the pediatric age group is being recognized with increasing frequency. Renal artery stenosis is second only to coarctation of the aorta as a cause of surgically remediable hypertension in children. A number of centers recently have reported on their experience with renovascular hypertension in children.[23, 45-47] A few points are noteworthy. First, screening by IVP has been uniformly disappointing. Only 24% of the patients of Stanley and Fry[23] and 42% of those of Lawson et al.[45] had an abnormal IVP. All authors believe the arteriogram to be the primary diagnostic tool and recommend an aggressive surgical approach in all hypertensive children with demonstrated renal artery lesions. Renal vein renin assays have been positive in a large proportion of cases. Eleven of the pediatric hypertensive patients of Fry et al.[47] had renal vein renin determinations and these were abnormal on the involved side in

TABLE 1. – PEDIATRIC RENOVASCULAR HYPERTENSION –
OPERATIVE RESULTS

STUDY	NO. PATIENTS	CURED (%)	IMPROVED (%)	FAILURE (%)
Vanderbilt[52]	25	68	24	8
University of Michigan[23]	27	89	7	4
University of California[46]	14	93	0	7

each. The most common lesion in this group is fibromuscular dysplasia. Generally good results can be expected (Table 1).

Surgical repair of these lesions must take into account the small size of the vessels, the necessity for growth in the reconstructed segments and the need for durable repair. Most of the lesions in children are treated by bypass grafting, using either autogenous artery or saphenous vein. We prefer the former. A review of the University of California experience by Stoney, Cooke and String has shown the hypogastric artery to be a durable graft.[46] There was minimal dilatation in one graft used in their pediatric group. All the remaining grafts appeared to grow with the child and have remained patent. This represents the only abnormal change in over 73 hypogastric autografts used in various locations with follow-up periods extending up to 17 years. Fry and coworkers have used the saphenous vein with good results, though they did report graft dilatation in 2 of 27 patients, 130% and 150% compared to their original size.[47] Neither the Michigan nor the Vanderbilt group has reported vein stenosis in its pediatric series.

Results of surgical treatment are excellent in this group (see Table 1). Nephrectomy previously had been used in cases not believed to be amenable to surgical repair. However, with the advent of ex vivo techniques these lesions may now be managed almost uniformly without sacrifice of renal tissue.

Surgical management of atherosclerotic lesions of the renal arteries has as its goal the reversal of hypertension and the prevention of renal artery thrombosis. Since most patients with atherosclerotic renovascular hypertension are asymptomatic, the ultimate objective of operation in this group is to improve longevity. Thus the most ideal candidates are those younger than 60 years old without life-threatening atherosclerosis at other sites, or patients of any age with progressive uremia and bilateral advanced renal artery lesions.

The two techniques most commonly used in the treatment of atherosclerotic lesions are endarterectomy and bypass grafting. We prefer the former technique for the following reasons. More than 60% of atherosclerotic patients will have bilateral involvement. Twenty percent will have more than a single artery to each kidney. When multiple lesions are present, it often is difficult to determine with accuracy which of the lesions is responsible for the hypertension. Also, since atherosclerosis is a progressive disease a minimally stenotic lesion may progress and eventually may restrict blood flow. Transaortic endarterectomy has proven to be an excellent method to deal with each of these problems.

Bypass grafts customarily are anastomosed to the side of the infrarenal aorta or to an aortic prosthesis, if associated aortic disease requires aortectomy. They are extended to the undersurface of the renal artery with an end-to-side anastomosis or are anastomosed end-to-end to the transected stump. The most commonly used graft materials have been tubular fabric grafts or saphenous vein segments. There are several major drawbacks to these types of grafting operations for atherosclerotic disease. The thickened aortic wall makes it almost mandatory to use an oversized graft (one larger than the renal artery) if satisfactory proximal anastomosis is to be accomplished. Distally, the disparity in graft-artery size is conducive to graft thrombosis, as a result of accumulation of mural thrombus within the larger graft.[48] Proximally, the predictable advance of aortic disease favors closure of the proximal anastomosis. Turbulence within a retrograde graft also is conducive to thrombosis.

Early enthusiasm for the saphenous vein as a durable conduit has been tempered by the finding that an increasing number of saphenous veins, when used in this position, undergo eventual degeneration leading to fibrotic constriction or aneurysm. Autogenous arterial grafts, which have been highly successful in patients with fibromuscular dysplasia, would appear to be superior but it is difficult to find an undiseased donor artery in atherosclerotic patients.

Transaortic renal endarterectomy for atherosclerotic stenosis appears to have several advantages over bypass grafting in most patients. It restores a slightly greater than normal lumen. Contralateral and accessory artery lesions can be removed in one maneuver within the ischemic tolerance time for both kidneys (see Fig 1). Its only disadvantage is the dissection time required for adequate mobilization of the aorta.

The technique used is illustrated in Figure 3. Mobilization of the suprarenal aorta is facilitated greatly by transection of the muscular ligamentous bands of the crura of the diaphragm, which encase the posterior half of the aorta. These can be palpated as firm ridges closely adherent to the aortic wall. They are avascular and can be simply divided with scissors. The small

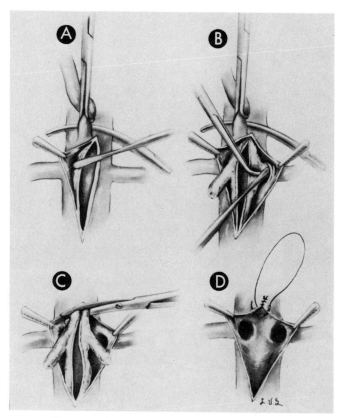

Fig 3. — Technique for transaortic endarterectomy.

arteries to each adrenal gland arising from the side of the aorta at the level of the superior mesenteric artery are identified and divided. Blind finger dissection to the level of the celiac artery frees the lateral and posterior aortic surfaces. (The single pair of lumbar arteries at this level is easily palpable and is preserved.) Mobilization of the anterior surface of the aorta requires partial resection of the dense mass of neural tissue that constitutes the celiac plexus, lying between the celiac and superior mesenteric artery origins.

Clamps are applied to the aorta, one at the infraceliac level and the other at the level of the inferior mesenteric artery, to both renal arteries and to the superior mesenteric artery. A single long, straight arterial clamp can be passed cephalad behind the aorta to occlude the lumbar arteries. The aortotomy is made on the anterior surface of the aorta beginning at the level of the inferior aortic clamp and curved to the left of the superior mesenteric artery at the proximal end. A circumferential incision is made in the aortic intima distal to the renal arteries at a level where the intima is thinnest. The resulting ledge distally remains in its normal position. We have never encountered a problem with postoperative subintimal dissection of the aorta. The dissection plane is developed superiorly to remove a sleeve of the full circumference of the aortic intima. Insofar as possible, the dissection into the renal orifices should be avoided until the aortic intima has been separated and transected proximally immediately caudad to the orifice of the superior mesenteric artery. Traction on the aortic specimen combined with circumferential dissection in each renal orifice individually extracts the renal lesions. In this maneuver the renal artery tends to prolapse into the aortic lumen until the end of the lesion is reached. At this point the specimen breaks away cleanly without separation of the distal intima. At the distal end of the renal dissection where the diseased intima involves only a portion of the arterial circumference, care should be taken to limit the action of the dissection to pushing away only that portion of the media subjacent to the thickened intima. The tip of the dissector should never be out of view.

After reduction of the prolapsed renal artery, a curved hemostat is introduced into the lumen and the end point is inspected as the jaws are spread to insure the absence of an intimal flap. After closure of the aortotomy, the clamps are removed. The renal clamps are the last to be removed to avoid possible microembolization into the renal parenchyma. The total ischemia time after closure of the aortotomy and release of the clamps rarely exceeds 15 minutes.

An operative arteriogram is performed by reapplication of the superior mesenteric and aortic clamps and by injection of contrast solution into the aorta between them (Figs 3 and 4). In the rare event that a stenotic zone secondary to platelet aggregation or intimal flap is demonstrated, the lesion may be removed without interrupting blood flow in the aorta and to the renal artery. A transverse arteriotomy is made in the artery distal to the area

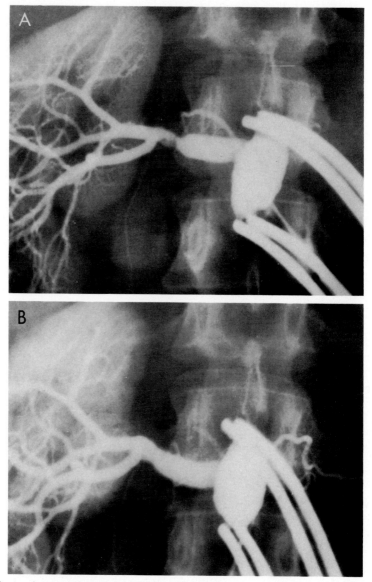

Fig 4. — **A,** operative arteriogram demonstrating an intimal defect at the endarterectomy endpoint. **B,** subsequent arteriogram after removal of a distal intimal flap through a distal arteriotomy.

of stenosis. The posterior intima is incised and by retrograde endarterectomy a sleeve of intima is removed to the previous end point.

The operative arteriogram frequently discloses diffuse or spotty zones of profound stenosis in secondary and tertiary renal artery branches. These arteries are particularly susceptible to vasoconstriction in the immediate postoperative period and, except for instrumental dilatation of obvious clamp defects, they require no further attention. In patients who have had a followup arteriogram after recovery from operation, the arteries have returned to their normal size.

Approximately 20% of patients with atherosclerotic renal artery stenosis will have obstructive lesions in the distal aorta or iliac arteries requiring removal. These can be managed by conventional endarterectomy or bypass techniques after flow has been restored to the renal arteries. If a bypass operation is selected and an end-to-end aortic anastomosis is to be used, it is preferable to transect the aorta distal to the end of the aortotomy and to extract the residual aortic intima.

In patients with frank aortic aneurysmal disease with associated renal artery lesions for which renal revascularization is clearly indicated (usually not the case in view of the criteria described earlier), the perirenal aortic intima usually does not lend itself to endarterectomy. For these patients the preferred technique is the use of sidearm grafts from the aortic prosthesis used to replace the aneurysm.

In the rare patient with the type of necrotic intimal degeneration in the aorta described earlier, we have used an alternate technique for aortic occlusion. The proximal aortic clamp is applied cephalad to the celiac artery above the area of intimal necrosis. This portion of the aorta is readily accessible by an approach through the gastrohepatic ligament followed by splitting of the posterior fibers of the diaphragm. Clamping at this level provides an almost bloodless field where the aortotomy is made and avoids the risk of embolization of intimal fragments into the renal arteries.

Results from this procedure have been satisfactory, as outlined in Tables 2 and 3. There were six deaths early in our series as a result of technical errors. There have been no deaths in the last 100 operations. Two patients have developed recurrent ste-

TABLE 2. – RENOVASCULAR HYPERTENSION
(ATHEROSCLEROSIS) – OPERATIVE MORTALITY RATE

Cooperative study[52]	9.3%
Michigan[23]	3.0%
Vanderbilt[49]	5.0%
UCSF*[56]	1.2%

*1963 – 1975 only

nosis at the operative site 8 and 10 years after revascularization.

Foster at Vanderbilt and Fry at Michigan, together with their colleagues, also have had considerable experience with renovascular reconstructions for atherosclerosis.[23, 49, 50] Their results are also displayed in Tables 2 and 3. Both of these groups preferentially have used bypass techniques using the saphenous vein.

All authors have noted a poor prognosis when atherosclerosis is generalized. In Stanley and Fry's review of their series, there were no deaths except in patients with generalized disease. The late mortality rate was twice as great in patients with generalized as opposed to focal renal artery atherosclerosis.[23, 51]

The treatment of fibromuscular dysplasia has proven to be more rewarding than treatment of patients with atherosclerosis.[23, 52-56] The percentage of cured and improved patients is greater in the former group.

We prefer to treat fibromuscular dysplasia by bypass grafting using autogenous tissue, preferably the hypogastric artery.[48, 57] The size of this artery closely approximates the renal artery and is harvested easily from the abdominal approach. If bilateral grafts are necessary, the common iliac artery, together with its

TABLE 3. – RENOVASCULAR HYPERTENSION
(ATHEROSCLEROSIS) – OPERATIVE RESULTS

STUDY	NO. PATIENTS	CURED	IMPROVED	FAILURES
Michigan[23]				
Focal renal atherosclerosis	54	31%	60%	9%
Generalized atherosclerosis	51	26%	47%	27%
Vanderbilt[49]	78	53%	36%	11%
UCSF*[56]	117	38%	31%	31%

*In the UCSF series the resulting criteria are those described earlier. All operations were transaortic endarterectomies performed over a 15-year period. The recorded result is based upon the most recent blood pressure in patients whose follow-up period exceeds six months.

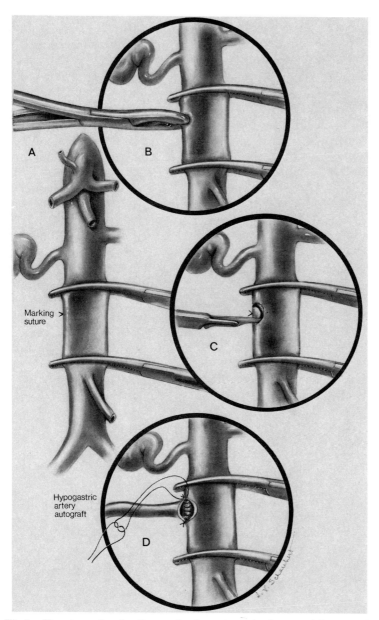

Fig 5.—Steps in performing the proximal anastomosis of an arterial autograft.

internal and external iliac branches, can be used. The common iliac segment is anastomosed end-to-side to the infrarenal aorta and the iliac arms are extended in a cephalad direction to the renal arteries. Arterial continuity to the extremity is then reestablished with a Dacron graft. It is not advisable in males to use both hypogastric arteries.

Particular care should be taken in performing the end-to-side anastomosis to the aorta (Fig 5). A single graft should take off from the aorta at a point midway between the superior and inferior poles of the kidney. Since the renal artery tends to course posteriorly, the origin of the graft from the aorta should be made just posterior to the equator of the aorta. It is advisable to place a marking stitch denoting proper placement for the graft orifice before the application of clamps so that the proper orientation will not be lost. Partially occluding clamps are not desirable as they coapt the aortic walls and make it more difficult to anastomose the graft properly. The proximal anastomosis is made first to minimize renal ischemia time. The distal anastomosis is made end-to-end to nondiseased distal renal artery. Grafts to the right renal artery are placed in a retrocaval location.

Results with patients with fibromuscular dysplasia generally are better than with atherosclerosis. Tables 4 and 5 demonstrate the results at the University of California and compares them with results from Michigan and Vanderbilt.

TABLE 4.—RENOVASCULAR
HYPERTENSION (FIBROMUSCULAR
DYSPLASIA)—OPERATIVE
MORTALITY

Cooperative study[52]	1.2%
Vanderbilt[49]	2.3%
Michigan[23]	0.0%
UCSF[56]	1.2%

TABLE 5.—RENOVASCULAR HYPERTENSION (FIBROMUSCULAR
DYSPLASIA)—OPERATIVE RESULTS

	NO. PATIENTS	CURED (%)	IMPROVED (%)	FAILURE (%)
Michigan[23]	132	57	39	4
Vanderbilt[49]	44	72	24	4
UCSF[56]	45	49	42	9

Renal artery stenosis and subsequent hypertension also may be produced by blunt abdominal trauma.[58-60] This is believed to be due, in most cases, to stretching of the renal artery at the time of a decelerating injury. Several cases have been treated successfully by revascularization.[59, 60] We have had one patient in our series in whom renal artery stenosis was believed to be secondary to blunt trauma. This entity should be suspected in any patient with unexplained hypertension and a past history of trauma, particularly in anyone who does not fit into the classic atherosclerotic or fibromuscular dysplasia group. These lesions usually involve the proximal portion of the right renal artery and are best treated by graft replacement using autogenous tissue.

Renovascular hypertension may also occur secondary to complete renal artery occlusion. There are multiple reports in the surgical literature of renal artery occlusion associated with acute onset of renal failure and sudden or rapidly progressive hypertension.[61-64] This may occur in association with infrarenal aortic occlusions with proximal propagation of clot.[65, 66] Besarab et al. reported three patients in whom vascular reconstruction was performed as late as seven to 29 days after the onset of renal failure, with return to normal renal function in each case.[63] One of the three was cured of hypertension; the other two were improved.

There is a characteristic clinical picture that suggests occlusive disease of the renal arteries as the cause of acute oliguric renal failure: (1) recent onset of severe hypertension or acceleration of prior hypertension; (2) signs and symptoms of associated atherosclerotic disease; (3) abdominal bruit; (4) rapidly progressive oliguric renal failure without evidence of obstructive uropathy; and (5) urinalysis showing minimal proteinuria and no red blood cell casts indicative of glomerulitis or vasculitis. Roentgenographic features suggesting that renal artery revascularization may restore normal renal function include: (1) normal-sized kidney; (2) nephrogram; and (3) incomplete renal artery occlusion or adequate collateral to a kidney with a complete renal artery occlusion. It would appear that the best results can be expected in patients with slowly progressive occlusive disease whose kidneys are protected by collateral formation. Sudden renal artery occlusion without collateralization rarely will permit delayed revascularization.

One of the major advances in renovascular surgery in the past decade has been the development of ex vivo renal artery reconstructions. Renal autotransplantation was first successfully performed for renovascular hypertension by Woodruff et al. in 1965.[67] Ota et al. first reported nephrectomy with ex vivo reconstruction and successful autotransplantation in 1967.[68] The use of continuous extracorporeal hypothermic perfusion first was described in laboratory animals by Belzer and colleagues in 1970.[69] Subsequently, several authors have reported using ex vivo techniques for renal artery reconstructions.[70-73]

Twenty-two patients have undergone 24 renal artery reconstructions in our institution using this technique. Uncontrollable hypertension was the indication for surgery in all but two patients who had symptomatic renal artery aneurysms involving the artery to a solitary kidney. Our technique involves mobilization of the involved kidney along with its artery and vein. After division of the artery and vein, the kidney is moved to a perfusion platform on the lower abdominal wall. The ureter is left intact. Renal washout is performed using Ringer's lactate solution at 4C. Perfusion preservation using a miniature Belzer preservation apparatus is then initiated using cryoprecipitated plasma. The use of multiple cannulae during perfusion allows for perfusion of all vessels except the one being reconstructed. With continuous perfusion of the remainder of the kidney, the renal core temperature can be maintained at 10–13C throughout the procedure. In our series, all reconstructions were performed using autogenous hypogastric artery. The branches of this artery usually have been ample to allow for end-to-end anastomosis between the hypogastric artery and the nondiseased distal branches of the renal artery. If not, anastomoses can be constructed to the side of the hypogastric artery.

In our early experience, the ureter was divided and the kidney was moved to a separate table for the reconstruction. We now perform the reconstruction on a dissection platform on the lower abdominal wall. In the last 18 cases, kidneys have been repaired without division of the ureter. Retrograde bleeding into the kidney is prevented by an elastic tourniquet around the ureter.

Of the 20 patients who underwent ex vivo renal artery reconstruction for hypertension, 15 were cured, 4 improved and there was 1 failure due to graft occlusion. The graft was autogenous artery in each case. The hypogastric artery was used in 22 reconstructions, the splenic artery was used in one and the common iliac and its branches were used in one bilateral procedure. The total number of anastomoses per kidney ranged from 2 to 5, averaging 2.7.

Iodine-131 hippurate renal scintiphotography was performed on the first postoperative day on each of the patients. There was no evidence of acute tubular necrosis in any of the patients, thus attesting to the efficacy of ex vivo perfusion.

There are five distinct advantages to the use of continuous hypothermic perfusion in ex vivo renal artery reconstructions: (1) dissection around branch vessels is simplified because the vessels are distended; (2) any injury occurring to minute vessels during the dissection can be identified and repaired accurately; (3) a maintenance of constant core temperature eliminates ischemic time limitations; (4) at the end of the procedure, perfusion pressure can be set at the patient's normal systolic pressure and vessel leaks can be identified and repaired before reimplantation; and (5) postoperative acute tubular necrosis is avoided. In our experience the ureter can be left intact except in those cases necessitating removal of the kidney to a separate operating area, e.g., to permit in situ reconstruction of the contralateral kidney.

The primary indication for ex vivo renal artery reconstruction remains uncontrollable hypertension due to lesions that are inoperable by standard in situ techniques. Primary among these is extensive fibromuscular dysplasia in young females. Nephrectomy should be reserved for cases of severe renal atrophy, especially in older patients in whom the chance of progression of disease in the opposite kidney is unlikely.

A remaining controversial issue relative to renovascular surgery is the choice of grafting material when an aortorenal bypass is performed, particularly in the management of fibromuscular dysplasia where fabric grafts are difficult to apply. Most surgeons use the saphenous vein as an autogenous graft. However, recent long-term evaluation of these grafts has demonstrated a substantial rate of degenerative abnormalities. Studies by Stanley and colleagues and by Dean and coworkers have been addressed to this problem.[74, 75] The Michigan group noted abnormalities in 60% of grafts in patients followed for 1 – 12 years. These included dilatation in 44%, frank aneurysm formation in 8% and stenosis in 9%. In the Vanderbilt series

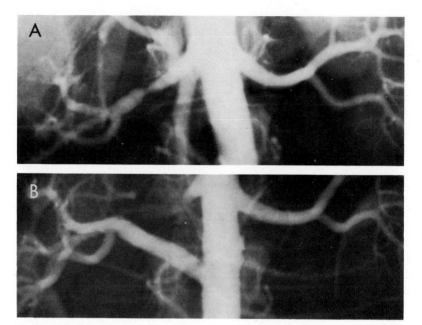

Fig 6.—Preoperative (A) and postoperative (B) aortograms in a patient with fibromuscular dysplasia of the right renal artery in whom a hypogastric artery autograft was used to bypass the lesion.

these numbers were 20, 5 and 17%, respectively. In Szilagyi's report of 260 saphenous vein grafts used in femoropopliteal bypasses, 2.6% developed aneurysmal dilatation and 29% developed stenosing lesions.[76] It is therefore apparent that there is a significant degeneration rate with saphenous vein grafts. At present, a number of investigators are examining methods to better handle vein grafts prior to implantation in an effort to reduct graft degeneration or fibrosis.

We prefer to use the autogenous artery[77-80] (Fig 6). In most cases, the internal iliac artery is used, which does not require replacement due to the rich collateral circulation in the pelvis. If bilateral grafts are necessary the common iliac artery, with its bifurcation branches, is resected and used. The iliac system is then replaced with a Dacron tube graft. The common iliac artery can be anastomosed to the anterior surface of the aorta and one branch can be used to revascularize each kidney.

In a late arteriographic appraisal of 73 arterial autografts used in a variety of circumstances (59 of them renal) with follow-ups extending to 17 years, there was one early graft occlusion, no late graft occlusions, slight graft dilatation in one child, but no other graft abnormalities. It would appear that the arterial autograft has several advantages: (1) it is an arterial graft; (2) the size of the internal iliac artery closely approximates that of the renal artery both in adults and children; (3) the internal iliac artery usually terminates in several branches, which is particularly useful when doing distal renal artery reconstructions, e.g., ex vivo reconstructions; (4) the iliac arteries are accessible in the same operative field; (5) the arterial autografts appear to do well in children and their growth parallels that of their host; and (6) the arterial autograft appears to be more durable than saphenous veins. The major contraindication to the use of an arterial graft is the presence of atherosclerosis in the donor artery. A relative contraindication exists in the use of bilateral hypogastric arteries in males, as this may be associated with impotence. Two females with unilateral hypogastric artery grafts have undergone uneventful pregnancies and normal vaginal deliveries.

Summary

In summary, renovascular surgery has evolved during the past 20 years to become a highly efficacious therapeutic modality provided proper patient selection is practiced. Surgical techniques are now well established, and with the advent of ex vivo techniques practically any extraparenchymal renal artery lesion may be repaired. At present, much investigative work is in progress in an attempt to develop better means of selecting patients who will benefit from renovascular surgery. The newer modifications of renal vein renin assays may permit better patient selection.

Many factors must be weighed when considering medical versus surgical management of hypertension. Paramount among these must be the quality of life of the patient. The inconstancy of pressure control and the frequency of undesirable side effects in the more extreme medical regimens are the primary disadvantages of nonsurgical management. An aggressive surgical approach appears to be warranted in selected patients with atherosclerosis and in almost all patients with fibromuscular dysplasia.

REFERENCES

1. Tigerstedt, R., and Bergman, P. C.: Skand. Arch. Physiol. 8:223, 1898.
2. Page, I. H., and Helmer, O. M.: A crystalline pressor substance (angiotonin) resulting from the reaction between renin and renin-activator, J. Exp. Med. 71:29, 1940.
3. Goldblatt, H., Lynch, J., and Hanzal, R. E.: Studies on experimental hypertension I. The production of persistent elevation of systolic blood pressure by means of renal ischemia, J. Exp. Med. 59:347, 1934.
4. Butler, A. M.: Chronic pyelonephritis and arterial hypertension, J. Clin. Invest. 16:889, 1937.
5. Barker, N. W., and Walters, W.: Hypertension associated with unilateral chronic atrophic pyelonephritis: treatment by nephrectomy, Mayo Clin. Proc. 13:118, 1938.
6. Boyd, C. H., and Lewis, L. G.: Nephrectomy for arterial hypertension: Preliminary report, J. Urol. 39:627, 1938.
7. Perry, C. B.: Malignant hypertension cured by unilateral nephrectomy, Br. Heart J. 7:139, 1945.
8. Goodman, H. L.: Malignant hypertension with unilateral renal-artery occlusion, N. Engl. J. Med. 246:8, 1952.
9. DeCamp, P. T., and Birchall, R.: Recognition and treatment of renal artery stenosis associated with hypertension, Surgery 43:134, 1958.
10. Poutasse, E. F., Humphries, A. W., McCormack, L. J., and Corcoran, A. C.: Bilateral stenosis of renal arteries and hypertension: treatment by arterial homografts, JAMA 161:419, 1956.
11. Smith, H. W.: Unilateral nephrectomy in hypertensive disease, J. Urol. 76:685, 1956.
12. Russell, R. P.: Renal hypertension, Surg. Clin. North Am. 54:349, 1974.
13. Hunt, J. C., and Strong, C. G.: Renovascular hypertension: mechanisms, natural history and treatment, in Laragh, J. H. (ed.): *Hypertension Manual: Mechanisms, Methods, Management* (New York: Yorke Medical Books, 1974).
14. Macgregor, A. M. C., and Cade, J. R.: Renal hypertension, Surg. Gynecol. Obstet. 140:97, 1975.
15. Edwards, J. C.: *Management of Hypertensive Disease* (St. Louis: C. V. Mosby, 1960), p. 21.
16. Wilber, J. A., and Barrow, J. G.: Hypertension – A community problem, Am. J. Med. 52:653, 1972.
17. Correa, R. J., Jr., Conway, J., Hoobler, S. W., and Stewart, B. H.: Renalvascular disease as a cause of hypertension. Selection of patients for aortographic studies, Mich. State Med. Soc. J. 61:1361, 1962.
18. Fry, W. J., Dean, R. H., Stanley, J. C., and Wylie, E. J. Symposium on renovascular hypertension, Contemp. Surg. (in preparation).
19. Dustan, H. P., and Page, I. H.: Unilateral renal disease and hypertension, DM 8:December, 1962.
20. Burbank, M. K., Hunt, J. C., Tauxe, W. N., and Maher, F. T.: Radioisotopic renography. Diagnosis of renal arterial disease in hypertensive patients, Circulation 27:328, 1963.
21. Grim, C. E., Weinberger, M. H., Higgins, J. T., and Kramer, N. J.: Diagno-

sis of secondary forms of hypertension: A comprehensive protocol, JAMA 237:1331, 1977.

22. Bookstein, J. J., Abrams, H. L., Buenger, R. E., Lecky, J., Franklin, S. S., Reiss, M. D., Bleifer, K. H., Klatte, E. C., Varady, P. D., and Maxwell, M. H.: Radiologic aspects of renovascular hypertension. Part 2. The role of urography in unilateral renovascular disease, JAMA 220:1225, 1972.

23. Stanley, J. C., and Fry, W. J.: Surgical treatment of renovascular hypertension, Arch. Surg. 112:1291, 1977.

24. Dustan, H. P. (ed.): Renal arterial stenosis and parenchymal diseases, in Page, I. H., and McCubbin, J. W. (eds.): *Renal Hypertension* (Chicago: Year Book Medical Publishers Inc., 1968).

25. dos Santos, M. R., Jamas, M. M., and Caldos, R. J.: L'arteriogoraphie des membres, de l'aorte et de ses branches abdominale, Soc. Natl. Chir. Bull. Mem. 55:587, 1929.

26. Seldinger, S. I.: Catheter replacement of the needle in percutaneous arteriography. A new technique, Acta Radiol. 39:368, 1953.

27. Dean, R. H., Burko, H., Wilson, J. P., Mulherin, J. H., and Foster, J. H.: Deceptive patterns of renal artery stenosis, Surgery 76:872, 1974.

28. Bookstein, J. J., Walter, J. F., Stanley, J. C., and Fry, W. J.: Pharmacoangiographic manipulation of renal collateral blood flow, Circulation 54:328, 1976.

29. Howard, J. W., and Connor, T. B.: Hypertension produced by unilateral renal disease, Arch. Intern Med. 109:8, 1962.

30. Stamey, T. A., Nudelman, I. J., Good, P. H., Schwentker, F. N., and Hendricks, F.: Functional characteristics of renovascular hypertension, Medicine (Baltimore) 40:347, 1961.

31. Dean, R. H., and Foster, J. H.: Criteria for diagnosis of renovascular hypertension, Surgery 74:926, 1973.

32. Oparil, S., and Haber, E.: The renin-angiotensin system, N. Engl. J. Med. 291:389, 1974.

33. Skeggs, L. T., Dorer, F. E., Kahn, J. R., Lentz, K. E., and Levine, M.: The biochemistry of the renin-angiotensin system and its role in hypertension, Am. J. Med. 60:737, 1976.

34. Couch, N. P., Sullivan, J., and Crane, C.: The predictive accuracy of renal vein activity in the surgery of renovascular hypertension, Surgery 79:70, 1976.

35. Ernst, C. B., Daugherty, M. E., and Kotchen, T. A.: Relationship between collateral development and renin in experimental renal artery stenosis, Surgery 80:252, 1976.

36. Schambelan, M., Gickman, M., Stockigt, J. R., and Biglieri, E. G.: Selective renal-vein renin sampling in hypertensive patients with segmental renal lesions, N. Engl. J. Med. 290:1153, 1974.

37. Stanley, J. C., Gewertz, B. L., and Fry, W. J.: Renal:systemic renin indices and renal vein renin ratios as prognostic indicators in remedial renovascular hypertension, J. Surg. Res. 20:149, 1976.

38. Vaughan, E. D., Jr., Buhler, F. R., Laragh, J. H., Sealey, J. E., Baer, L., and Bard, R. H.: Renovascular hypertension: Renin measurements to indicate hypersecretion and contralateral suppression, estimate renal plasma flow, and score for surgical curability, Am. J. Med. 55:402, 1973.

39. Baer, L., Parra-Carrillo, J. Z., Radichevich, I., and Williams, G. S.: Detection of renovascular hypertension with angiotensin II blockade, Ann. Intern. Med. 86:257, 1977.
40. Marks, L. S., Maxwell, M. H., and Kaufman, J. J.: Renin, sodium, and vasodepressor response to saralasin in renovascular and essential hypertension, Ann. Intern. Med. 87:176, 1977.
41. Palubinskas, A. J., and Ripley, H. R.: Fibromuscular hyperplasia in extrarenal arteries, Radiology 82:451, 1969.
42. Harrison, E. G., and McCormack, L. J.: Pathologic classification of renal arterial disease in renovascular hypertension, Mayo Clin. Proc. 46:161, 1971.
43. Meaney, T. F., Dustan, H. P., and McCormack, L. J.: Natural history of renal arterial disease, Radiology 91:881, 1968.
44. Sottiurai, V. S., Fry, W. J., and Stanley, J. C.: Ultrastructural characteristics of experimental arterial fibroplasia induced by vasa vasorum occlusion, J. Surg. Res. (in press).
45. Lawson, J. D., Boerth, R., Foster, J. H., and Dean, R. H.: Diagnosis and management of hypertension in children, Arch. Surg. 112:1307, 1977.
46. Stoney, R. J., Cooke, P. A., and String, S. T.: Surgical treatment of renovascular hypertension in children, J. Pediatr. Surg. 10:631, 1975.
47. Fry, W. J., Ernst, C. B., Stanley, J. C., and Brink, B.: Renovascular hypertension in the pediatric patient, Arch. Surg. 107:692, 1973.
48. Wylie, E. J., Ehrenfeld, W. K. and Stoney, R. J.: Atlas of Vascular Surgery (New York: Springer-Verlag [in preparation]).
49. Foster, J. N., Dean, R. N., Pinkerton, J. A., and Rhamy, R. K.: Ten years experience with the surgical management of renovascular hypertension, Ann. Surg. 177:755, 1973.
50. Ernst, C. B., Stanley, J. C., Marshall, F. F., and Fry, W. J.: Autogenous saphenous vein aortorenal grafts. A ten year experience, Arch. Surg. 105:855, 1972.
51. Ernst, C. B., Stanley, J. C., Marshall, F. F. and Fry, W. J.: Renal revascularization for arteriosclerotic renovascular hypertension: prognostic implications of focal renal arterial vs. overt generalized generalized arteriosclerosis, Surgery 73:859, 1973.
52. Foster, J. H., Maxwell, M. M., Franklin, S. S., Bleifer, K. H., Trippel, O. H., Julian, O. C., DeCamp, P. T., and Varady, P. T.: Renovascular occlusive disease. Results of operative treatment, JAMA 231:1043, 1975.
53. Foster, J. N., Oates, J. A., Rhamy, R. K., Klatte, E. C., Burko, H. C., and Michelakis, A. M.: Hypertension and fibromuscular dysplasia of the renal arteries, Surgery 65:157, 1969.
54. Fry, W. J., Brink, B. E., and Thompson, N. W.: New techniques in the treatment of extensive fibromuscular disease involving the renal arteries, Surgery 68:959, 1970.
55. Stanley, J. C., and Fry, W. J.: Renovascular hypertension secondary to arterial fibrodysplasia in adults, Arch. Surg. 110:922, 1975.
56. Stoney, R. J., Swanson, R. J., Carlson, R. E., and Perloff, D. L.: Operative treatment of renovascular hypertension, in Varco, R. L., and Delaney, J. P. (eds.): Controversy in Surgery (Philadelphia: W. B. Saunders Co., 1976).
57. Wylie, E. J.: Endarterectomy and autogenous arterial grafts in the surgi-

cal treatment of stenosing lesions of the renal artery, Urol. Clin. North Am. 2:351, 1975.

58. Sechas, M. N., Plessas, S. N., and Skalkeas, G. D.: Post-traumatic renovascular hypertension, Surgery 76:666, 1974.
59. Depner, T. A., Sullivan, M. J., Ryan, K. G., Winn, D. F., Jr., McCusker, J. J. and Yamauchi, H.: Post-traumatic renal artery stenosis, Arch. Surg. 110:1150, 1975.
60. Gewertz, B. L., Stanley, J. C., and Fry, W. J.: Renal artery dissections, Arch. Surg. 112:409, 1977.
61. Spanos, P. K., Terhorst, T. R., and Sako, Y.: Acute prolonged renal arterial infarction. Return of function after thromboendarterectomy, Am. J. Surg. 129:579, 1975.
62. Magilligan, D. J., Jr., DeWeese, J. A., May, A. G. and Rob, C. G.: The occluded renal artery, Surgery 78:730, 1975.
63. Besarab, A., Brown, R. S., Rubin, N. T., Salzman, E., Wirthlin, L., Steinman, T., Atlia, R. R., and Skillman, J. J.: Reversable renal failure following bilateral renal artery occlusive disease. Clinical features, pathology, and the role of surgical revascularization, JAMA 235:2838, 1976.
64. Heaney, D., Kupor, L. R., Noon, G. P., and Suki, W. N.: Bilateral renal artery stenosis causing acute oliguric renal failure. Report of a case corrected by renovascular surgery, Arch. Surg. 112:641, 1977.
65. Starrett, R. W., and Stoney, R. J.: Juxtarenal aortic occlusion, Surgery 76:890, 1974.
66. Hertzer, N. R., Montie, J. E. Hall, P. M., and Banowsky, L. H.: Revascularization of the kidney after occlusion of the aorta and both renal arteries, Surgery 79:52, 1976.
67. Woodruff, M. F. A., Doig, A., Donald, K. W., and Nolan, B.: Renal autotransplantation, Lancet 1:433, 1966.
68. Ota, K., Mori, S., Awane, Y., and Ueno, A.: Ex-situ repair of renal artery for renovascular hypertension, Arch. Surg. 94:370, 1967.
69. Belzer, F. O., Keaveny, T. V., Reed, T. W., and Pryor, J. P.: A new method of renal artery reconstruction, Surgery 68:619, 1970.
70. Lim, R. C., Eastman, A. B. and Blaisdell, F. W.: Renal autotransplantation. Adjunct to repair of renal vascular lesions, Arch. Surg. 105:847, 1972.
71. Belzer, F. O., Salvatierra, O., Perloff, D. L., and Grausz, H.: Surgical correction of advanced fibromuscular dysplasia of the renal arteries, Surgery 75:31, 1974.
72. Belzer, F. O., Salvatierra, O., Palubinskas, A., and Stoney, R. J.: Ex vivo renal artery reconstruction, Ann. Surg. 182:456, 1976.
73. Salvatierra, O., Olcott, C., and Stoney, R. J.: Ex-vivo renal artery reconstruction utilizing perfusion preservation, J. Urol. (in press).
74. Stanley, J. C., Ernst, C. B., and Fry, W. J.: Fate of 100 aortorenal vein grafts: characteristics of late graft expansion, aneurysmal dilatation and stenosis, Surgery 74:931, 1973.
75. Dean, R. H., Wilson, J. P., Burko, H. and Foster, J. H.: Saphenous vein aortorenal bypass grafts: serial arteriographic study, Ann. Surg. 180:469, 1974.
76. Szilagyi, D. E., Elliott, J. P., Hageman, J. H., Smith, R. F., and Dell'omo,

C. A.: Biologic fate of autogenous vein implants as arterial substitutes: clinical, angiographic and histopathologic observations in femoro-popliteal operations for atherosclerosis, Ann. Surg. 178:232, 1973.

77. Wylie, E. J.: Vascular replacement with arterial autografts, Surgery 57: 14, 1965.

78. Wylie, E. J., Perloff, D. L. and Stoney, R. J.: Autogenous tissue revascularization technics in surgery for renovascular hypertension, Ann. Surg. 170: 416, 1969.

79. Stoney, R. J. and Wylie, E. J.: Arterial autografts, Surgery 67:18, 1970.

80. Lye, C. R., String, S. T. and Wylie, E. J.: Aortorenal arterial autografts. Late observations, Arch. Surg. 110:1321, 1975.

Therapeutic Techniques in Diagnostic Radiology

ERIK BOIJSEN, M.D. AND ANDERS
LUNDERQUIST, M.D.

Department of Diagnostic Radiology, University Hospital, Lund, Sweden

The traditional techniques of diagnostic radiology, fluoroscopy and film documentation, have not changed; however, new equipment and accumulated experience have changed the radiologist's role in the clinical team approach. To some extent, the radiologist has always taken active part in therapy (e.g., in correction of fractures or treatment of intussusception), but during the past few years a marked change has occurred. The radiologist is now assuming an increasingly important role in the treatment of a variety of disorders. This is especially so in the management of patients for whom other therapeutic alternatives are less attractive or impossible.

One of the most important steps in the direction of therapy in diagnostic radiology was the development of the percutaneous needle technique. Introduced in 1929 by Dos Santos for lumbar aortography, in 1953 it was refined by Seldinger for percutaneous vessel catheterization. The radiologist soon became aware of the potentials of this method, especially when radiopaque catheters became available. Soon a catheter could be introduced into almost any of the larger vessels of the body. Improved catheters, as well as fluoroscopic and recording equipment, made examinations safe and reliable.

With the advent of abdominal echography and computerized axial tomography (CAT scanning), angiography became less

0065-3411/78/0012-0259$03.75

important as a diagnostic tool, particularly in tumor diagnosis. The experience gained from angiography, however, was not in vain because it formed the basis for the development of a new technique developed during the 1970s. This may be called therapeutic technique in diagnostic radiology, a method whereby radiologic experience and equipment are used for treatment of a variety of diseases. Some of the lesions treated are in patients who are regarded as inoperable, but others are in poor-risk patients who could be brought to an operable condition. It has become obvious that many patients do not require any further treatment. There is no doubt that in the future these methods will change the therapeutic approach to a variety of disease entities, and that we have just entered the era of therapeutic technique in diagnostic radiology.

Methods

Most of the methods presented here are still experimental, but they have been used in clinical trials; some of them, however, have been used in only a few cases. A short survey of the various methods will be given. They may be classified as follows: (1) intravascular therapy; (2) draining of ducts, cysts and abscesses; and (3) extraction of stones.

INTRAVASCULAR THERAPY

Many methods have been developed for the obstruction of blood flow, most of them to stop bleeding or to destroy a tumor. The method chosen in a given case depends on the indications for the treatment. Thus a brief obstruction of flow is meaningful in a hemorrhage where one can expect that the normal healing procedure later will cure the patient, or where operation later will be the preferred therapy.

The most frequently used method for an effect of short duration is infusion of a vasoconstrictor. This has been particularly effective in gastrointestinal hemorrhage and in postoperative bleeding.[1-6] Vasopressin has been used most frequently but epinephrine also has proven helpful when combined with propranolol. The ideal control of a bleeding artery is acquired by using a balloon catheter. The technique of balloon introduction via arteriotomy has been used for years, but the percutaneous technique for control of bleeding has only recently been developed.[7, 8] If necessary, the balloon can be inflated and deflated intermittently to preserve organ function.[9] The site of bleeding is defined and operation can be performed electively. If operation is found unreasonable and bleeding proceeds after deflation of the balloon, embolization can be performed with the balloon inflated. This method has also been used to prevent embolic material from passing into the systemic circulation.[10] Balloon catheters also have been used for occlusion of arteriovenous fistulas and aneurysms not accessible for surgery, and for infusion of chemical substances.[9, 11] A detachable balloon for permanent occlusion has been devised by Serbinenko.[9]

Embolic occlusion of arteries may be obtained using different methods. Irrespective of reason and site of lesion, the percutaneously introduced catheter should be as close as possible to the vessel supplying the lesion. Specially devised catheters with small, tapered tips are suggested in order to reach as far out as possible in the arteries to avoid spill-over of embolic material.[12] Magnetically guided Silastic rubber tubings,[13] flow-guided balloon catheters and coaxial catheters have been developed for this purpose.

It has been shown repeatedly that an injected embolus finds its way to the vessel that has the greatest flow, i.e., the artery that is bleeding or feeding an arteriovenous fistula. When the flow begins to decrease because of embolization, some embolic material will always pass to adjacent normal vessels; thus, permanent damage to adjacent normal structures must always be expected.

The type of embolic material used depends on the clinical situation and on plans for further therapy. A patient who is expecting to be operated on as soon as possible after embolization should have an embolus that causes as small an infarction as possible and that also causes only temporary occlusion. The most suitable embolus in this respect is the autogenous clot, which is prepared by withdrawing 10 – 20 cc of blood immediately before angiography. It is injected in 0.5 – 1.0-ml increments and adapts easily to the vessel, but often is fragmented and passes far out in the small arteries.[14] The advantage with a blood clot is that it may disappear within a few hours.[14, 15] However, experimental studies on pigs, which have fibrinolytic activity similar to that in man, have shown that the autogenous clot causes partial or complete occlusion for at least 48 hours and that many arteries are still occluded 14 days later.[16] A prolonged effect of the clot has been observed when mixed with epsilon-aminocaproic acid. This reacts with plasmin to form fibrin, which has an increased resistance to fibrinolysis. In animal experiments, these prepared emboli undergo lysis within 24 hours but may stay longer.[17] Addition of oxycel (oxidized cellulose) to the clot also has been used in patients in whom deficient clotting is present, a frequently observed phenomenon in those receiving multiple blood transfusions.[18] This substance promotes coagulation and increases clot durability.

Autologous muscle and subcutaneous fat are used for more definitive vascular occlusion. A piece of muscle tissue injected intra-arterially after arteriotomy was, in fact, the first embolic material used for a carotid-cavernous fistula in 1930 by Brooks.[19] It was later used extensively in cerebral arterial lesions. When homogenized preparations of crushed muscle or muscle fragments have been injected together with a contrast medium, it has been observed that the material passes far out in the small vessels. Later controls have presented complete or almost complete occlusion of the vessels.[20-22] Muscle tissue has been used for tumor occlusion as well as for bleeding with this transcatheter technique.[20, 22-24] Fat has been used in a few cases to stop bleeding or to occlude the feeding artery of an arteriovenous fistula.[25]

Gelfoam and other sponge materials are used most commonly for embolization via catheters today. Gelfoam has the advantage that it can be cut into sizes varying from 1 – 10 mm in length and 1 – 2 mm in width. These pieces can be compressed easily and thus can be injected through small-bore catheters, which is of specific importance for superselective catheterization.[12] The Gelfoam is a gelatin sponge, most of which is absorbed within 48 hours when injected intra-arterially, but blood clots are formed in the framework of the sponge and occlusion therefore is more persistent than with blood clot alone. Recanalization of vessels occluded by Gelfoam, however, has been observed.[26, 27]

Polyvinyl alcohol (Ivalon), another sponge material, has interesting properties in that it absorbs water and is easily compressible when wet, with excellent plastic memory when allowed to expand.[28, 29] The material is more difficult to handle than Gelfoam, and misplacement has occurred experimentally.

It has good biocompatibility, however, and causes a permanent occlusion. If injected distal to a balloon occlusion, the risk of misplacement is small.

Solid emboli of a large variety of materials also have been tested. These have been used in angiomatous malformations that are notoriously difficult to treat surgically. Particularly in these lesions it is important to have a distal occlusion of the feeding arteries. However, the particles may not be too small because they may then pass through the malformation and cause pulmonary embolization. The essential drawback common to the solid particles is that they are unmalleable. Thus, they may be too small for the lesion when they can pass through a catheter and too large for the catheter when they are adequate for the lesion. An advantage is that they usually are radiopaque and the position can be checked later by plain films. Solid materials tested for vascular occlusion include Silastic and silicone balls,[30] methacrylate spheres,[31] stainless steel pellets[32] and plastic microspheres.[33, 34] These are all inert and nonantigenic. In several experiments it has been shown, however, that the spheres may cause complications. Therefore, these have not been recommended for use in humans.[33] With increasing vascular resistance as a result of injected microspheres, reflux to the aorta will occur at the end of the injection. A balloon catheter may reduce this risk, but with increasing numbers of spheres there is another risk, i.e., the vessel may rupture distal to the balloon because of the increased pressure.[34] Another variety of solid particles is used in the injection of radioactive gold seeds.[35]

Since it may be impossible to achieve the occlusion of large arteries with the techniques reported above, wool coils have been introduced[36] (Fig 1). Woolen strands are attached to a tightly coiled 5-cm long segment of a steel guide wire. The combination of peripheral embolization with Gelfoam or cotton threads and the wool coil has been quite successful for permanent occlusion of larger arteries and their branches.[37]

Another approach to vascular occlusion is the use of different kinds of glue, which through polymerization causes instant occlusion of a vessel when the glue comes in contact with blood. Methylcyanoacrylate was the first homologue used as a tissue adhesive, but it has irritating properties. Increasing the length of the carbon chain shortens polymerization time and decreases tissue damage. Isobutyl-2-cyanoacrylate therefore is the me-

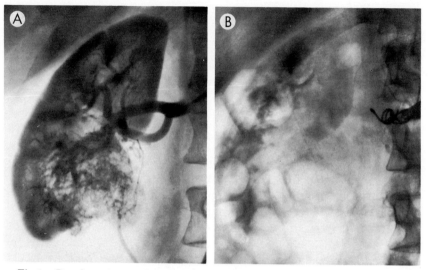

Fig 1. — Renal carcinoma of right kidney in 59-year-old man. Tumor was not operable because of lung metastases. Selective right renal angiography before (A) and after (B) occlusion with steel coil.

dium chosen most often because it is nonirritating and it polymerizes in approximately one second. It therefore will occlude even high-flow arteriovenous shunts.[38, 39] The monomer solution is easy to inject but cannot be allowed to come in contact with blood or saline in the catheter. Glucose, on the other hand, will not cause polymerization. Therefore, a coaxial catheter filled with dextrose or glucose solution is introduced.[39, 40] One-half to 2 ml of the monomer usually is adequate for complete and fast occlusion of the vessel (Fig 2). Addition of a tantalum powder will make clear the extent of occlusion. The vascular thrombus will adhere to the wall and cause a permanent occlusion. For venous occlusion in portal hypertension, neither this material nor hypertonic glucose alone or combined with etolein and Gelfoam is a definite solution.[27, 41] Complications with this technique have been observed experimentally and clinically. The catheter may be fixed to the polymerized mass,[26, 34] and reflux of material may occur to the aorta, causing embolization of vessels not intended to be embolized.[34] Incomplete polymerization with resultant pulmonary infarcts may occur.[42] However, these risks seem nonexistent with proper technique and adequate material.

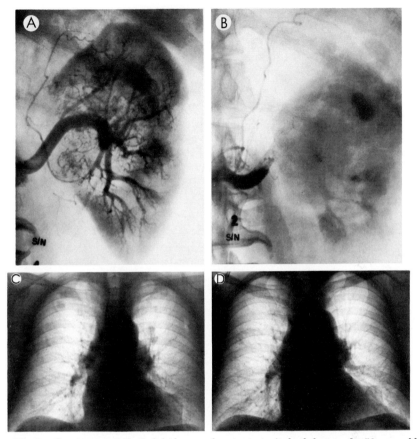

Fig 2.—Carcinoma of the left kidney and metastases in both lungs of a 59-year-old man. Left renal angiography before (**A**) and after (**B**) occlusion with bucrylate. Chest examinations before (**C**) and 17 months after occlusion of the renal artery (**D**) show that metastases have disappeared.

Because of the instantaneous polymerization of isobutyl-2-cyanoacrylate, mainly large arteries are occluded. In the treatment of tumors or angiomatous malformations that cannot be removed surgically, the precapillary branches of the lesions should be occluded; if not, collateral feeding arteries will soon replace the occluded ones. For this reason, silicone rubber has been selected. It is inert, which is well known from the use of this elastomer in prosthetic and cosmetic inplants.[43] The polymerization reaction is different from that with isobutyl-2-cyanoacrylate and starts already when mixed outside the body. When injected intra-arterially it is without toxic effects.[34, 43] Mixed with tantalum and diluted with silicone fluid, the peripheral as well as the main stem of the renal vessels in dogs are filled. The silicone rubber forms a cast of the vessels without adhesion to the walls. To avoid reflux to the aorta or embolization to the lungs, iron particles are added to the silicone rubber and a superconducting magnet directs the preparation to the organ or part of organ intended to be destroyed.[44] The ferrosilicon reaches the terminal arterioles and some capillary vessels before vulcanization. No ferrosilicon passes over into veins. This technique thus is promising and has been effective in humans but the necessary powerful magnets are not available in many hospitals.

Electrocoagulation via catheter is a method for vascular occlusion extensively practiced in experimental models.[34, 45] So far it is not a clinically well-established method despite its use in a few cases. Alternating high-frequency current is said to be too difficult to control and causes damage to the vessel wall, with risk of rupture. Direct current applied by catheter-placed electrodes is feasible. Clot formation probably is induced both by intimal damage and by attachment of platelets to the positively charged electrode. Thus, a localized occlusion of the vessel is achieved. One drawback that so far has not been overcome is that it takes more than 30 minutes to occlude vessels larger than 5 mm.

As mentioned previously, occlusion of arterial systems is bound to cause complications in terms of infarction and necrosis. The extent of these complications usually cannot be predicted because they depend on the site of occlusion and the presence of collateral arterial supply. It is therefore advisable to perform every attempt at embolization with extreme care, and to proceed only in patients who refuse operation or for whom the prognosis of operation is deemed to be poor. The potential complications of embolization must be placed in proper relation to the complications of surgery or other methods available for therapy. In most cases, embolization should be followed by surgery.

In venous occlusion therapy the same methods have been used as for arterial occlusion. For partial occlusion of the inferior vena cava, a special technique has been devised by Mobin-

Uddin, McLean and Jude[46] Vasodilatation is another field of intravascular therapy included in therapeutic diagnostic radiology. Two main methods can be recognized, i.e., pharmacologic and mechanical dilatation of vessels.

A variety of vasodilating substances have been injected intraarterially immediately before angiography to enhance the accumulation of contrast medium in the capillary phase and increase the density of the contrast medium in the veins. Because of the local application, the vasodilating effect may be obtained without changes in systemic circulation. This experience has been used for intra-arterial therapy in nonocclusive bowel ischemia and also in ischemia of the extremities in, for example, severe peripheral vascular disease. Mechanical dilatation of stenosed arteries is a therapeutic technique that was introduced in diagnostic radiology in 1964 by Dotter and Judkins.[47] Later improvements with balloon catheters appear to give effective dilatation of severely stenosed iliac arteries with slight complications.

INTRA-ARTERIAL INFUSION OF CYTOTOXIC SUBSTANCES. — Intraarterial infusion of cytotoxic substances is not a new approach since Bierman et al., as early as 1950, infused nitrogen mustard in the hepatic artery for liver metastases after cut-down catheterization from the brachial artery.[48] The indwelling catheter is placed percutaneously from the femoral or, most often, left brachial artery. The time of infusion varies depending on what is to be treated and what type of anticarcinogenic agent is used. In order to potentiate the effect of cytotoxic substances, agents may be infused with polysaccharide microspheres, which are dissolved by the normal enzymes of the body after a period of one hour or longer. Some preliminary experimental and clinical studies have given promising results.[49] A combination of radioactive infarct implants and intra-arterial chemotherapy has been used in patients with renal carcinoma with gratifying results.[35] To reduce perfusion to normal tissue and increase it to the tumor, intra-arterial injection of epinephrine has been combined with chemotherapy infusion.[35]

It is logical to assume that intra-arterial chemotherapy should be more effective than intravenous or oral administration. Various techniques and drugs therefore are tested for percutaneous intra-arterial therapy of tumors in the abdomen, pelvis, lung, and head and neck.[50-53] Because of the difficulty in predicting the prognosis of the single case, the results of this new therapy are not yet available.

DRAINAGE OF CAVITIES

The technique for percutaneous drainage of ducts, cysts and abscesses is based on an as exact radiologic localization of the ducts or lesions as is possible. Different approaches are used for various indications; these will be discussed in sections on separate organs. For puncture and drainage of ducts and cysts, the same technique as for arterial catheterization is used. It is of definite advantage to use biplane fluoroscopy. A straight approach to the lesion or duct is always to be recommended. After local anesthesia, a needle (outside diameter [OD], 0.9 mm) is advanced toward the lesion or duct and a small amount of contrast medium is injected as soon as some fluid can be aspirated from the needle. This is followed by insertion of a larger needle with a Teflon sheath. A guide wire is introduced through the sheath as soon as the needle is withdrawn. When the guide wire is in position, the sheath is withdrawn and the drainage catheter is pushed over the guide wire to its final position.

Intra-abdominal, intrahepatic and retroperitoneal abscesses may be drained in a similar manner but the lesion usually is approached directly, with the needle covered by the Teflon sheath. Ultrasound and CAT scanning are playing an increasing role in the management of these lesions for more exact and faster approach.

EXTRACTION OF STONES

Extraction of stones retained in the bile ducts at operation was introduced a few years ago[54] but has already received worldwide attention. For details of the extraction procedure the reader is referred to the inventor's detailed description.[55] Percutaneous pyelolithotomy is another recently introduced radiologic technique.[56]

OTHER METHODS

Other methods, more or less ingenious, could be mentioned. We will consider only one new method, which is at the experimental stage but may be of interest for future tumor destruction. A 3-mm positive electrode of platina is introduced percutaneously in the lung and a cathode of stainless steel is placed below the skin.[57] When a 12 ma and 6 v current is passed through the electrodes, chlorine gas is formed at the anode from the saline in the tissues and destroys the lung tissue; at 100 coulomb, a 1×1-cm destruction is noted; and at 200 coulomb, a 2×1-cm destruction is noted. The radiologist has good training in performing biopsy during fluoroscopy. A similar technique with electrodes will show whether this method will be of importance in tumor therapy.

Clinical Applications

NEURORADIOLOGY

Angiomatous lesions and tumors of the brain and spinal cord have been treated by embolization either by direct injection of embolizing material into the main feeding artery[13, 32, 58] or into the carotid or vertebral arteries.[31, 59] The latter method is, of course, hazardous; but in cases of inoperable arteriovenous malformations, the increased flow through the fistula usually is so high that the embolic material follows the main stream to the lesion. In this way a malformation can be reduced in size and the lesion can become operable. So far no intracranial lesion has been healed by embolization. Recent development with flow-directed balloon catheters, detachable balloons and the use of isobutyl-2-cyanoacrylate may make this type of therapy more efficient.[9, 39, 60, 61] Various methods of treatment of carotid-cavernous sinus fistulas with embolizing material and balloon catheters have been reported after the first attempt by Brooks in 1930.[19] The most wellknown is the detachable balloon technique of Serbinenko.[9]

Many intracranial lesions, especially angiomatous malformations and meningeomas, have been treated with Gelfoam via the external carotid artery, when it has been proven angiographically that the lesion is supplied from this artery.[62, 63] Since the risks of intracranial complications are relatively few, the method has been proven to be of definite value in that it diminishes considerably the risks of hemorrhage during surgery. The external carotid artery usually is included in the neuroradiologic speciality; and particularly in this area, intense activity occurs for intra-arterial treatment both by cytostatic agents and embolization of tumors and arteriovenous malformations.[64] In most cases, Gelfoam has been used and even if complete success cannot be expected, remarkable regression of the lesions may be observed at least for some time. Embolization immediately before operation has been of definite value. The method is not without risk; everyone active in this field has had cases with serious complications because of embolization to cerebral arteries. The importance of an almost wedge position of a small bore catheter is a prerequisite to avoid these complications. As expected, necroses and ulcerations have been observed within the territory of the embolized artery but with insufficient severity to warrant abandoning this method. On the contrary, many enthusiastic reports, especially by French authors and particularly by Djindjian and his group,[12, 58, 64] speak strongly in favor of more widespread use of this method.

Severe epistaxis from a tumor may be one reason for embolization but idiopathic epistaxis also may be treated effectively with Gelfoam embolization of the maxillary artery.[65]

THORACIC RADIOLOGY

Embolization of bronchial arteries because of severe hemoptysis has been reported mainly by French authors.[66, 67] In most cases hemoptysis is secondary to tuberculosis, aspergilloma, bronchiectasis or carcinoma. It has been proven that the hemorrhage is of systemic origin but it is rarely life-threatening. Gelfoam has been shown to be effective in most cases and is thus worthwhile to try in severe hemoptysis. However, several complications can be expected because the bronchial arteries are small and an adequate catheter position is difficult to keep. Reflux of embolic material has been reported.[66] If the spinal artery is observed at right bronchial arteriography, embolization is contraindicated. Local bronchial-wall necrosis has been observed but no detectable signs of pulmonary ischemia have appeared. In order to prevent an overflow of blood to the contralateral bronchus during massive hemoptysis, a balloon catheter may be introduced into the main bronchus.[68]

Mediastinal adenoma of the parathyroid glands has been successfully embolized by autogenous blood clot and Gelfoam.[69]

This is another field where therapeutic diagnostic radiology may be helpful after unsuccessful neck exploration for hyperparathyroidism.

Bronchogenic carcinoma has been treated with intra-arterial infusion of cytostatic agents with some success. New anticarcinogenic drugs seem to have a remarkable effect in some cases. In our own series, in patients treated with a single dose of 10 mg mitomycin-C diluted in saline, we observed complete regression of tumor in 2 of 9 patients with squamous cell carcinoma who later had operations.[53] Of the remaining patients, rather marked regression was observed in 5, and only slight regression in 2 (Fig 3). In more than 40 patients treated so far, we have observed no severe complications from the infusion, which in several patients, has been repeated three or four times. Similar experience has been observed by others. The long-term effect of this method so far is unknown, but in light of the poor prognosis of surgery or combination of surgery and cytostatic agents given intravenously or orally, there is reason to try new methods of treatment.

Pulmonary arteriovenous fistulae should be accessible for embolization but thus far no attempt has been reported. Other lesions available for catheter therapy are vena cava filter to

Fig 3.—Low differentiated squamous cell carcinoma of the right lower lobe in 61-year-old man. The richly vascularized tumor is demonstrated at bronchial angiography (A). Chest radiographs taken before (B) and four weeks after infusion of 10 mg mitomycin-C into bronchial artery (C) show marked regression of tumor.

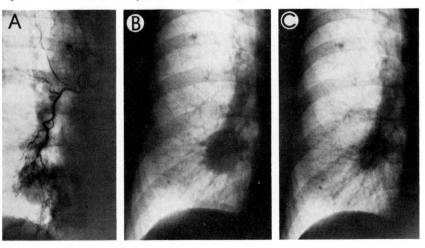

prevent pulmonary emboli. The Rashkind balloon catheter for palliative septostomy in transposition of the great vessels, and the Porstman method for percutaneous occlusion of a patent ductus[28] are other methods in which diagnostic radiology plays an important therapeutic role. The latter method has proven quite successful in skilled hands. Despite the fact that large catheters are used, complications at the puncture site are small.

GASTROINTESTINAL RADIOLOGY

Gastrointestinal Tract

ARTERIAL HEMORRHAGE. — Localization of the site of bleeding from the upper gastrointestinal tract usually is tried first by endoscopy and, if this is not successful, arteriography is performed. Experimental studies have shown bleeding of 0.5–1.3 ml/minute to be demonstrable by arteriography through extravasation of contrast media.

Selective injection of a contrast medium into the left gastric artery, common hepatic artery or gastroduodenal artery has made it possible to diagnose bleeding from Mallory-Weiss tears, peptic ulcers and gastritis. Selective injection of contrast medium into the superior or inferior mesenteric artery can localize bleeding from the small intestine and colon. Nusbaum and colleagues introduced intra-arterial infusion of vasopressin in 1968 to control gastrointestinal hemorrhage. The technique and effectiveness of this method in various gastrointestinal disorders causing bleeding was reviewed four years ago in this series.[1] Therefore, we will comment only briefly upon the technique.

When the site of bleeding has been found at selective injection of a contrast medium, vasopressin infusion through a catheter is started at the rate of 0.2 units/minute. Twenty minutes after the beginning of the infusion the angiogram is repeated to check if the bleeding has stopped. If this is the case, the infusion is continued at the same rate for 12–24 hours. If there is no clinical evidence of continued hemorrhage, the infusion rate is decreased to 0.1 unit/minute for another 12–24 hours, after which vasopressin is replaced by saline for another 12 hours. The catheter can then be removed. Vasoconstrictive therapy is most effective in capillary bleeding and bleeding from small arteries,[3, 5] whereas treatment of peptic ulcer hemorrhage often fails.[4] One reason for failure is that the bleeding may occur in an area with dual supply through a vascular arcade, which is particularly often present in the descending duodenum or splenic flexure of the colon. Proximal occlusion of one limb of an arcade by vasopressin can permit continuation of bleeding through collateral channels.[70] Infusion of both limbs will then often give effective treatment.

Complications from prolonged vasopressin infusion are rare. The drawback with infusion therapy is that the catheter must be in the vessel for at least 48 hours for continuous infusion. This may cause complications because of clot formation and occlusion of the superior mesenteric artery,[71] for example. Other complications such as bacterial peritonitis and thrombosis of superior mesenteric vein with bowel infarction have been reported.[72, 73] Intra-arterial infusion of vasopressin should be performed in selected cases, but not until the intravenous route has been tested. In patients bleeding from esophageal varices, intravenous infusion appears to be as effective as intra-arterial infusion.[74] Adverse myocardial effects of vasopressin are present with both techniques but probably more so with the intravenous method.

The bleeding artery may be so large that vasopressin is not effective. In such cases transcatheter embolic control of the hemorrhage or balloon occlusion of the artery has been tried when, for one reason or another, surgery could not be performed.[14, 70, 75-79] The most commonly used embolic material has been autogenous clot or its modifications, with the addition of Gelfoam or oxidized cellulose (Oxycel). The results are, on the whole, successful; but it has been stressed repeatedly that it is important to be very close to the site of bleeding to avoid reflux of embolic material or unnecessary widespread infarction. Even if a few investigators have reported no complications, most have experienced some unintentional infarctions.[18, 75, 79, 80] Thus, duodenal and gastric-wall necroses are reported with this technique.

VENOUS HEMORRHAGE. — Intravenous vasopressin infusion has long been used together with the Sengstaken-Blakemore tube in the control of bleeding varices in patients with portal hypertension. Intra-arterial vasopressin infusion was found to lower the portal vein pressure by 35–50%,[1, 81] and control of variceal bleeding was achieved in 80–90% of patients. Recent studies,

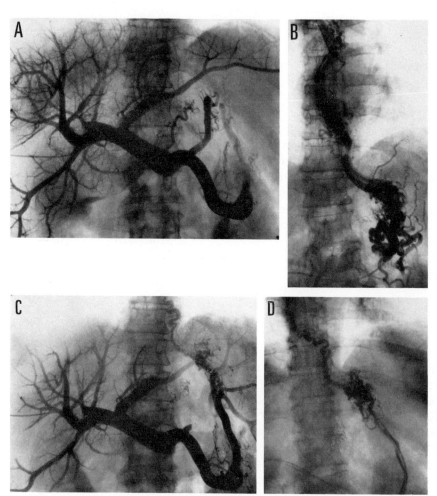

Fig 4. – Portal hypertension and bleeding esophageal varices in 63-year-old woman. Percutaneous transhepatic portography. **A,** portal vein pressure at 40 cm H_2O with retrograde filling of two coronary veins. **B,** at selective catheterization of the wider of the two veins, wide esophageal varices are filled. **C,** obliteration of the two coronary veins with bucrylate followed by portography reveals that the varices are now filled from short gastric veins. **D,** the short gastric veins were later catheterized and obliterated with bucrylate.

however, have shown that intra-arterial vasopressin infusion causes systemic effects and that the portal vein pressure is reduced to almost the same degree as by venous infusion.[74, 81]

Catheterization and obliteration of veins feeding esophageal varices after transhepatic access to the portal vein was introduced by Lunderquist and Vang in 1974[82] (Fig 4). This obliteration originally was performed with hypertonic glucose, thrombin and Gelfoam. The method has since been tried in smaller and larger groups of patients with portal hypertension. Usually Gelfoam has been used as an embolization agent, but nonabsorbable material such as isobutyl-2-cyanoacrylate also has been tried. When thrombin and Gelfoam are used, recanalization almost always occurs.[27] Nonabsorbable material has not been shown to prevent recanalization, but when this is the case the recanalized veins have a much reduced diameter.[41] Moreover, new collaterals between the portal vein and the esophageal varices can open up, which is why the procedure has not been used as permanent treatment but rather as a way to stop bleeding and prevent emergency portacaval shunt operation.

ISCHEMIA. — An embolus of the superior mesenteric artery may cause spasms of branches proximal and distal to the occlusion. These can be released with tolazoline.[83] Preoperative superior mesenteric angiography followed by vasodilating substances given intra-arterially will improve the prognosis. Also, in patients with nonocclusive bowel ischemia, intra-arterial vasodilatation has become successful. This previously fatal disease probably is caused by an intense vasoconstriction, which can be converted if intra-arterial vasodilatation starts before signs of peritonitis occur. Angiography is essential to prove the presence of intense vasoconstriction and to rule out other causes of bowel ischemia, such as an embolus or venous thrombosis.[84] When the characteristic angiogram is obtained and no peritonitis is present, papaverine diluted with normal saline is injected at a rate of 3 mg/minute for 15–20 minutes.[84] Finally, an additional bolus of 30 mg papaverine is given rapidly and the superior mesenteric angiogram is repeated. If a positive response is observed, papaverine is infused at a constant rate of 30–60 mg/hour for a varying period of time depending on the clinical situation. When the papaverine test fails, tolazoline, phenoxybenzamine[85] or prostaglandin E_1[86] should be tested.

IDIOPATHIC ULCERATIVE COLITIS. — Steroids given orally have

long been used in the treatment of ulcerative colitis, sometimes with a reasonably good effect. It was recently reported that injection of prednisolone into superior and inferior mesenteric arteries in patients with ulcerative colitis often causes marked clinical improvement of the condition.[87] We have tested this method of treatment in patients with exaggerated symptoms of ulcerative colitis but have found only temporary improvement. For patients with toxic dilatation we would like to stress the risk of perforation during the steroid treatment.

Liver

HEMOBILIA AND BLEEDING FROM HEPATIC TRAUMA. — Bleeding through the bile ducts into the gastrointestinal tract may occur from blunt hepatic trauma, aneurysms of the hepatic artery secondary to liver biopsy, and liver tumors. To control this kind of hemorrhage, extensive surgery often is necessary, with lobectomy or ligation of the hepatic artery. Recently a nonsurgical method of treatment was performed by transcatheter embolization of the right hepatic artery with Gelfoam in a patient with postbiopsy hemobilia.[88] Several other reports have demonstrated the successful arterial embolization of hemobilia and massive bleeding from blunt hepatic trauma.[89-91] In at least one case the embolization was lifesaving. In another patient treated with hepatic embolization, planned surgery never became necessary because of complete control of bleeding.

Hepatic function has been studied after experimental hepatic-artery embolization in dogs.[92] Hepatocellular damage was produced and liverfunction test results were not normalized until after six weeks. To reduce hepatic necrosis it was suggested that antibiotics be administered and that the presence of adequate portal blood supply to the liver be ascertained before embolization. Since about 70% of the blood supply to the normal liver comes from the portal vein, liver necrosis is supposed to develop if the hepatic artery is occluded when portal blood flow is insufficient from portal vein thrombosis or liver cirrhosis.

After embolization of the hepatic artery, rapid revascularization develops from arteries in the hepatoduodenal ligament and from the inferior phrenic artery. Gallbladder infarction, however, has occurred after hepatic artery embolization.[93, 94]

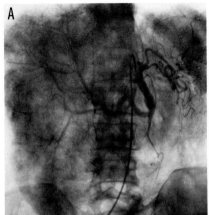
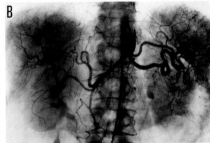
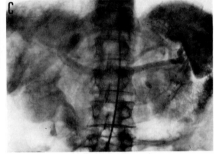

Fig 5. — Liver metastases from carcinoma of the colon in a 65-year-old woman. A, at celiac angiography the liver is enormously enlarged and filled with metastases. B and C, repeat angiography four months later after transbrachial 5-fluorouracil treatment with catheter into common hepatic artery, shows the liver to be of normal size. Multiple biopsies at exploratory laparotomy could not demonstrate viable tumor cells.

ARTERIAL INFUSION OF ANTICARCINOGENIC DRUGS. — Many different methods currently are used to control tumor growth in the liver including radiation, liver resection, liver dearterialization, cytostatic therapy and combinations of these. Cytostatic therapy can be administered orally, intravenously, intraportally or intra-arterially. As liver malignancies are supplied mainly by hepatic arteries, regional intra-arterial infusion should be the best way to administer the cytostatic drug. This has been tried for many years and has shown an increased survival time of the patients in comparison with that of nontreated patients. Tumor regression was confirmed angiographically in about 50% of cases[97] (Fig 5). The presence of liver metastasis is shown and the hepatic vascular anatomy is defined by celiac and superior mesenteric angiography, after which the infusion catheter is introduced into the left brachial artery about 10 cm proximal to the antecubital fossa. The radiopaque catheter (OD-inside diameter [ID], 1.58/1.14) is positioned with the tip in the proper or common hepatic artery. The most commonly used anticarcinogenic drug is 5-fluorouracil which is infused in a daily dose of 500 mg. The period of infusion varies between a few weeks and several months, depending on the clinical situation.

The percutaneously introduced catheter frequently is passed from the left brachial artery,[95-98] but some workers prefer the femoral route.[99] Complications from an indwelling catheter are common. Thus, occlusion of the brachial artery frequently is observed when the catheter is extracted at the end of intra-arterial infusion. No severe complications due to brachial artery thrombosis have been observed, however. Thrombus formation at the tip of the catheter with secondary hepatic embolization, occlusion of the common hepatic artery and marked wall irregularities have been noted. These complications occur despite the fact that the patients received systemic heparinization.[99] Aneurysm formation in the common hepatic artery also has been observed probably because the tip of the catheter, together with the drug, causes an intimal lesion. Infection at the puncture site and mycotic emboli have occurred. Cracking and leakage of the catheters are frequent problems with a long infusion period.[98] The tendency, at the present time, is to shorten the infusion time and perform repeated infusions at intervals depending on the patient's general condition.

ARTERIAL EMBOLIZATION. — Hepatic dearterialization through ligation of the arteries supplying the liver has been tried for many years as a palliative method of therapy and also has been combined with chemotherapy. The patient can be spared the surgical procedure necessary for ligation of the vascular supply of the liver if transcatheter embolization of the hepatic artery is performed. Furthermore, the emboli pass far out and come close to the metastases. This seems to be more effective than hepatic artery ligation, where collateral channels soon open up to compensate the ligation.

After arterial Gelfoam embolization, liver metastases decrease in size.[37, 100] Patients often are relieved of pain. To prevent recanalization of the arteries, additional obliteration with a stainless steel coil has been suggested.[37] The materials reported are too small and follow-up has been too short to evaluate the long-term effect of this kind of treatment. The combination of cytostatic agents and short- or long-term occlusion is another way to attack the problem.[49, 100]

As in patients previously reported on who were treated for

hepatic hemorrhage, complications may occur such as gangrene of the gallbladder or renal infarctions.[94] Contraindications for hepatic embolization are portal hypertension and hepatic insufficiency.[100]

DRAINAGE OF ABSCESSES AND CYSTS.—The percutaneous technique used for angiography is now also available for drainage of hepatic abscesses and cysts.[101, 102] Radiologic or ultrasonic localization of the lesion is followed by percutaneous drainage after injection of contrast medium to define the size and extent of the lesion. In many instances the method can replace exploration and drainage, and in other cases it can make the surgical exploration easier.

PERCUTANEOUS BILE DRAINAGE IN PATIENTS WITH OBSTRUCTIVE JAUNDICE.—Percutaneous transhepatic cholangiography first was performed as a diagnostic procedure for detection of obstructive jaundice immediately before surgery. Later, the procedure was combined with the introduction of a catheter into the bile ducts for external drainage until operation.[103, 104] In this way, external drainage could be established for one to two weeks preoperatively, during which time the condition of the patient improved; or the drainage could continue up to one year in patients with nonresectable tumors.[105]

For drainage of bile ducts, a 15-cm needle (OD, 0.9 mm) is inserted during fluoroscopy with the Shiba-needle technique from the right midaxillary line parallel to the table top and directed toward the estimated position of the hilum of the liver.[106] During retraction of the needle, contrast medium is slowly injected. When the contrast medium passes into dilated bile ducts, retraction is stopped and the bile ducts are filled. The needle is then withdrawn and radiographs are taken for location of site and, if possible, extent of obstruction. For decompression and bile drainage the opacified bile ducts are punctured again from the right midaxillary line with a 25-cm needle coated with a radiopaque polyethylene catheter (OD/ID, 1.6/1.1 mm). The bile duct is punctured during fluoroscopy and the needle is withdrawn. A 0.9-mm guide wire with a slightly curved, soft tip is introduced and is passed to the site of the obstruction. If the obstruction is not complete the guide wire is allowed to pass to the duodenum. The catheter is withdrawn and replaced with a final drainage catheter (OD/ID, 2.2/1.4 mm) which is passed, if possible, over the guide wire into the duodenum. Multiple side holes in the

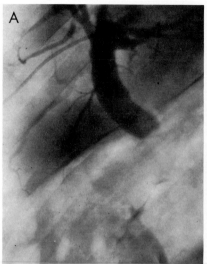
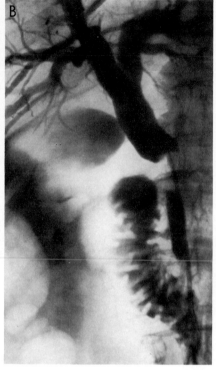

Fig 6. – Seventy-five-year-old man with jaundice. **A,** percutaneous transhepatic cholangiography, dilated bile ducts were present and common bile duct was occluded. Percutaneous biopsy: cholangiocarcinoma. **B,** catheter with several side-holes was passed through the obstruction down into the duodenum for combined internal-external drainage.

catheter positioned above as well as below the stricture can provide internal drainage[106-108] (Fig 6).

Occasionally, the obstruction cannot be passed by the catheter. After a few days of drainage and irrigation of the bile ducts, another attempt is made to pass the obstruction and is then often successful. Daily checkups of the catheter position are made and readjustment often is required during the first few days.

Transhepatic introduction of endoprosthesis also has been performed successfully after removal of the external drainage catheter.[109, 110] Complications from the transhepatic drainage procedure are few, including bile leakage, cholangitis and intraabdominal hemorrhage.[105, 107] To reduce these complications, one or two chunks of Gelfoam can be introduced into the liver parenchyma just below the capsule when the catheter is extracted.

EXTRACTION OF RETAINED BILIARY TRACT STONES. – In spite of

intraoperative cholangiography, retained stones in bile ducts after surgery are not an unusual finding at postoperative cholangiography; a large number of patients therefore must undergo reoperation each year. Burhenne in 1972[54] introduced a new technique of nonoperative stone extraction. His first report included 20 patients with retained stones, in whom stone removal was possible in 19 without any complication. Only in one patient was the procedure unsuccessful, necessitating surgical removal.

Nonoperative extraction of retained stones is now an established procedure that involves very few complications. Burhenne[111] reviewed the complications of stone extraction encountered in 612 patients at 38 institutions in the United States. No fatalities occurred. Reoperation for failure of stone extraction was necessary in 9% of patients. A large number of patients were treated as outpatients. The author reports that most important for a successful result is that the indwelling T tube is large enough (larger than 4 mm OD) and kept in place for ten weeks in order to form a fibrous wall of the sinus tract. After removal of the T tube, a "steerable" catheter is introduced with the tip pointing at the stone. A Dormia stone basket is introduced and the stone is retracted. Stones larger than 10 mm usually cannot pass the sinus tract but they usually can be fragmented by forceful traction of the open basket into the sinus tract or by closure of the basket. Complications are rare but septicemia may follow prolonged and difficult instrumentation.

Pancreas

Percutaneous aspiration biopsy has been a valuable adjunct in the diagnosis of malignancy in the bile ducts and pancreas.[105] When an avascular pancreatic lesion is observed at angiography, this procedure is immediately followed by percutaneous puncture for cytology. If fluid is withdrawn, the diagnosis of a pancreatic pseudocyst can be made both by cytology and by contrast medium injection. We have found it valuable in these cases to decompress the cyst either by immediate aspiration of its content or by drainage of the cyst through a percutaneously introduced catheter.

Pseudoaneurysm of the pancreas may cause severe gastrointestinal hemorrhage and sometimes may cause hemobilia. One patient has been successfully treated percutaneously by electrocoagulation through a guide wire with alternating current,[112] and several others have been treated by embolization, balloon catheter or vasopressin infusion.[113]

Spleen

Splenic artery ligation has been tried in an attempt to reduce the portal blood flow in patients with portal hypertension and bleeding esophageal varices. When splenic artery ligation was performed in cirrhotic patients with hypersplenism, platelet counts were found to increase markedly.[114] The advantage with splenic artery ligation in cirrhotic patients with hypersplenism thus was twofold: first, the portal blood flow was reduced with maintained liver circulation; and second, thrombocytopenia was reduced.

Nonsurgical occlusion with transcatheter embolization of the splenic artery with autologous blood clots, Gelfoam, fibrinfoam, silicone spheres and steel coils combined with Gelfoam has been performed experimentally and clinically.[17, 37, 115-120] The problem of splenic abscess formation has been severe both in experimental and clinical series.[37, 116, 118] At our institution we have treated 11 patients with portal hypertension and hypersplenism with embolization of the splenic artery with Gelfoam (Fig 7). A splenic abscess usually was formed when the splenic artery was obliterated completely. However, in patients in whom one-third to one-fourth of the spleen was infarcted, no abscess developed and the procedure could be repeated several times with one- to two-month intervals, successively reducing the size of the spleen. Marked increase in platelet counts followed each embolization procedure, which confirms findings in other reports. Experimentally as well as clinically it has been observed that even "complete" dearterialization does not result in a completely atrophic and nonfunctional spleen.

In severely ill patients with portal hypertension, where other conservative attempts to stop variceal bleeding were unsuccessful and emergency shunt operation was impossible to carry out, embolization of the splenic artery was performed as an alternative method.[120] The bleeding could be stopped for some time so that an interval was obtained during which liver function could improve and surgery could become possible.

Experimental[117, 119] and clinical[26] experience of splenic artery

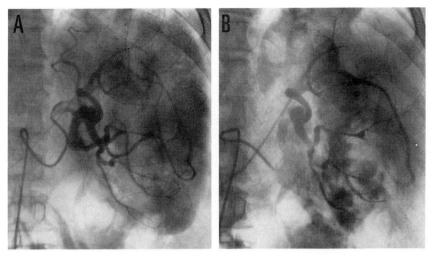

Fig 7.—Hypersplenism in a 61-year-old man with portal hypertension. Selective splenic angiogram before (**A**) and after (**B**) 50% embolization of the spleen with Gelfoam.

embolization in trauma have been reported with Amicar-mixed blood clots, Gelfoam and silicone spheres. It appears that Gelfoam or silicone spheres should be used if a longer duration of the occlusion is desired.

Without doubt, splenic artery embolization has a place in those cases where angiography has demonstrated a ruptured spleen. Emergency angiography often is performed in order to localize the site and define the extent of bleeding. If a ruptured spleen is found, embolization of the splenic artery is a reasonable way to prevent further hemorrhage until surgical splenectomy is performed.

UROGENITAL RADIOLOGY

Kidney

BENIGN CYSTS.—Benign solitary renal cysts usually are asymptomatic and are discovered accidentally at urography in about 2% of cases. Symptoms are rare, but flank discomfort and hematuria are supposed to be related to the cysts. Complications are few and may include hypertension and caliceal obstruction. When simple percutaneous aspiration of the cyst is performed, very soon the cyst will return to its previous size. As early as 1939 Fish[121] reported his experience with instillation of 50% dextrose as a sclerosing agent for treating benign cysts. Also, injection of a hypertonic contrast medium to verify the urographic diagnosis is said to cause a reduction in size and, sometimes, disappearance of the cyst. The first extensive report on percutaneous treatment of benign renal cysts was published

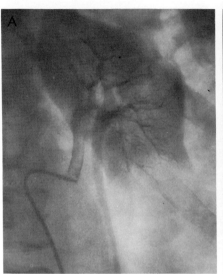
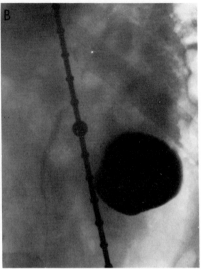
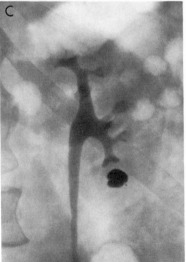

Fig 8.—Benign cyst of the lower pole of the kidney demonstrated at selective left renal angiography (**A**) in a 55-year-old man. **B**, percutaneous puncture of the cyst with injection of contrast medium plus 2 ml of Pantopaque. **C**, urography six years later showed marked reduction of the size of the cyst.

by Vestby,[122] who injected isophendylate (Pantopaque) into the cysts of 20 patients with a follow-up of 2–46 months. In all patients the cysts either decreased in size or disappeared (Fig 8). A control series on 71 patients has shown that Pantopaque instillation is superior to simple aspiration.[123]

The clinical importance of this kind of treatment can be discussed, since symptoms related to the presence of the cyst are few or nonexisting unless the cyst is of remarkable size or is compressing the renal pelvis. A cystic lesion observed at urography, ultrasonography, angiography or CAT scan must be punctured for diagnostic reasons to exclude malignancy. The cyst fluid is extracted and is examined by cytology for its histochemical content. Contrast medium is injected for demonstration of any wall irregularities that could signify cancer. Systematic treatment combined with these tests by injection of a sclerosing agent is advantageous. The complications are few in experienced hands and occur mainly in puncture of upper-pole cysts, when pneumothorax may occur.

PERCUTANEOUS PYELOSTOMY. – In cases of hydronephrosis of malignant origin, surgery with cutaneous pyelostomy to improve the renal parenchyma was the rule, later followed by surgical repair of the obstruction. Total obstruction of the urine outflow from the kidney will soon produce irreparable damage to the organ if not relieved. Percutaneous puncture of the renal pelvis with introduction of a catheter (Fig 9) therefore has been used widely in recent years to relieve acute infectious obstruction as well as various types of chronic obstruction.[124-128] In emergency cases, nephrostomy was mainly performed because of azotemia, infection or sepsis, or when the clinical condition precluded surgical correction.[125, 127] Another advantage with the method is that the antegrade pyelogram is technically superior to the urogram and will give helpful information on the cause of obstruction. With the assistance of CAT scanning it appears to be a rather simple method to reach the renal pelvis in patients in whom no hydronephrosis is present.[128] When this technique is not available, puncture with the guidance of fluoroscopy or ultrasound is possible. If the kidney is still functioning, contrast medium is injected to localize the renal pelvis. If the kidney is silent – which most often is the case – the patient is placed prone and the kidney is localized with a survey film or ultrasound. The renal pelvis is punctured with a 15-cm needle (OD, 0.9 mm) and

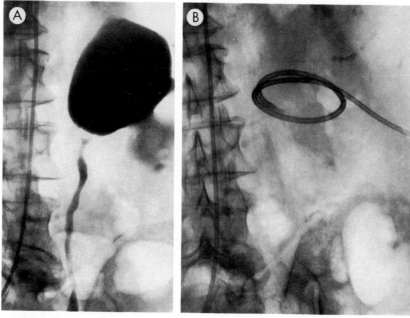

Fig 9. — Seventy-six-year-old woman with pyonephrosis. **A,** left renal pelvis injected with contrast medium through percutaneous puncture. **B,** catheter with multiple side-holes introduced percutaneously and coiled in the renal pelvis for drainage.

contrast medium is injected during fluoroscopy. For the percutaneous drainage a posterolateral approach is taken. The same catheter-needle combination as for bile drainage is selected. With the aid of biplane fluoroscopy one can easily find the dilated renal pelvis. After withdrawal of the needle, a guide wire is introduced followed by a catheter in the same manner previously described for the bile ducts — with the tip, if possible, in the ureter. Daily checkup during the first few days is required to check the position of the tubing, which is replaced after a few days by a larger catheter with multiple side holes (OD/ID, 3.0/1.8 mm). Depending on the indications, a nephropyelostomy tube may be kept in place for a week or for several months. For permanent pyelostomy, a Foley catheter should be installed. This can be accomplished by widening the canal using larger tubes over a period of several days or weeks.[124]

Percutaneous puncture of the renal pelvis has also been an incentive for percutaneous pyelolithotomy.[56] The same technique that is used for pyelostomy is used. The sinus tract is dilated daily with increasing sizes of Couvelaire catheters. When the adequate diameter is obtained the catheter is left in place for 14 days. The stone is extracted with Dormia stone baskets or stone-grasping forceps.

TRANSCATHETER OCCLUSION OF THE RENAL ARTERY. — Most often the indication for renal artery embolization is massive hematuria secondary to trauma, arteriovenous fistula, pseudoaneurysm or tumor. In renal carcinoma intractable pain and inoperability also have been reasons for embolization. Other indications have been therapeutic renal infarction in end-stage renal disease in patients who require nephrectomy.[129] Experimental studies have shown injection of autogenous blood clots into the renal artery to be useful to stop hemorrhage from a traumatized kidney.[130] Without doubt, this is a nonsurgical alternative to nephrectomy or resection.[131, 132] It also may be the treatment of choice in a patient with multiple trauma whose general condition makes surgery hazardous.

Iatrogenic trauma from renal biopsy or surgery can produce pseudoaneurysms or arteriovenous fistulae causing hematuria, hypertension and even heart failure. Surgical treatment of these lesions without nephrectomy may be difficult or impossible. Transcatheter embolization of the segmental artery feeding the lesion is a feasible alternative in preserving the function of at least part of the kidney. Different embolization agents have been used including autologous clots,[15] Gelfoam,[131] steel coils[37] and cyanoacrylate.[133]

Theoretically, renal hypertension can be produced from ischemia peripheral to the embolized artery. This has not been possible to prove by experimental studies.[130] In clinically treated patients, hypertension has not been found to be a problem.[133, 134] In fact, hypertension caused by segmental renal artery stenosis has been treated by injection of sterile barium and Gelfoam.[135]

In cases of embolization for nonmalignant hemorrhages, autogenous clots seem to be preferred to other embolization agents because of their relatively short duration of occlusion.

Resectable as well as nonresectable renal tumors have been treated with renal artery embolization. As early as 1971 Lang did clinical experiments with radioactive gold particles to produce a radiation nephrectomy.[35] The reasons for embolization of resectable renal tumors are to achieve a preoperative reduction of tumor size and to facilitate surgery by reduced bleeding.[134] The indications for embolization of nonresectable tumors are: (1) treatment of hematuria, (2) reduction of tumor size, (3) pain relief, and (4) influence on the immunologic response of the body.

Even if there is no convincing proof thus far of an immunoresponse, metastases have been seen to be reduced in size or disappear after embolization of the primary tumor (see Fig 2). When the renal artery supplying the tumor is embolized, a long-lasting occlusion is desirable; autogenous clot or Gelfoam thus is less suitable. Wallace et al.[37] introduced a steel coil with wool strands that could cause permanent occlusion of the renal artery (see Fig 1). Isobutyl-2-cyanoacrylate is another agent that is reputed to produce permanent vascular occlusion which has been used in the renal artery.[133, 136]

Occlusion of the renal artery with a balloon catheter is another method used to facilitate operation of a renal carcinoma.[10, 137] The inflatable balloon is placed in the renal artery and is inflated just before operation. This seems to be the preferred method since it will not produce the complications that can be expected with embolization. Another indication for renal artery occlusion with balloon catheters not mentioned previously is in cases of extensive pyelolithotomy or other complicated surgical procedures to be performed in the kidney.[137] Temporary balloon occlusion with continuous perfusion of the kidney with hypothermic solutions (4 C) is an advantage for several reasons. One is that the ischemic period can be much longer; another is that the renal pedicle need never be dissected and traumatized during operation. In the future, balloon catheters may also be used for percutaneous dilatation of renal artery stenosis.

Side effects from renal artery embolization may occur. Severe pain lasting for 4–8 hours is common. Depending on the size of the embolized tumor, fever of one to several days' duration is seen as a reaction to the tissue necrosis. When Gelfoam, autogenous clot or cyanoacrylate is used, complications with spillover into the aorta of the embolization material easily occur, with embolization into the contralateral kidney or peripheral arteries. Spinal cord infarction also has been reported.[138] In order to prevent these serious complications as a result of spillover of embolic material, a balloon catheter might be helpful.[139]

LOWER URINARY TRACT AND GENITAL ORGANS. — Bladder tumors have been treated with radioactive spheres injected into the hypogastric arteries.[35] Since the particles cannot be placed selectively into the vesical arteries, the method does not seem to have been taken up by other authors. Infusion of cytostatic agents in the hypogastric arteries for bladder and gynecologic tumors[52] probably will be a future alternative to surgical and radiotherapeutic procedures.

Embolization of vesical and genital vessels are on record for therapy of massive bleeding from the bladder and urethra[23, 101, 140] and pelvic malignancies.[101, 141] Bleeding from arteries after genitourinary tract surgery also can be managed by occlusive therapy.[142]

RADIOLOGY OF TRUNK AND LIMBS

Trauma

Angiography has been proven to be of great value in assessing the extent and degree of parenchymatous lesions in abdominal trauma. As previously mentioned, embolization has been performed in extravasation due to hepatic, splenic or renal rupture. The same is true for any extravasation due to trauma. Thus in uncontrollable hemorrhage from intercostal arteries[143] and from lacerated branches of the internal iliac arteries secondary to pelvic fracture or surgical trauma,[144, 145] embolization has been performed. The site of bleeding can be localized by selective angiography; and to prevent the forming of overly massive hematomas and loss of blood, embolization of the lacerated artery with blood clots, Gelfoam or steel coils can be performed (Fig 10). Balloon catheters also have been proven to be highly effective in this respect.[8]

Vascular Lesions

VASCULAR OCCLUSION THERAPY. — Embolization of vascular malformations of trunk and limbs with Gelfoam has been performed with definite immediate success.[146] It is too soon at the present time to discuss the prognosis for embolization in vascular malformations of the limbs, as well as in other treated vascular malformations. However, embolization should never be regarded as an alternative to surgery, but rather as an adjunct to future surgery.

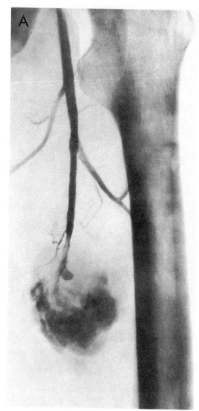
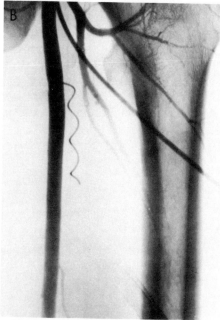

Fig 10.—A, profuse bleeding from mycotic aneurysm of a branch of left deep femoral artery demonstrated at arteriography of deep femoral artery. B, after occlusion with a steel coil, repeat angiography with injection into common femoral artery shows no further extravasation.

Aortic rupture is another condition for which radiologic assistance in the future will be an important support.[147] A Fogarty catheter may be introduced via the left axillary artery after arteriotomy. This acts as a tamponade for the aorta above the rupture until it is possible to perform surgical repair.

Partial occlusion of the inferior vena cava to prevent embolization from iliac and lower-leg thrombosis has become an established procedure.[46] The miniature umbrella introduced from a cut-down on the internal jugular vein via a catheter has replaced the original surgical ligation of the vena cava. A new method is now available where a pliable wire of mitinol is passed through a percutaneously introduced catheter.[148] The wire has unique thermal-shaped memory properties. Straight in room temperature, it becomes coiled at body temperature and acts as a filter when it becomes fixed in the inferior vena cava.

VASCULAR DILATATION. — In ischemic conditions of the limbs, certain vasodilators have been found to be quite efficient intraarterially. Thus reserpine has proven to be effective for frostbite,[149] sodium nitroprusside, for ergotism[150] and prostaglandin E_1, for severe peripheral vascular disease.[151]

Mechanical dilatation of stenosed arteries has changed somewhat since its introduction in 1964[47] but the technique is basically the same. A guide wire first is passed through the stenosed area followed by a small Teflon catheter. When this has passed through the stenosis, a wider Teflon catheter (OD, 4 mm) is passed over the first one and forced through the stenosed area in the same way as dilatation of stenosed regions is performed during surgery. A Teflon catheter with a small, tapered tip and gradually increasing diameter is a recent modification.[152] Thus only the guide wire and one catheter are used for recanalization of the femoropopliteal area. Both methods have certain drawbacks, including the risk that a large-bore catheter may cause complications in terms of hemorrhage at the puncture site, and the risk of embolization because of the technique. The main purpose of the recanalization technique is to force, by dilatation, arteriosclerotic materials into the wall of the arteries. This is now better accomplished with the recent development of a distensible segment of polyvinyl chloride, which is placed on a double lumen catheter[153] (OD/ID, 2.8/1.2 mm). When compared with other balloon catheters made of latex, the distensible segment is extremely rigid and can resist high pressures. The diameter of the distensible part is 4 – 5 mm when the superficial femoral artery is catheterized. Stenosed iliac arteries can be distended to a diameter of 8 mm. If anticoagulation and exercise are included in the treatment, the effect of the dilatation is remarkably high.[154] The results thus are promising and attempts are now also being made to correct renal artery stenosis with this method.

REFERENCES

1. Baum, S., Athanasoulis, C. A., Waltman, A. C., and Ring, E. J.: Angiographic diagnosis and control of gastrointestinal bleeding, in Welch, C. (ed.): *Survey of the Stomach and Duodenum*, Vol. 7 (Chicago: Year Book Medical Publishers, Inc., 1973.), pp. 149 – 198.

2. Baum, S., and Nusbaum, M.: The control of gastrointestinal hemorrhage by selective mesenteric arterial infusion of vasopressin, Radiology 98: 497, 1971.
3. Baum, S., Rösch, J., Dotter, C. T., et al.: Selective mesenteric arterial infusions in the management of massive diverticular hemorrhage, N. Engl. J. Med. 288:1269, 1973.
4. Rösch, J., Dotter, C. T., and Antonovic, R.: Selective vasoconstrictor infusion in the management of arterio-capillary gastrointestinal hemorrhage, Am. J. Roentgenol. Radium Ther. Nucl. Med. 116:279, 1972.
5. Athanasoulis, C. A., Brown, B., and Shapiro, J. H.: Angiography in the diagnosis and management of bleeding stress ulcers and gastritis, Am. J. Surg. 125:468, 1973.
6. Athanasoulis, C. A., Waltman, A. C., Ring, E. J., et al.: Angiographic management of postoperative bleeding, Radiology 113:37, 1974.
7. Wholey, M. H., Stockdale, R., and Hung, T. K.: A percutaneous balloon catheter for the immediate control of hemorrhage, Radiology 96:65, 1970.
8. Paster, S. B., Van Houten, F. X., and Adams, D. F.: Percutaneous balloon catheterization; a technique for the control of arterial hemorrhage caused by pelvic trauma, JAMA 230:573, 1974.
9. Serbinenko, F. A.: Balloon catheterization and occlusion of major cerebral vessels, J. Neurosurg. 41:125, 1974.
10. Marberger, M., and Georgi, M.: Balloon occlusion of the renal artery in tumor nephrectomy, J. Urol. 114:360, 1975.
11. Wholey, M. H., Kessler, L., and Boehnke, M.: A percutaneous balloon catheter technique for the treatment of intracranial aneurysm, Acta Radiol. [Diagn.] (Stockh.) 18:286, 1972.
12. Manelfe, C., and Djindjian, R.: Techniques de l'embolisation thérapeutique par cathéterisme percutané, J. Neuroradiologie 2:11, 1975.
13. Hilal, S. K., Michelsen, W. J., Driller, J., and Leonard, E.: Magnetically guided devices for vascular exploration and treatment. Laboratory and clinical investigations, Radiology 113:529, 1974.
14. Rösch, J., Dotter, C. T., and Brown, M. J.: Selective arterial embolization: New method for control of acute gastrointestinal bleeding, Radiology 102:303, 1972.
15. Bookstein, J. J., and Goldstein, H. M.: Successful management of postbiopsy arteriovenous fistula with selective arterial embolization, Radiology 109:535, 1973.
16. Osterman, F. A., Bell, W. R., Montali, R. J., and White, R. I.: Natural history of blood clot embolization in swine, Invest. Radiol. 11:267, 1976.
17. Chuang, V. P., and Reuter, S. R.: Experimental diminution of splenic function by selective embolization of splenic artery, Surg. Gynecol. Obstet. 140:715, 1975.
18. Bookstein, J. J., Chlosta, E. M., Foley, D., and Walter, J. F.: Transcatheter hemostasis of gastrointestinal bleeding using modified autogenous clot, Radiology 113:277, 1974.
19. Brooks, B.: The treatment of traumatic arteriovenous fistula, South. Med. J. 23:100, 1930.
20. Almgård, L. E., Fernström, I., Haverling, M., and Ljungqvist, A.: Treat-

ment of renal adenocarcinoma by embolic occlusion of the renal circulation, Br. J. Urol. 45:474, 1973.
21. Lalli, A. F., Bookstein, J. J., and Lapides, J.: Experimental renal infarction in dogs, Invest. Urol. 8:516, 1971.
22. Steckenmesser, R., Bayindir, S., Rothauge, C. F., et al.: Embolisation maligner Nierentumoren, Fortschr. Röntgenstr. 125:251, 1976.
23. Hald, T. and Mygind, T.: Control of life-threatening vesical hemorrhage by unilateral hypogastric artery muscle embolization, J. Urol. 112:60, 1974.
24. Hekster, R. E. M., Luyendijk, W., and Matricali, B.: Transfemoral catheter embolization: a method of treatment of glomus jugulare tumors, Neuroradiology 5:208, 1972.
25. Rizk, G. K., Atallah, N. K., and Bridi, G. I.: Renal arteriovenous fistula treated by catheter embolization, Br. J. Radiol. 46:222, 1973.
26. Katzen, B. T., Rossi, P., Passariello, R., and Simonetti, G.: Transcatheter therapeutic arterial embolization, Radiology 120:523, 1976.
27. Lunderquist, A., Simert, G., Tylén, U., and Vang, J.: Follow-up of patients with portal hypertension and esophageal varices treated with percutaneous obliteration of gastric coronary vein, Radiology 122:59, 1977.
28. Porstmann, W., Wierny, L., Warnke, H., et al.: Catheter closure of patent ductus arteriosus, Radiol. Clin. North. Am. 9:203, 1971.
29. Tadavarthy, S. M., Moller, J. H., and Amplatz, K.: Polyvinyl alcohol (Ivalon)–a new embolic material, Am. J. Roentgen. Radium Ther. Nucl. Med. 125:609, 1975.
30. Fleischer, A. S., Kricheff, J., and Ransohoff, J.: Postmortem findings following the embolization of an arteriovenous malformation, J. Neurosurg. 37:606, 1972.
31. Luessenhop, A. J., and Spence, W. T.: Artificial embolization of cerebral arteries; report of use in a case of arteriovenous malformation, JAMA 172:1153, 1960.
32. Doppman, J. L., Di Chiro, G., and Ommaya, A.: Obliteration of spinal cord arteriovenous malformation by percutaneous embolization, Lancet 131:477, 1968.
33. Bischoff, W., Kauffmann, R., Rohrbach, R., and Wenzel, G.: Permanent stop of renal circulation by embolization with microspheres. Angiographic and histologic findings, Urol. Res. 5:38, 1977.
34. Kauffmann, G., Bischoff, W., Wimmer, B., and Roth, F.-J.: Die wertigkeit experimenteller Arterienverschlüsse unter besonderer Berücksichtigung ihrer Komplikationen. Fortschr. Röntgenstr. 125:445, 1976.
35. Lang, E. K.: Superselective arterial catheterization as a vehicle for delivering radioactive infarct particles to tumors, Radiology 98:391, 1971.
36. Gianturco, C., Anderson, J. H., and Wallace, S.: Mechanical devices for arterial occlusion, Am. J. Roentgenol. Radium Ther. Nucl. Med. 124:428, 1975.
37. Wallace, S., Gianturco, C., Anderson, J. H., et al.: Therapeutic vascular occlusion utilizing steel coil technique. Clinical applications, Am. J. Roentgenol. Radium Ther. Nucl. Med. 127:381, 1976.
38. Zanetti, P. H., and Sherman, F. E.: Experimental evaluation of a tissue

adhesive as an agent for the treatment of aneurysms and arteriovenous anomalies, J. Neurosurg. 36:72, 1972.
39. Kerber, C.: Experimental arteriovenous fistula. Creation and percutaneous catheter obstruction with cyano-acrylate, Invest. Radiol. 10:10, 1975.
40. Dotter, C. T., Goldman, M. L., and Rösch, J.: Instant selective arterial occlusion with isobutyl-2-cyanoacrylate, Radiology 114:227, 1975.
41. Lunderquist, A., Börjesson, B., Owman, T., and Bengmark, S.: Isobuthyl-2-cyanoacrylate (Bucrylate) in obliteration of gastric coronary vein and esophegeal varices, Am. J. Roentgenol. Radium Ther. Nucl. Med. 130:1, 1978.
42. Bücheler, E., Hupe, W., Hertel, E. U., und Klosterhalfen, H.: Katheterembolisation von Nierentumoren, Fortschr. Röntgenstr. 124:134, 1976.
43. Doppman, J. L., Zapol, W., and Pierce, J.: Transcatheter embolization with a silicon rubber preparation; experimental observations, Invest. Radiol. 6:304, 1971.
44. Mosso, J. A., and Rand, R. W.: Ferromagnetic silicone vascular occlusions. A technique for selective infarction of tumors and organs, Ann. Surg. 178:663, 1973.
45. Phillips, J. F.: Transcatheter electrocoagulation of blood vessels, Invest. Radiol. 8:295, 1973.
46. Mobin-Uddin, K., Mc Lean, R., and Jude, J. R.: A new catheter technique of interruption of inferior vena cava for prevention of pulmonary embolism, Ann. Surg. 35:889, 1969.
47. Dotter, C. T., and Judkins, M. P.: Transluminal treatment of arteriosclerotic obstruction. Description of a technique and a preliminary report of its application, Circulation 30:654, 1964.
48. Bierman, H. R., Byron, R. L., Jr., Miller, E. R., and Shimkin, M. V.: Effects of intra-arterial administration of nitrogen mustard, Am. J. Med. 8: 535, 1950.
49. Rothman, U., Lindell, B., Aronsen, K. F., and Boijsen, E.: Unpublished data.
50. Miley, A. L., Jr., Wirtanen, G. W., Ansfield, F. J., and Ramirez, G.: Combined intra-arterial actinomycin D and radiation therapy for surgically unresectable hypernephroma, J. Urol. 114:198, 1975.
51. Suzuki, T., Kawabe, K., Imamura, M., et al.: Percutaneous double catheter infusion technique for the treatment of carcinoma in the abdomen, Surg. Gynecol. Obstet. 134:403, 1972.
52. Miyamoto, T., Tabake, Y., Watanabe, M., and Terasima, T.: Drastic remission effect of a sequential combination of bleomycin and mitomycin-C (B-M) on advanced cervical cancer, Cancer Chemother. Rep. 4:273, 1977.
53. Hellekant, C., Boijsen, E., and Svanberg, L.: Preoperative infusion of mitomycin-C in the bronchial artery in patients with squamous cell carcinoma of the lung, Acta Radiol. [Diagn.] (Stockh.), in press.
54. Burhenne, H. J.: Non-operative retained biliary tract stone extraction: A new roentgenologic technique, Am. J. Roentgenol. Radium Ther. Nucl. Med. 117:388, 1972.
55. Burhenne, H. J.: The technique of biliary duct stone extraction. Experience with 126 cases, Radiology 113:567, 1974.

56. Fernström, I., and Johansson, B.: Percutaneous pyelolithotomy. A new extraction technique, Scand. J. Urol. Nephrol. 10:257, 1976.
57. Samuelsson, L., and Olin, T.: Electrolytic Destruction of Lung Tissue. Paper presented at meeting of Swedish Society of Medical Radiology, November, 1977.
58. Djindjian, R., Cophignon, J., Theron, J., et al.: Embolization by super-selective arteriography from the femoral route in neurology; review of 60 cases. I. Techniques, indications, complications, Neuroradiology 6:20, 1973.
59. Kricheff, I. I., Madayag, M., and Braunstein, P.: Transfemoral catheter embolization of cerebral and posterior fossa arteriovenous malformations, Radiology 103:107, 1972.
60. Pevsner, P. H.: Micro-balloon catheter for superselective angiography and therapeutic occlusion, Am. J. Roentgenol. Radium Ther. Nucl. Med. 128:225, 1977.
61. Kerber, C.: Intracranial cyanoacrylate. A new catheter therapy for arteriovenous malformation, Invest. Radiol. 10:536, 1975.
62. Picard, L., André, J. M., Roland, J., et al.: L'embolisation dans les malformations vasculaire, méningo-cranio-cutanées complexes, J. Neuroradiologie 2:233, 1975.
63. Manelfe, C., Espagno, J., Guiraud, B., et al.: Embolisation thérapeutique des tumeurs cranio-cérébrales, J. Neuroradiologie 2:257, 1975.
64. Djindjian, R.: Indications, contre-indications, accidents, incidents dans l'embolisation de la carotide externe, J. Neuroradiologie 2:173, 1975.
65. Sokoloff, J., Wickbom, I., McDonald, D., et al.: Therapeutic percutaneous embolization in intractable epistaxis, Radiology 111:285, 1974.
66. Remy, J., Arnaud, A., Fardou, H., et al.: Treatment of hemoptysis by embolization of bronchial arteries, Radiology 122:33, 1977.
67. Helenon, C., Jacri, P., Akoun, G., et al.: Le traitment des hémoptysies par embolisation des artères systémiques, J. Radiol. Electrol. Med. Nucl. 57:487, 1976.
68. Wholey, M. H., Chamorro, H. A., Rao, G., et al.: Bronchial artery embolization for massive hemoptysis, JAMA 236:2501, 1976.
69. Doppman, J. L., Marx, S. J., Spiegel, A. M., et al.: Treatment of hyperparathyroidism by percutaneous embolization of a mediastinal adenoma, Radiology 115:37, 1975.
70. Ring, E. J., Oleaga, J. A., Freiman, D., et al.: Pitfalls in the angiographic management of hemorrhage: hemodynamic considerations, Am. J. Roentgenol. Radium Ther. Nucl. Med. 129:1007, 1977.
71. Berts, C., and Maddison, F. E.: Partial mesenteric arterial occlusion with subsequent ischemic bowel damage due to Pitressin infusion, Am. J. Roentgenol. Radium Ther. Nucl. Med. 126:829, 1976.
72. Bar Meir, S., and Conn, H. O.: Spontaneous bacterial peritonitis induced by intraarterial vasopressin therapy, Gastroenterology 70:418, 1976.
73. Renert, W. A., Button, K. F., Fuld, S. L., and Casarella, W. J.: Mesenteric venous thrombosis and small bowel infarction following infusion of vasopressin into the superior mesenteric artery, Radiology 102:299, 1972.
74. Athanasoulis, C. A., Waltman, A. C., Novelline, R. A., et al.: Angiogra-

phy: Its contribution to the emergency management of gastrointestinal hemorrhage, Radiol. Clin. North Am. 14:265, 1976.
75. Prochaska, J. M., Flye, M. W., and Johnsrude, J. S.: Left gastric artery embolization for control of gastric bleeding, Radiology 107:521, 1973.
76. Reuter, S. R., Chuang, V. P., and Bree, R. L.: Selective arterial embolization for control of massive upper gastrointestinal bleeding, Am. J. Roentgenol. Radium Ther. Nucl. Med. 125:119, 1975.
77. Bradley, E. L. III, and Goldman, M. L.: Gastric infarction after therapeutic embolization, Surgery 79:421, 1976.
78. Goldstein, H. M., Medellin, H., Ben-Menachem, Y., and Wallace, S.: Transcatheter arterial embolization in the management of bleeding in the cancer patient, Radiology 115:603, 1975.
79. Goldman, M. L., Land, W. C., Bradley, E. L., and Anderson, J.: Transcatheter therapeutic embolization in the management of massive upper gastrointestinal bleeding, Radiology 120:513, 1976.
80. Goldberger, L. E., and Bookstein, J. J.: Transcatheter embolization for treatment of diverticular hemorrhage, Radiology 122:613, 1977.
81. Barr, J. W., Lakin, R. C., and Rösch, J.: Similarity of arterial and intravenous vasopressin on portal and systemic hemodynamics, Gastroenterology 69:13, 1975.
82. Lunderquist, A., and Vang, J.: Transhepatic catheterization and obliteration of the coronary vein in patients with portal hypertension and esophageal varices, N. Engl. J. Med. 291:646, 1974.
83. Aakhus, T., and Braband, G.: Angiography in acute superior mesenteric arterial insufficiency, Acta Radiol. [Diagn.] (Stockh.) 6:1, 1967.
84. Boley, S. J., Sprayregen, S., Veith, F. J., and Siegelman, S. S.: An aggressive roentgenologic and surgical approach to acute mesenteric ischemia, Surg. Ann. 5:355, 1973.
85. Athanasoulis, C. A., Wittenberg, J., Berstein, R., and Williams, L. F.: Vasodilatory drugs in the management of nonocclusive bowel ischemia, Gastroenterology 68:146, 1975.
86. Davis, L. J., Anderson, J., Wallace, S., and Jacobson, E. D.: Experimental use of prostaglandin E_1 in nonocclusive mesenteric ischemia, Am. J. Roentgenol. Radium Ther. Nucl. Med. 125:99, 1975.
87. Hiramatsu, K., Asakura, H., and Baba, S.: Selective intraarterial steroid injection in ulcerative colitis, Acta Radiol. [Diagn.] (Stockh.) 17:299, 1976.
88. Walter, J. F., Paaso, B. T., and Cannon, W. B.: Successful transcatheter embolic control of massive hematobilia secondary to liver biopsy, Am. J. Roentgenol. Radium Ther. Nucl. Med. 127:847, 1976.
89. Merino-de Villa Sante, J., Alvarez-Rodriquez, R. E., and Hernandez-Ortiz, J.: Management of postbiopsy hemobilia with selective arterial embolization, Am. J. Roentgenol. Radium Ther. Nucl. Med. 128:668, 1977.
90. Rubin, B. E., and Katzen, B. T.: Selective hepatic artery embolization to control massive hepatic hemorrhage after trauma, Am. J. Roentgenol. Radium Ther. Nucl. Med. 129:253, 1977.
91. Jander, H. P., Laws, H. L., Kogutt, M. S., and Mihas, A. A.: Emergency embolization in blunt hepatic trauma, Am. J. Roentgenol. Radium Ther. Nucl. Med. 129:249, 1977.

92. Kyung, J. C., Reuter, S. R., and Schmidt, R.: Effects of experimental hepatic artery embolization on hepatic function, Am. J. Roentgenol. Radium Ther. Nucl. Med. 127:563, 1976.
93. DeJode, L. R., Nicholls, R. J., and Wright, P. L.: Ischemic necrosis of the gallbladder following hepatic artery embolism, Br. J. Surg. 63:621, 1976.
94. Tegtmeyer, C. J., Smith, T. H., Shaw, A., et al.: Renal infarction: a complication of gelfoam embolization of a hemangioendothelioma of the liver, Am. J. Roentgenol. Radium Ther. Nucl. Med. 128:305, 1977.
95. Wirtanen, G. W.: Percutaneous transbrachial infusion catheter techniques, Am. J. Roentgenol. Radium Ther. Nucl. Med. 117:696, 1973.
96. Antonovic, R., Rösch, J., and Dotter, C. T.: Complications of percutaneous transaxillary catheterization for arteriography and selective chemotherapy, Am. J. Roentgenol. Radium Ther. Nucl. Med. 126:386, 1976.
97. Forsberg, L., Hafström, L. O., Lunderquist, A., and Sundquist, K.: Arterial changes during treatment with intrahepatic arterial infusion of 5-fluorouracil, Radiology 126:49, 1978.
98. Clouse, M. E., Ahmed, R., Ryan, R. B., et al.: Complications of long-term transbrachial hepatic arterial infusion chemotherapy, Am. J. Roentgenol. Radium Ther. Nucl. Med. 129:799, 1977.
99. Goldman, M. L., Bilbao, M. K., Rösch, J., and Dotter, C. T.: Complications of indwelling chemotherapy catheters, Cancer 36:1983, 1975.
100. Doyon, D., Mouzon, A., Jourde, A.-M., et al.: L'embolisation artérielle hépatique dans les tumeurs malignes du foie, Ann. Radiol. 17:593, 1974.
101. Wallace, S.: Interventional radiology, Cancer 37:517, 1976.
102. Grønvall, J., Grønvall, S., and Hegedüs, V.: Ultrasound-guided drainage of fluid containing masses using angiographic catheterization technique, Am. J. Roentgenol. Radium Ther. Nucl. Med. 129:997, 1977.
103. Zinberg, S. S., Berk, J. E., and Plasencia, H.: Percutaneous transhepatic cholangiography; its use and limitations, Am. J. Dig. Dis. 10:154, 1965.
104. Marions, O., and Wiechel, K. L.: Percutaneous transhepatic cholangiography; indications, technique, complications, and diagnostic criteria, Opusc. Med. (suppl. 32), 1974.
105. Tylén, U., Hoevels, J., and Vang, J.: Percutaneous transhepatic cholangiography with external drainage of obstructive biliary lesions, Surg. Gynecol. Obstet. 144:13, 1977.
106. Hoevels, J., Lunderquist, A., and Ihse, I.: Percutaneous transhepatic intubation of bile ducts for combined internal-external drainage in preoperative and palliative treatment of obstructive jaundice, Gastrointest. Radiol. 3:23, 1978.
107. Molnar, W., and Stockum, A. E.: Relief of obstructive jaundice through percutaneous transhepatic catheter; a new therapeutic method, Am. J. Roentgenol. Radium Ther. Nucl. Med. 122:356, 1974.
108. Burcharth, F., Christiansen, L., Nielbo, N., and Stage, P.: Percutaneous transhepatic cholangiography in diagnostic evaluation of 160 jaundiced patients, Am. J. Surg. 133:559, 1977.
109. Burcharth, F.: A new endoprosthesis for non-operative intubation of the biliary tract in malignant obstructive jaundice, Surg. Gynecol. Obstet. 146:76, 1978.

110. Baum, S., and Ring, E. J.: Personal communication.
111. Burhenne, H. J.: Complications of nonoperative extraction of retained common duct stones, Am. J. Surg. 131:260, 1976.
112. Gold, R. E., Blair, D. C., Finlay, J. B., and Johnston, D. W. B.: Transarterial electrocoagulation therapy of a pseudoaneurysm in the head of the pancreas, Am. J. Roentgenol. Radium Ther. Nucl. Med. 125:422, 1975.
113. Walter, J. F., Chuang, V. P., Bookstein, J. J., et al.: Angiography of massive hemorrhage secondary to pancreatic disease, Radiology 124:336, 1977.
114. Witte, C. L., Witte, M. H., Renert, W., et al.: Splenic artery ligation in selected patients with hepatic cirrhosis and in Sprague-Dawley rats, Surg. Gynecol. Obstet. 142:1, 1976.
115. Maddison, F. E.: Embolic therapy in hypersplenism, Invest. Radiol. 8:280, 1975.
116. Castaneda-Zuinga, W. R., Hammerschmidt, D. E., Sanchez, R., and Amplatz, K.: Nonsurgical splenectomy, Am. J. Roentgenol. Radium Ther. Nucl. Med. 129:805, 1977.
117. Guilford, W. and Scatliff, J. H.: Transcatheter embolization of the spleen for control of splenic hemorrhage and in situ splenectomy: an experimental study using silicone spheres, Radiology 119:549, 1976.
118. Anderson, J. H., Vu Ban, A., Wallace, S. et al.: Transcatheter splenic arterial occlusion: an experimental study in dogs, Radiology 125:95, 1977.
119. Chuang, V. P. and Reuter, S. R.: Selective arterial embolization for the control of traumatic splenic bleeding, Invest. Radiol. 10:18, 1975.
120. Bücheler, E., Thelen, M., Schirmer, G., et al.: Katheterembolisation der Miltzarterien zum Stopp der akuten Varizenblutning, Fortschr. Röntgenstr. 122:224, 1975.
121. Fish, G. W.: Large solitary serous cysts of the kidney, JAMA 112:514, 1939.
122. Vestby, G. W.: Percutaneous needle puncture of renal cysts. New method in therapeutic management, Invest. Radiol. 2:449, 1967.
123. Rashken, M., Poole, O., Roen, S., and Viamonte, M.: Percutaneous management of renal cysts, Radiology 115:551, 1975.
124. Almgärd, L. E. and Fernström, I.: Percutaneous nephropyelostomy, Acta Radiol. [Diagn.] (Stockh.) 15:288, 1974.
125. Barbaric, Z. L., Davis, R. S., Frank, I. N., et al.: Percutaneous nephropyelostomy in the management of acute pyohydronephrosis, Radiology 118:567, 1976.
126. Stables, D. P., Holt, S. A., Sheridan, H. M., and Donohue, R. E.: Permanent nephrostomy via percutaneous puncture, J. Urol. 114:684, 1975.
127. Barbaric, Z. L., and Wood, B. P.: Emergency nephropyelostomy: Experience with 34 patients and review of the literature, Am. J. Roentgenol. Radium Ther. Nucl. Med. 128:453, 1977.
128. Haga, J. R., Zelch, M. G., Alfidi, R. J., et al.: CT-guided antegrade pyelography and percutaneous nephrostomy, Am. J. Roentgenol. Radium Ther. Nucl. Med. 128:621, 1977.
129. Mc Carron, D. A., Rubin, R. J., Barnes, B. A., et al.: Therapeutic bilateral renal infarction in end-stage renal disease, N. Engl. J. Med. 12:652, 1976.
130. Chuang, V. P., Reuter, S. R., and Schmiet, R. W.: Control of experimental

traumatic renal hemorrhage by embolization with autogenous blood clot, Radiology 117:55, 1975.
131. Chuang, V. P., Reuter, S. R., Walter, J., et al.: Control of renal hemorrhage by selective arterial embolization, Am. J. Roentgenol. Radium Ther. Nucl. Med. 125:300, 1975.
132. Richman, S. D., Green, W. M., Kroll, R., and Casarella, W. J.: Superselective transcatheter embolization of traumatic renal hemorrhage, Am. J. Roentgenol. Radium Ther. Nucl. Med. 128:843, 1977.
133. Kerber, C. W., Freeny, R. C., Cromwell, L., et al.: Cyano-acrylate occlusion of a renal arteriovenous fistula, Am. J. Roentgenol. Radium Ther. Nucl. Med. 128:663, 1977.
134. Goldstein, H. M., Medellin, H., Beydoun, T., et al.: Transcatheter embolization of renal cell carcinoma, Am. J. Roentgenol. Radium Ther. Nucl. Med. 123:557, 1975.
135. Reuter, S. R., Pomeroy, P. R., Chuang, V. P., and Cho, K. J.: Embolic control of hypertension caused by segmental renal artery stenosis, Am. J. Roentgenol. Radium Ther. Nucl. Med. 127:389, 1976.
136. Thelen, M., Brühl, P., Gerlach, F., and Biersack, H. J.: Katheterembolisation von metastasierten Nierenkarzinomen mit Butyl-2-Cyanoacrylat, Fortschr. Röntgenstr. 124:232, 1976.
137. Bischoff, W. and Goertler, U.: Ballonverschluss der Nierenarterie in der Urologie, Radiologe 17:498, 1977.
138. Gang, D. L., Dole, K. B., and Adelman, L. S.: Spinal cord infarction following therapeutic renal artery embolization, JAMA 237:2841, 1977.
139. Woodside, J., Schwarz, H., and Bergreen, P.: Peripheral embolization complicating renal infarction with gelfoam, Am. J. Roentgenol. Radium Ther. Nucl. Med. 126:1033, 1976.
140. Merland, J. J., Le Guillou, M., Lepage, T., et al.: Artériographie hypersélective et embolisation en pathologie génito-vesicale chez l'homme, Ann. Radiol. 17:611, 1974.
141. Miller, F. J., Jr., Mortel, R., Mann, W. J., and Jahshan, A. E.: Selective arterial embolization for control of hemorrhage in pelvic malignancy: femoral and brachial approaches, Am. J. Roentgenol. Radium Ther. Nucl. Med. 126:1028, 1976.
142. Smith, J. C., Jr., Kerr, W. S., Athanasoulis, C. A., et al.: Angiographic management of bleeding secondary to genitourinary tract surgery, J. Urol. 113:89, 1975.
143. Barbaric, Z. L., and Luka, N. L.: Angiographic demonstration and transcatheter embolic control of post-traumatic intercostal arterial hemorrhage, Surgery 81:409, 1977.
144. Ring, E. J., Athanasoulis, C., Waltman, A. C., et al.: Arteriographic management of hemorrhage following pelvic fracture, Radiology 109:65, 1973.
145. Halpern, A. A., Rinsky, L. J., and Burton, D. S.: Selective arterial embolization for hemorrhage following hip arthroplasty, Clin. Ortop. 124:144, 1977.
146. Stanley, R. J., and Cubillo, E.: Nonsurgical treatment of arteriovenous malformations of the trunk and limb by transcatheter arterial embolization, Radiology 115:609, 1975.

147. Ng, A. C., and Ochsner, E. C.: Use of Fogarty catheter tamponade for ruptured abdominal aortic aneurysms, Am. J. Roentgenol. Radium Ther. Nucl. Med. 128:31, 1977.
148. Simon, M., Kaplow, R., Salzman, E., and Freiman, D.: A vena cava filter using thermal shaped memory alloy, Radiology 125:89, 1977.
149. Gralino, B. J., Porter, J. M., and Rösch, J.: Angiography in the diagnosis and therapy of frostbite, Radiology 119:301, 1976.
150. O'Dell, C. W., Davis, G. B., Johnson, A. D., et al.: Sodium nitroprusside in the treatment of ergotism, Radiology 124:73, 1977.
151. Carlson, L. A., and Eriksson, I.: Femoral-artery infusion of Prostaglandin E_1 in severe peripheral vascular disease, Lancet 1:155, 1973.
152. van Andel, G. J.: *Percutaneous transluminal angioplasty (the Dotter procedure)* (Amsterdam: Excerpta Medica, 1976).
153. Grüntzig, A.: Die perkutane Rekanalisation chronischer arterieller Verschlüsse mit einem doppellumigen Dilatationskatheter (Dotter-Prinzip), Fortschr. Röntgenstr. 124:80, 1976.
154. Grüntzig, A.: *Die perkutane transluminale Rekanalisation chronischer Arterienverschlüsse mit einer neuen Dilatationstechnik* (Baden Baden: Verlag G. Witzstrock, 1977).

Surgical Management of Parotid Tumors

OLIVER H. BEAHRS, M.D., JOHN E. WOODS, M.D.
AND LOUIS H. WEILAND, M.D.

Mayo Clinic and Mayo Foundation, Rochester, Minnesota

Parotid gland tumors are being managed adequately today more often than they were several decades ago. Previously, even though the anatomy of the facial nerve was appreciated, techniques for parotidectomy were not well established; hence, often the tumor was inadequately removed or the facial nerve was iatrogenically injured, or both. The severity of the cosmetic deformity associated with damage to the facial nerve led to conservatism or delay in the treatment of disease. Today the anatomy of the nerve has been discussed frequently and several technical approaches to surgical parotidectomy have become widely accepted, so that tumors are being treated earlier, more adequately and with better results. Several decades ago, the long-term recurrence rate was 10–40% after enucleation or excision of even benign tumors and was greater for malignant ones.[4, 5, 10]

The pathology of salivary gland tissue is complex; tumors are congenital, inflammatory and benign or malignant. The biologic behavior of various tumors differs and must be understood for the most appropriate surgical treatment to be used for a particular lesion.

Pathology

The salivary glands have a greater variety of tumor types than do most other organs. All of the many tumors that occur in

301

0065-3411/78/0012-0301$03.75

the major and minor salivary glands can arise in the parotid gland. Some, such as Warthin's tumor, have a striking preference for the parotid gland. In Caucasian populations, about 75% of all salivary gland tumors occur in the parotid gland.[7] A knowledge of the clinical presentations and the likelihood of occurrence of the different tumors is a tremendous aid in the preoperative diagnosis of parotid gland enlargements. Certainly, not all salivary enlargements are due to neoplasm. Localized or diffuse parotid swelling also may be due to one of many inflammatory processes known to occur in salivary glands.

On the basis of microscopic morphology, most parotid gland tumors appear to arise from the epithelium or myoepithelium, or both, of the salivary gland duct. The exceptions to this origin are acinic cell carcinoma and, possibly, oncocytoma. This relationship between ductal tumors and tumors of the secreting portion of the organ is similar to that in the breast and pancreas, organs with which the salivary glands share morphologic or functional similarities. Most of the tumors maintain easily recognized epithelial qualities; some, such as mixed tumor and occasionally adenoid cystic carcinoma and adenocarcinoma, possess the "double layering" of epithelium and myoepithelium found in the normal salivary gland duct. A few are nearly pure myoepithelial cell proliferations that can mimic neurogenic, fibrogenic or myogenic spindle cell neoplasms.

Gross examination of parotid gland tumors can provide clues to histopathologic diagnosis. Cartilaginous and myxoid tissues make a diagnosis of mixed tumor very likely. Necrosis usually implies malignancy. Most benign tumors are encapsulated. All malignant tumors eventually develop infiltrating borders. This peripheral invasion, particularly in adenoid cystic carcinoma, rather commonly spreads to the adjacent facial nerve or its branches, producing clinical signs and symptoms that are valuable clues to the nature of the tumor. A cystic lesion is likely to be a retention cyst, Warthin's tumor, mucoepidermoid carcinoma, or, rarely, acinic cell carcinoma, mixed tumor or basal cell adenoma. In patients with bilateral parotid gland tumors, Warthin's tumor, oncocytoma, and, rarely, acinic cell carcinoma should be considered.

CLASSIFICATION

All meaningful classifications of salivary gland tumors are based on histopathology. The classifications are many, ranging from the complicated and detailed[7] to the simplified categorization of "benign" or "malignant." We consider any classification to be valid if it has consistent practicality for pathologic diagnosis and if the diagnoses are of clinical usefulness to the surgeon. The classification used at the Mayo Clinic is as follows:

Adenomas
  Pleomorphic (mixed tumor)
  Monomorphic
    Cystadenoma (Warthin's tumor)
    Oncocytoma
    Basal cell (and variants)
Carcinomas
  Adenoid cystic
  Mucoepidermoid
  Acinic cell
  Adenocarcinoma
  Squamous cell
  Undifferentiated
  Carcinoma arising in a pleomorphic adenoma
    (malignant mixed tumor)
Sarcomas
Metastatic tumors
Tumefacient inflammation

This classification encompasses nearly all tumors. It differs from many others in that it designates mucoepidermoid and acinic lesions as malignant. There are very few new tumors in parotid gland nomenclature. In the American literature, basal cell adenoma is one of these.[1] Oat cell carcinoma might be a distinct tumor entity.[11] This name tends to be confusing because of its application to certain lung tumors. It is unlikely that it is identical to the bronchial tumor.[14] Undoubtedly, this tumor has been classified previously as undifferentiated carcinoma or malignant lymphoma. Tumors that arise from the mesenchymal and lymphoreticular structures of the parotid gland should not be considered true salivary gland neoplasms. These soft-tissue tumors and malignant lymphomas are parotid tumors by anatomic location only. They do not behave differently from the same tumors occurring elsewhere in the body.

BENIGN TUMORS

MIXED TUMORS. — Mixed tumors are peculiar in having both epithelial and mesenchymal tissue components. This blend allows for ease of recognition in the typical case. Because of a high recurrence rate, many early studies on this tumor considered it malignant. Although mixed tumors are well encapsulated, the periphery is frequently lobulated. Incomplete removal of portions of these lobules results in recurrences that frequently consist of multiple nodules. Since by definition mixed tumors have both epithelial and mesenchymal tissue components, one of these elements might predominate and create diagnostic confusion. The greatest problem is in the differential diagnosis of the cellular variety of mixed tumor in which the epithelial component nearly excludes the typical chondroid, myxoid or fibrous portion. Other serious considerations include adenocarcinoma, monomorphic adenoma and, occasionally, cylindroma. Very cellular mixed tumors, especially those in which mitoses are present, have been shown to have slightly different behavior from an ordinary mixed tumor and may even metastasize.[12] Benign mixed tumors account for well over half of all parotid gland tumors.[6, 8, 12] We retain the term "mixed tumor" while agreeing that "pleomorphic adenoma" is more accurately descriptive. Whether the epithelial and mesenchymal portions are unilateral or bilateral is obviously important, but not in the planning of surgical treatment for patients with this tumor.

WARTHIN'S TUMOR. — Warthin's tumor is less tongue-twisting than its synonym, "papillary adenocystoma lymphomatosum." The gross features of a typical Warthin's tumor often allow its identification at the operating table. It is cystic and, on sectioning, exudes a thick, tan-gray, semiliquid mucoid material. The cut surface is geographic, with broad bands of dark tan tissue intermingling with pools of mucus. Warthin's tumor is now restricted to the parotid gland. Similar tumors without the lymphoid elements (cystadenomas) may, however, occur in other salivary gland tissues. This tumor has a notable tendency to occur in males and in the lower pole of the superficial parotid lobe. Malignancy developing in Warthin's tumor is rare and need not be considered in planning treatment. Metachronous multicentricity certainly can take place and should not be considered to be recurrence of an excised tumor.

ONCOCYTOMAS. – Oncocytomas are distinctive tumors containing large cells with abundant eosinophilic cytoplasm. Individually similar cells may be found in the normal ductal epithelium and are called "oncocytes." These cells have microscopic features that are reminiscent of hepatocytes, and oncocytomas frequently have the red-brown color of hepatic tissue. The epithelial cells of Warthin's tumor and occasionally some of those in mixed tumors may be similar or identical. Differential diagnosis includes the aforementioned tumors and acinic cell carcinoma. Occasionally, the oncocytes of ductal epithelium proliferate to form microscopic foci, or "microtumors." Often one must decide arbitrarily whether this proliferation represents hyperplasia or neoplasia. Malignancy in oncocytic tumors is almost nonexistent and, for practical purposes, may be considered as such.

BASAL CELL ADENOMA. – Basal cell adenoma is one of the more recently described salivary gland tumors. Batsakis[1] has advanced its recognition in this country. Basal cell adenoma and other variants of monomorphic adenoma are benign tumors. They are similar to mixed tumors in clinical presentation, except that they tend to occur in older age groups. Microscopically they are like mixed tumors that lack a mesenchymal component and may easily be mistaken for the cellular forms of mixed tumor. Undoubtedly, the reason they were not diagnosed frequently in this country before a decade ago is that they were classified as mixed tumors. The problem, however, is not as serious as it sounds. Their behavior is probably less aggressive than is that of a mixed tumor; treatment that is appropriate for one is appropriate for the other.

MALIGNANT TUMORS

ADENOID CYSTIC CARCINOMA. – The term *"adenoid cystic carcinoma"* is preferable to "cylindroma," since it connotes the malignant nature of this tumor. The lesions are unencapsulated and have a remarkable propensity to invade their surroundings, including the potential space around peripheral nerves. The microscopic diagnosis of adenoid cystic carcinoma is not always easy, since the tumor has some features in common with mixed tumor and basal cell adenoma. Experience is required in correctly identifying confusing cases. The fact that adenoid cystic carcinoma can be mistaken for benign tumors attests to its relative lack of cytologic anaplasia, deceptive of its true behavior. Because of the infiltrative tendency, the gross margins of tumor resection can be misleading. It is not unusual to find a microscopic tumor well removed from that seen grossly. Surgical margins are best examined microscopically by frozen-section techniques.

MUCOEPIDERMOID CARCINOMA. — Mucoepidermoid carcinoma is recognized microscopically by its mixture of mucus-producing cells and cells relating to epidermoid differentiation. Like mixed tumor, it is an example of the multipotential nature of ductal cells. Mucoepidermoid carcinomas may be cystic; they usually are not encapsulated. We consider mucoepidermoid tumors carcinomas[13] and do not acknowledge the existence of a benign variant. It is likely that some of the well-differentiated tumors are in fact benign. The problem lies in the inability, on microscopic examination, to differentiate these tumors from those that recur and lead a malignant course. It seems more reasonable, especially for purposes of treatment, to consider all of these tumors as having malignant potential. The spectrum of differentiation can be striking. The well-differentiated lesions are likely to be cystic and to have an abundance of mucus-producing cells. The poorly differentiated growths are likely to be solid and to have a predominance of epidermoid epithelium, with relatively little mucus production by the appropriate cells.

ACINIC CELL CARCINOMA. — Acinic cell carcinoma is the only tumor of the salivary glands with generally accepted origin from the acinus. We consider all acinic cell tumors, like mucoepidermoid lesions, to have malignant potential and designate them "carcinomas" for the same reasons as previously stated. This tumor is frequently encapsulated, soft and tan-yellow. Microscopically, the well-differentiated tumors have a striking resemblance to normal serous acinar structures. In most cases, the likeness to normal serous cells provides convincing evidence of origin from these cells. Histochemical stains provide further proof. Acinic cell carcinomas are all relatively well differentiated. If a poorly differentiated and highly malignant form of this tumor exists, it is not recognized as such and probably is classified as an adenocarcinoma.

ADENOCARCINOMA. – Adenocarcinoma includes all carcinomas of the salivary glands that have a glandular microscopic pattern and cannot be classified as mucoepidermoid carcinoma, acinic cell carcinoma or adenoid cystic carcinoma. The frequency of salivary gland adenocarcinomas depends somewhat on how rigidly one adheres to the criteria for the diagnosis of the previously described tumors. The morphologic features of adenocarcinoma can vary from papillary to tubular. The tumor cells may be oxyphilic, but such tumors should not be considered to be malignant oncocytomas. These are significant malignancies whose behavior usually can be suspected from gross and microscopic examination. While their aggressiveness is somewhat like that of adenoid cystic carcinoma, it is greater than that of the average acinic cell carcinoma or mucoepidermoid carcinoma. Therefore, the correct diagnosis of adenocarcinoma is of some importance.

SQUAMOUS CELL CARCINOMA. – Squamous cell carcinoma of the parotid gland is rare. The differential diagnosis includes benign squamous metaplasia, metastatic squamous cell carcinoma to intraparotid and paraparotid lymph nodes, mucoepidermoid carcinoma and squamous carcinoma developing in a mixed tumor. When all of these possibilities have been excluded, a small percentage of tumors will fill the criteria for primary squamous cell carcinoma of salivary glands. Such cancers probably arise from the ductal epithelium, perhaps after it has undergone benign squamous metaplasia. A similar situation exists in the lung, where most bronchial tumors are squamous cell in type and have their origin in nonsquamous epithelium.

CARCINOMA ARISING IN MIXED TUMORS. – Carcinoma arising in mixed tumors (malignant mixed tumor) has been written about extensively. Whether some mixed tumors are malignant from their beginning or whether malignancy develops within a previously benign mixed tumor is difficult or impossible to ascertain. From a practical and logical point of view, the latter situation usually applies. If a firm lump has been in the parotid gland for many years and suddenly begins to grow rapidly, the concept that malignancy has occurred in a previously benign tumor seems justifiable. To maintain some consistency, the following criteria for the diagnosis of malignancy in a mixed tumor are reasonable: (1) microscopic evidence of benign mixed tumor somewhere in the tumor is undeniable; and (2) evidence of malignancy is unequivocal, the malignant portion usually being sharply delineated from the benign portion. This definition does not adequately cover the occasional mixed tumor that has a benign microscopic appearance (such as some cellular mixed tumors) yet has an undeniably malignant course.

The carcinoma that develops in mixed tumors is usually adenocarcinoma of moderate differentiation, sometimes undifferentiated carcinoma and rarely squamous cell carcinoma or mixtures of the other types. Taken by themselves, the malignant portions do not differ appreciably from the same tumors arising without the benign mixed tumor background. The same is probably true of their behavior. The finding of a malignant mesenchymal component in a mixed tumor is exceptionally rare.[2]

UNDIFFERENTIATED CARCINOMA. — Undifferentiated carcinoma is a diagnosis made when the other forms of carcinoma have been excluded. The cells lack squamous or glandular morphology and usually are easily recognized as epithelial growths. However, if they grow in solid sheets, differentiation from malignant lymphoma can be a problem. Undifferentiated carcinomas most likely have their origin in ductal elements. To consider these tumors a distinct entity seems unreasonable; further studies should uncover a variety of neoplasms. The small-cell undifferentiated carcinoma[11] has some features that make it similar to oat cell carcinoma of bronchial type that has been found in minor salivary glands. At least some of the small-cell tumors arise in the parotid gland and have ultrastructural features of myoepithelial cells.[14] Argentaffin cells have been noted in canine species.[9] If such cells exist in human salivary glands, neoplasia could occur. Tumors arising from neuroendocrine cells of this type would be expected to resemble carcinoid tumors or undifferentiated bronchical carcinoma, and might even produce hormones. Further studies will help in documenting or disproving this speculation.

Treatment

For highly selected small tumors located at the inferior pole or the border of the inferior portion of the parotid gland, local excision can be considered if the surgeon judges the facial nerve not to be in jeopardy. Should the tumor prove to be malignant on frozen-section study, the operation can be extended into parotidectomy. Tumors in these regions amenable to local treatment most likely would be lymphadenoma of the subparotid or infraparotid lymph nodes, papillary adenocystoma lymphomatosum (Warthin's tumor) or mixed tumor. Otherwise, the minimal procedure should be subtotal parotidectomy with preservation of the nerve.

If examination of fresh-frozen sections is not immediately available, one might consider preliminary needle or aspiration biopsy to establish a diagnosis before the definitive operation. The disadvantages of this procedure are possible seeding of the needle tract and the chance of obtaining inadequate or nonrepresentative tissue of the pathologic process. Preferably, the surgical environment should include frozen-section diagnosis, since the patient is best served in this manner.

Except for the few tumors that might be locally excised, the minimal surgical procedure for excisional biopsy or definitive treatment of a lesion superficial to the facial nerve should be subtotal (superficial) parotidectomy. The portion of the parotid gland superficial to the facial nerve is removed and the main trunk, two divisions and multiple branches of the nerve are identified. If the lesion is in the part of the gland that is deep to the nerve, subtotal parotidectomy should be done to identify the nerve before the remaining gland with the tumor is removed. If an invasive lesion is found, one must decide whether to excise part or all of the nerve en bloc with parotid tissue and tumor. This decision is based in part on the pathologic interpretation of the tumor.

Fortunately, about 80% of the parotid parenchyma is superficial to the nerve and removal of this portion of the gland removes about 80% of the tumors. The part of the gland deep to the nerve after subtotal parotidectomy is almost always disconnected from the ductal system. It continues to excrete some saliva after the operation until fibrosis and atrophy set in. This secretion often delays primary healing of the operative site for days or weeks. Although not essential, for this reason one should almost always remove most of the parenchyma from beneath the nerve, completing the procedure as a total conservative (nerve preserved) parotidectomy. This can be simply done by removing the salivary tissue piecemeal by pinching it and "milking" it away from nerve and vessels. This way, the operative site heals primarily without significant drainage. A suction drain is left in place for 24 – 48 hours to evacuate blood, serum and exudate and to draw the overlying skin flaps into the recess left after removal of the gland. An effective pressure dressing is difficult to apply in this anatomic region.

For recurrent chronic sialadenitis and calculus formation in the ductal system, total conservative parotidectomy is indicated. The dissection is somewhat difficult becuase of inflammation and fibrosis but can be done without damaging the nerve. If the parenchyma deep to the nerve is left in place, about 10% of patients will have persistent symptoms.[4]

Cavernous hemangiomas and lymphangiomas must also be totally removed. The parotid parenchyma is almost always replaced by the disease process. At times the nerve is difficult to dissect free from the tenacious tissue planes, but with care it can be preserved. The dissection is much simpler and safer if it is not preceded by an inadequate operation, by radiation treatment or by use of sclerosing agents. Mikulicz's disease, or diffuse lymphocytic infiltration of salivary tissue, as seen in Sjögren's syndrome, usually does not require surgical treatment unless there is a cosmetic reason for parotidectomy or excision of the submaxillary gland. Multiple glands are involved by these processes and if one gland is to be excised, usually several should be removed to obtain the desired cosmetic result. Whether or not salivary tissue is removed, "dry mouth" remains a problem for the patient.

For benign tumors – the mixed cell tumor, basal cell adenoma, papillary adenocystoma lymphomatosum (Warthin's tumor) and oncocytic adenocarcinoma – partial or subtotal parotidectomy should be done, assuming that the procedure completely circumscribes the lesion. If the tumor is in the deep part of the gland, this portion of the gland is removed and the procedure is completed as a total conservative parotidectomy. If the nerve closely approximates tumor, it can be freed from the tissue to be removed and can be preserved. In second operations, however, dense scar tissue may make the dissection very difficult and at times small nerve branches may have to be sacrificed.

In general, malignant tumors of the parotid gland can be divided into two groups for treatment: less malignant and highly malignant. Well-differentiated mucoepidermoid carcinoma, adenoid cystic carcinoma (cylindroma) and acinic cell carcinoma remain fairly well localized or even encapsulated, spreading into the adjacent salivary gland parenchyma or other tissues. In the patient with clinical evidence of facial nerve involvement who has not been operated on, the nerve must be considered involved by tumor. Total parotidectomy is done and the nerve is preserved unless a branch, a division or the trunk is involved by tumor. That portion of the nerve grossly involved by or closely approximating the tumor should be sacrificed. The whole nerve need not be sacrificed unless the trunk is involved or the tumor is so large that it jeopardizes the entire nerve.

This kind of tumor spreads infrequently to the regional lymphatics — probably in less than 10% of cases. For this reason, radical neck dissection is not often necessary and is indicated only if there is gross or microscopic evidence of metastasis in the infraparotid or subparotid lymph nodes or in those of the upper deep jugular region.[5] These nodes can be removed with the parotid gland or separately for histologic study. If metastasis is found, radical neck dissection is indicated.

Highly malignant tumors — malignant mixed tumor, undifferentiated mucoepidermoid carcinoma, adenocarcinoma, and so forth — are treated best by total radical parotidectomy with sacrifice of the facial nerve. A part of the nerve or, infrequently, the entire nerve may be preserved if it is widely separated from tumor and the surgeon judges that treatment of the cancer is not being jeopardized. In about 50% of these cases regional nodal metastasis will have occurred; hence, radical neck dissection should be considered as part of the definitive treatment for most of these lesions.[5]

In selected cases in which the entire facial nerve or a major division has been sacrificed, one should consider inserting a free nerve graft to bridge the defect. The great auricular nerve or another superficial cervical nerve can be used as the graft. Fine vascular silk should be used for the anastomoses. In 70–90% of patients, facial nerve function will return in about six months.[3]

Anatomy

Although parotidectomy should always be approached with respect, knowledge of the basic anatomy of the region should give the surgeon solid confidence in operating. The key structure is the facial nerve with its two divisions and five principal branches. Once the surgeon understands this unit and its relationships to other anatomic landmarks, the procedure becomes straightforward. A brief review of the anatomy is in order.

MUSCULOSKELETAL RELATIONSHIPS

The parotid gland is related in its various dimensions to several skeletal and muscular structures (Figs 1 and 2). Posteriorly it abuts the anterior surface of the mastoid process and posterosuperiorly, the cartilaginous (more superficial) and bony (deep) portions of the external auditory meatus. Anterosuperiorly, the recess in which the gland lies is bordered by the temporomandibular joint. The ramus of the mandible lies, in part, medial to

Fig 1.—Skeletal bed of parotid gland. (From Beahrs, O. H., and Adson, M. A.: The surgical anatomy and technic of parotidectomy, Am. J. Surg. 95:885, 1958. By permission of Dun-Donnelley Publishing Corporation.)

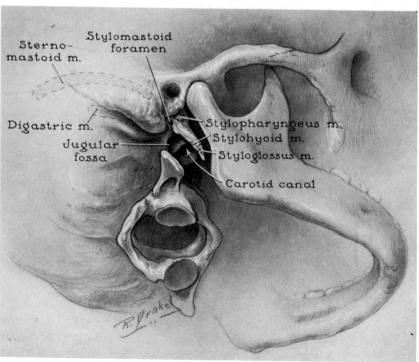

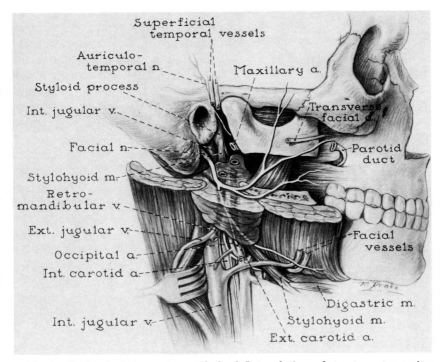

Fig 2.—Regional anatomy of parotid gland. Interrelations of structures traversing and lying deep to gland are emphasized. (From Beahrs, O. H., and Adson, M. A.: The surgical anatomy and technic of parotidectomy, Am. J. Surg. 95:885, 1958. By permission of Dun-Donnelley Publishing Corporation.)

the anterior portion of the superficial part of the gland, which may extend well below the angle of the jaw. Deep to the medial surface of the gland lies the styloid process superiorly, and more inferiorly is the tip of the transverse process of the atlas. Of importance in this area are the jugular foramen and carotid canal carrying the corresponding vein and artery. These lie deep to the styloid process. Attaching to or covering the bony structures forming the recess is the sternocleidomastoid muscle, which covers the mastoid process and relates to the posteroinferior portion of the gland. The masseter muscle, which covers the ramus mandibularis, lies deep to the anterior portion of the gland except in the most downward projection of the latter. The deeper portion of the gland as it wraps around the posterior border of the mandibular ramus is in relation to the insertions of the pterygoid muscles. More medially and posteriorly, the origin of the posterior belly of the digastric muscle arises from a notch medial to the tip of the mastoid process and passes obliquely downward, covering the surface of the transverse process of the atlas. Also forming a portion of the medial limits of musculoskeletal fossa are the stylohyoid, styloglossus and stylopharyngeus muscles, with their more or less common origins from the styloid process, although only the stylohyoid is easily seen in the course of the usual dissection.

THE PAROTID GLAND

The gland itself may vary considerably in size and configuration. It is roughly triangular, with its base lying parallel to the transverse zygomatic process and the apex extending below the angle of the jaw (Fig 3). It may extend forward close to the anterior margin of the masseter muscle or barely overlap its posterior portion. In most of our surgical dissections two thirds or more of the gland lay superficial to the facial nerve, although some tumors arising from the deep portion of the gland extend deep to the mandibular ramus into the parapharyngeal region.

Several tributaries converge at the anterior margin of the gland to form Stensen's duct, which passes across the masseter muscle to dive medially through the buccinator muscle and thence to its buccal orifice opposite the second upper molar.

THE FACIAL NERVE

The main trunk of the facial nerve, after emerging from the stylomastoid foramen, passes anterolaterally into the substance of the parotid gland at the midpoint of the mastoid process (Figs 4 and 5). Except when the nerve is distorted by an unusually large tumor, this location rarely varies in the adult. In the infant or child, it may take a somewhat more infero-oblique course. The main trunk is seen distal to the posterior auricular nerve. Shortly after entering the gland, the main trunk divides into two main divisions: the cervicofacial and the temporofacial. Although there are variations, most commonly the cervicofacial division divides into the buccal, mandibular and cervical branches; and the temporofacial division divides into the temporal and zygomatic branches (see Fig 5). These branches all pass

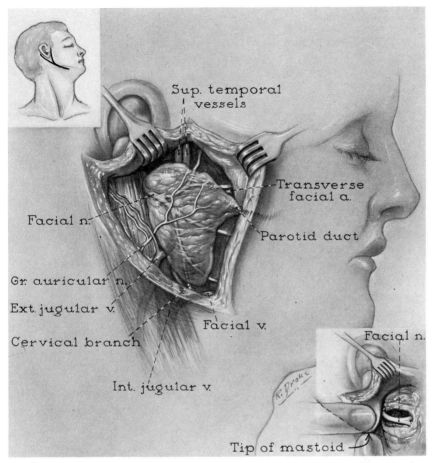

Fig 3. — Operative field after cutaneous flaps have been elevated. (Anterior flap has been mobilized more than is recommended at this stage of dissection.) **Upper inset,** incision. **Lower inset,** facial nerve is identified by its relation to mastoid process. (From Beahrs, O. H., and Adson, M. A.: The surgical anatomy and technic of parotidectomy, Am. J. Surg. 95:885, 1958. By permission of Dun-Donnelley Publishing Corporation.)

through the substance of the gland, emerging peripherally to penetrate and innervate the muscles of facial expression. The buccal branch, after leaving the cervicofacial division, travels forward inferior to the zygomatic branch to innervate the buccal and orbicularis oris muscles. There are commonly decussations, or cross linkages, between the buccal and zygomatic branches;

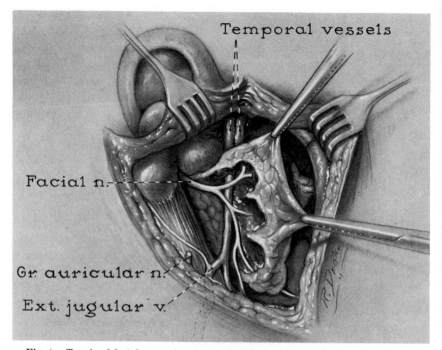

Fig 4.—Trunk of facial nerve has been identified and superficial portion of parotid gland is dissected free of nerve rami. (From Beahrs, O. H., and Adson, M. A.: The surgical anatomy and technic of parotidectomy, Am. J. Surg. 95:885, 1958. By permission of Dun-Donnelley Publishing Corporation.)

hence, damage to these branches results in less noticeable deficits in most instances. Typically, the mandibular branch travels forward along the masseter muscle just above the lower border of the mandible; the cervical branch passes downward to the platysma near the angle of the jaw. The temporal branch is the first and most posterior branch of the superior division and generally is 1 cm or more anterior to the anterior auricular sulcus. It passes over the zygomatic arch, supplying the frontalis and the facial muscles lying above the arch. The zygomatic branch usually divides into a smaller upper and a more substantial lower branch; the lower branch runs parallel with the transverse facial vessels to innervate muscles of the nose and upper lip.

The other nerve of significance in relation to the parotid gland is the great auricular nerve, which is usually the largest branch

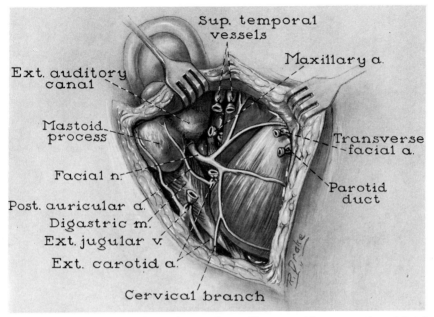

Fig 5.—Bed of parotid gland after total parotidectomy with preservation of facial nerve. (From Beahrs, O. H., and Adson, M. A.: The surgical anatomy and technic of parotidectomy, Am. J. Surg. 95:885, 1958. By permission of Dun-Donnelley Publishing Corporation.)

of the cervical plexus (see Fig 3). Most commonly, it curves around the posterior aspect of the sternocleidomastoid muscle, passing upward on its lateral surface often behind and parallel to the external jugular vein. It divides into mastoid, auricular, and facial branches at varying levels. It is most frequently identified 2–3 cm below the mastoid process in the course of exposing the gland and is divided routinely in parotidectomy.

REGIONAL BLOOD VESSELS

Although both arteries and blood vessels in the region of the parotid can be sacrificed without cause for concern, knowing the more important vessels facilitates dissection (see Figs 2 and 5).

The arteries, which are less variable than the veins, are all branches of the carotid system. The internal carotid artery, which lies medial and anterior to the internal jugular vein, runs deep to the musculoskeletal bed of the parotid gland.

The external carotid artery travels upward from beneath the anterior border of the sternocleidomastoid muscle behind the angle of the mandible and deep to the digastric and stylohyoid muscles. It then curves gently outward over the upper border of the stylohyoid muscle and enters the deep portion of the gland overlying and anterior to the styloid process. The artery may divide into its terminal branches either within this portion of the gland or on emerging from it, so that either the artery or its branches groove the medial surface of the parotid.

Of the anterior, posterior, ascending and terminal branches of the external carotid, only the last two branches are in direct relationship with the parotid gland. The posterior auricular artery, which arises near the upper border of the digastric muscle, passes posteriorly and superiorly along or superficial to its border to reach the space between the mastoid process and the external auditory canal. Its significance lies in its almost invariable exposure on the anterior surface of the mastoid process — a key landmark in the identification of the main trunk of the facial nerve.

The internal maxillary and superficial temporal arteries are the two terminal branches of the external carotid artery. The former passes forward deep to the ramus of the mandible and lies either superficial to or deep to the external pterygoid muscle. The superficial temporal artery passes upward deep to the parotid gland just in front of the tragus and superficial to and usually posterior to the temporomandibular joint. Its important branch, the transverse facial artery, travels forward superficial to the ramus mandibularis, just below the zygomatic arch on the surface of the masseter muscle.

The veins of the parotid region are more variable than the arteries. Most commonly, the superficial temporal and internal maxillary veins join to form the posterior facial vein. This, in turn, divides into two branches — an anterior and a posterior. The former joins the anterior facial vein to form the common facial vein, while the latter may unite with the small posterior auricular vein to form the external jugular vein.

The posterior facial vein is the vein of greatest significance in the parotid dissection because it often lies in close apposition to the cervical branch of the facial nerve. It frequently is divided and ligated to permit more direct visualization of this nerve and to facilitate its dissection downward. The anterior jugular vein usually is not in the operative field, lying anterior thereto. The internal jugular vein lies deep to the operative field as it exits from the skull through the jugular foramen just medial to the base of the styloid process, traveling on the lateral wall of the pharynx. It lies deep to the tip of the transverse process of the atlas and to the digastric and stylohyoid muscles.

Fascial Planes

Although deep and superficial fascial layers have been described as enclosing the parotid gland, these are not usually distinctly identifiable structures. They are more recognizable as septa passing in and among the lobules of the gland. Although rarely seen, discrete fascial layers facilitate dissection between subcutaneous tissue and gland surface as well as glandular dissection along the course of the individual branches of the facial nerve.

Surgical Technique

The present technique is a composite of aspects of many descriptions of methods of parotidectomy. Some surgeons prefer to base their dissections on peripheral identification of one of the facial nerve branches, but wide experience with tumors of all sizes and varieties has convinced us that identification of the main trunk is possible in essentially all instances. Furthermore, it is the key to a rapid and relatively straightforward and safe parotid dissection. For this reason, this description will be confined to that one technique, with modifications or variations in certain instances that require more radical procedures.

Preoperative Preparation

A thorough discussion of the procedure and its complications, including temporary or permanent nerve weakness and sensory nerve deficit to the earlobe, is mandatory before the decision to operate is made.

Blood transfusions rarely are needed in operations of the parotid, but the patient's blood group should be known, and a blood sample should be available for crossmatching in the unlikely event that transfusion is necessary.

The hair in front of the ear is shaved to the level of the upper extent of the auricle, as is any hair over the mastoid process. The patient is placed in the supine position on the operating table, with a footboard in place to allow for elevation of the head. A small pillow under the shoulders may facilitate rotation of the head to allow optimal positioning for the dissection, but this is not essential.

Two doubled orthopedic sheets placed beneath the patient's head provide a simple, highly satisfactory drape. The more superficial sheet is brought up around the mastoid process on the operative side and over the ear on the opposite side, and one side is snugly slamped to the other over a double sterile towel used to cover the endotracheal and esophageal stethoscope tubes. Two towels forming a V from below the ears to the middle of the neck complete the draping of the operative site, and a sterile sheet is added over the trunk and extremities. The patient's head is turned toward the nonoperative side and the corner of the mouth and the eye are exposed for easy visualization of any facial nerve stimulation.

THE OPERATION

The incision most commonly used by us is the so-called inverted T. The vertical limb is begun in front of the ear in the preauricular crease with the skin pulled forward, extended downward from the junction of the auricle and scalp to the earlobe, and curved gently backward to meet the oblique limb of the incision (Fig 6A). The oblique limb of the incision is extended down from just below the mastoid process to parallel the anterior border of the sternocleidomastoid muscle about two fingerbreadths below the angle of the jaw. The vertical limb of the incision should join the oblique limb at approximately right angles to avoid a narrow triangle of skin just below the earlobe.

Our practice is to make the vertical incision first, carrying it through skin down to the level of parotid fascia, which may or may not appear as a white layer of fibrous strands overlying the gland. Dissection using Jones scissors is carried out along this plane, parallel to the skin edge. The scissors are then directed anterosuperiorly, more or less parallel to the upper nerve branches, under and at right angles to the overlying skin, tunneling for a short distance and then spreading to lift and dissect

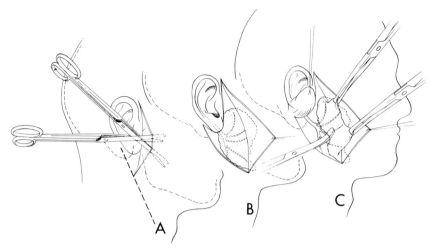

Fig 6. – A, Vertical limb of incision is made first. Scissor blades are directed perpendicular to underlying gland and traversing nerve branches. Axis of scissors is directed parallel to distribution of each branch as skin flap is freed up over it. B, Horizontal limb of incision is made well below angle of jaw, and skin flap is retracted anteriorly. Nerve emerges from stylomastoid foramen at level of midpoint of mastoid process just below ear at level of earlobe. C, When nerve trunk is exposed and gland is retracted upward, point of closed blades of scissors is used to separate gland up and off underlying branches of nerve. (From Woods, J. E., and Beahrs, O. H.: A technique for the rapid performance of parotidectomy with minimal risk, Surg. Gynecol. Obstet. 142:87, 1976. By permission.)

away skin from the underlying gland. Because the scissors are kept at right angles to skin and gland, the opening and closing of the blades does not injure nerve branches as the dissection proceeds peripherally (see Fig 6 A). As this dissecting motion is continued, the axis of the scissors is rotated around a pivotal point roughly over the mastoid process, so that the dissection continuously parallels the various branches of the facial nerve as they fan out from the main trunk. This is an additional safety factor in performing a rapid freeing-up of the anterior skin flap. The dissection is carried anteriorly until the masseter muscle can be identified readily by palpation or direct sight. Leaving the oblique limb of the incision until later facilitates dissection of the flap, since it is accomplished against countertraction. The skin thus is freed from its superior extent over the temporomandibular joint to its inferior limit at the proposed site of the oblique incision just over the sternocleidomastoid muscle.

The oblique incision then is made from behind the ear just

below the mastoid process, paralleling the underlying sterno-cleidomastoid muscle and extending downward to a point about two fingerbreadths below the angle of the jaw (see Fig 6 B). If the anterior flap has been appropriately freed-up, a stroke of the scissors along the anterior portion of the new incision will completely free up the anterior skin flap when the incision is carried down to subcutaneous tissue. Troublesome bleeders are treated with electrocautery, since the facial nerve is nowhere exposed except at the most peripheral anterior extremes of the operative field, where little bleeding occurs. The triangle of skin under the ear then is freed up, with care taken to preserve its underlying subcutaneous tissue to avoid postoperative necrosis of this skin. The mastoid process thus is exposed and from there the scissor points are directed upward to find a distinct plane above the cartilaginous portion of the external auditory meatus. Once identified, this plane, if followed with the scissor blades, allows ready separation of the posterior portion of the gland from the meatus and from the remaining tissue constituting the posterior portion of the vertical incision.

In order to identify the main trunk of the facial nerve, it is important to avoid working in a hole. Therefore, a wide trough is developed by dissecting the glandular tissue forward. The dissection can be accomplished readily by repeatedly spreading the scissor points between meatus and gland, so that the blade ends open parallel to the nerve. In the superior part of the dissection, the superficial temporal artery or vein may cause troublesome bleeding and ligation may be necessary. At this point, the sternocleidomastoid muscle is followed down from the mastoid process, with one blade of the scissors hooking under the most posterior extension of the gland to free it from the anterior border of the muscle. The great auricular nerve usually is encountered at this point and is divided. The external jugular vein also may be found in this area and may be divided and ligated. Once this has been accomplished, the gland is more widely separated from muscle by the spreading scissor ends until a plane deep to the gland, often including the posterior belly of the digastric muscle, is exposed. The gland thus is swept forward to the extent that a depression is established in which the nerve can be more readily identified. This depression is further widened by placing Allis clamps on the posterior border of the gland, providing forward traction.

At this point, the all-important landmark is the mastoid process, the key to identification of the facial nerve. The anticipated site of the main trunk is 1–2 cm anterior and deep to the midpoint of the mastoid process, as identified by placing a forward-pointing index finger upon it. It may be slightly inferior to this point in young children. As the trunk of the nerve is sought, it is important that an assistant continuously watch the exposed corner of the eye and mouth for any signs of stimulation and indicate such stimulation aloud each time it occurs. The most common difficulty in finding the nerve is that the surgeon expects to find it at a more superficial level than it is. It usually penetrates the gland at least 1 cm deep to the lateral surface of the mastoid process. The nerve trunk is actually identified by the same careful spreading of the scissor tips parallel to its anticipated transverse course. As the scissors are spread more widely to push the gland farther forward, almost inevitably definite stimulation will occur, indicating proximity of the trunk; or its usually white, glistening surface may be seen. Failure to find the nerve by use of the foregoing landmarks and technique is almost always a consequence of not carrying the search deep enough. Once the nerve is identified, the procedure is usually quite straightforward. From this juncture forward, moist sponges should be used to avoid trauma to the nerve in blotting (not rubbing) the field dry. Also, care should be taken to keep the sucker tip away from the nerve, since strong suction on the nerve may produce postoperative weakness. The Allis clamps may be replaced more deeply on the posterior border of the gland to afford better exposure of the nerve trunk by forward traction. Closed scissors or a small curved clamp then may be used to expose more of the nerve and identify the bifurcation by hooking and tearing the gland up and away from the nerve (see Fig 6 C). It is extremely important that the end of the instrument always be directed from a point on top of the nerve, rather than at its side or underneath, where damage to an unsuspected branch may occur. It is essential to understand that a gland will give more readily than will a nerve (if the nerve is not directly hooked) and that this characteristic provides for rapid and safe exposure of the branches.

Usually, exposure of the branches is most convenient following the cervicofacial division of the nerve. Having identified the bifurcation, the surgeon should follow the most proximal branch downward with the instrument point, tearing the gland away from it. The posterior facial vein may be found in close proximity to this branch and may be carefully separated from it, clamped, divided and ligated. The nerve passes down into the neck to innervate the platysma muscle. When the nerve has been followed to the lower limit of the operative field, the overlying tissue may be divided with the scissors, with the nerve branch safely and clearly in sight at all times. Next, the marginal branch is followed forward again as the gland is torn away. The buccal branch is similarly identified and followed forward, always with traction on the parotid parenchyma pulling it forward. The duct often is encountered close to the buccal branch. Our practice is to divide it without ligation, since it may provide decompression of the deeper portion of the gland when it is not removed. Troublesome arterial pumpers may be clamped with care to avoid nerve twigs, but for the most part, small bleeders are ignored, since such bleeding almost inevitably stops when the gland is removed at the end of the dissection.

The temporofacial division of the nerve is approached. The most proximal and posterior branch, the temporal, is often the smallest and is injured easily as it passes upward unless care is exercised. Following it beyond the superior extent of the gland is unnecessary, because the gland is dissected away. The upper and lower zygomatic nerves are larger and more easily identified and followed. As the dissection nears completion with the gland on traction, the final nerve twigs may be bowstringed up; the assistant providing traction must be careful not to tear these small branches, allowing them to be freed surgically from the remaining strands of gland.

With the superficial portion of the gland removed, the main trunk, principal divisions, and all branches should be easily identifiable (see Fig 5). A good rule is never to stimulate them deliberately. Stimulation is not necessary with the technique described, and the result may be facial weakness. After the specimen is removed, troublesome bleeding usually stops, although an occasional small artery may require ligation.

If the tumor is malignant or involves the deeper portion of the gland, total parotidectomy is performed. Nerve hooks are used to gently elevate individual nerve branches and glandular tissue is gently morcellated away until only masseter muscle remains beneath it. Again, it is extremely important that the assistant holding the nerve hooks avoid undue traction, with its undesired consequence of temporary or permanent injury to the nerve branches.

Should the tumor be malignant and adherent or infiltrative to the main trunk or one of its branches, radical parotidectomy may be carried out with sacrifice of the involved portion of the nerve or nerves, especially if the malignancy is high-grade. In patients with less aggressive tumors, sparing of the nerve and postoperative radiation may be acceptable. If the nerve or one of its branches is sacrificed, continuity may be reestablished at once, either by direct reapproximation or by nerve grafting with a portion of the great auricular nerve, which is readily available. Such anastomoses should be done under magnification and with fine suture material (8 – 0 to 10 – 0 nylon).

When parotidectomy is done in conjunction with radical neck dissection (for malignant melanoma, for example), our practice is to perform parotidectomy first. If a tumor is not obvious at the junction of the parotid and neck dissections, the gland may be removed separately and radical neck dissection may be done subsequently. If an in-continuity dissection is desirable, the gland may be left attached to the neck specimen by carrying out the upper (temporofacial) portion of the parotid dissection first and sweeping the gland downward as the lower portion of the dissection is completed. In our practice, neck dissection rarely is carried out for parotid tumors unless they are anaplastic.

After completion of parotidectomy, with hemostasis secured, a Penrose drain or suction catheter is used. The incision is closed with interrupted subcutaneous sutures and the skin closure of preference. A large fluff compression dressing is applied to complete the procedure. With the technique described, parotid dissection usually can be completed in less than 45 minutes, with minimal facial nerve weakness. Additional time is required for closure.

POSTOPERATIVE PERIOD

Drains usually are removed on the second or third postoperative day, with suture removal between the fifth and seventh days. It is wise to reassure the patient with temporary weakness that facial nerve function will return. Reassurance about numbness of the earlobe may also be appropriate.

After healing is complete, deformity usually is slight, except for a mild concavity in the preauricular region, and the scar is scarcely visible. Should Frey's syndrome develop, topical application of atropine or scopolamine ointment may provide adequate control. There are few other long-term complications after parotidectomy with the exception of recurrence.

REFERENCES

1. Batsakis, J. G.: Basal cell adenoma of the parotid gland, Cancer 29:226, 1972.
2. Batsakis, J. G.: *Tumors of the Head and Neck: Clinical and Pathological Considerations* (Baltimore: Williams & Wilkins Company, 1974).
3. Beahrs, O. H., and Chong, G. C.: Management of the facial nerve in parotid gland surgery, Am. J. Surg. 124:473, 1972.
4. Beahrs, O. H., Devine, K. D., and Woolner, L. B.: Parotidectomy in the treatment of chronic sialadenitis, Am. J. Surg. 102:760, 1961.
5. Beahrs, O. H., Woolner, L. B., Carveth, S. W., and Devine, K. D.: Surgical management of parotid lesions: Review of seven hundred sixty cases, Arch. Surg. 80:890, 1960.
6. Eneroth, C.-M.: Histological and clinical aspects of parotid tumours, Acta Otolaryngol. [Suppl.] (Stockh.) 191:15, 1964.
7. Evans, R. W., and Cruickshank, A. H.: Epithelial tumours of the salivary glands, Major Probl. Pathol. 1:1, 1970.
8. Foote, F. W., Jr., and Frazell, E. L.: Tumors of the major salivary glands, Cancer 6:1065, 1953.
9. Godlowski, Z. Z., and Calandra, J. C.: Argentaffine cells in the submaxillary glands of dogs, Anat. Rec. 140:45, 1961.
10. Kirklin, J. W., McDonald, J. R., Harrington, S. W., and New, G. B.: Parotid tumors: Histopathology, clinical behaviour, and end results, Surg. Gynecol. Obstet. 92:721, 1951.
11. Koss, L. G., Spiro, R. H., and Hajdu, S.: Small cell (oat cell) carcinoma of minor salivary gland origin, Cancer 30:737, 1972.
12. Ryan, R. E., Jr., DeSanto, L. W., Weiland, L. H., Devine, K. D., and Beahrs, O. H.: Cellular mixed tumors of the salivary glands (submitted for publication).
13. Thorvaldsson, S. E., Beahrs, O. H., Woolner, L. B., and Simons, J. N.: Mucoepidermoid tumors of the major salivary glands, Am. J. Surg. 120:432, 1970.
14. Wirman, J. A., and Battifora, H. A.: Small cell undifferentiated carcinoma of salivary gland origin: An ultrastructural study, Cancer 37:1840, 1976.

Ulcers of the Leg

F. B. COCKETT, M.S., F.R.C.S.

St. Thomas' Hospital; King Edward VII Hospital for Officers, London; and the University of London, London, England

Evidence that leg ulcers have plagued mankind is found from the beginnings of written history. Hippocrates (460–377 B.C.), the first to associate ulcers of the leg with enlarged veins, advised his patients not to stand too much. Two of the most famous leg ulcers in history belonged to Henry VIII of England (1509–47) and to his daughter Elizabeth I of England (1558–1603). Both monarchs were subject to this malady throughout their declining years, making them ill-tempered and difficult to manage.

The first thought on seeing an ulcer of the leg should be diagnosis. In general, ulcers of the leg can be divided into two broad categories: venous ulcers and nonvenous ulcers.

Venous Ulcers

The basic cause of venous ulcers is abnormal venous hypertension in the lower third of the ankle and dorsum of the foot. The terms "varicose ulcer," "post-thrombotic ulcer" and "gravitational ulcer" all have been used to describe ulcers in the past. These terms suffer from the defect of focusing on only one cause of the venous hypertension. The term varicose ulcer is a particularly poor one, suggesting an association with large surface varicose veins, which is true only in a relatively small percentage of cases. These ulcers should all be termed "venous ulcers," which embraces all the causes of venous hypertension and is the original name suggested by Gay[1] in 1867.

0065-3411/78/0012-0327 $03.75

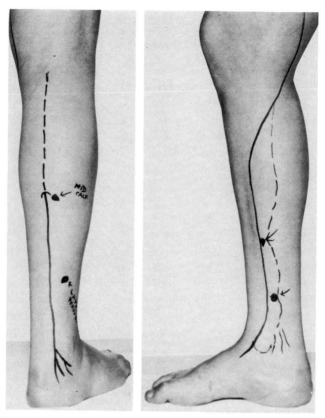

Fig 1.—Position of the four important direct ankle-perforating veins.

In the erect position, the ankle region normally is protected from sustained gravitational venous hypertension by muscle movement. When the calf pump and main deep veins are normal, even the slightest movement empties the superficial veins of the ankle region into the deep calf veins and dramatically lowers the superficial venous pressure.[2] The main pathway of venous drainage of the ankle skin in the erect exercising limbs is via the direct ankle perforating veins (Fig 1); therefore, when the valves in and near these veins become damaged, the worst and most concentrated effects of local venous hypertension in their immediate vicinity are seen. Thus, broadly speaking, the causes of abnormal venous hypertension at the ankle in the erect exercising limb fall into three groups:

1. The localized and explosive venous hypertension due to destruction of ankle perforating vein valves (seen at its most typical in the peripheral type of post-thrombotic syndrome, and complicating the more advanced cases of primary varicose veins) (Fig 2).
2. The more generally diffused type of hypertension seen when the main deep veins are obstructed anywhere from the popliteal vein to the cava.
3. The diffuse gravitational hypertension seen in an immobile or partly paralyzed dependent limb (seen in paraplegics, post-polio paralysis or atrophy of calf muscles in older people with stiff limbs and knees where muscle movement is at a minimum).

Fig 2. — The typical localized ankle perforator ulcer, with ankle flare below the ulcer, as seen in the type 1 post-thrombotic syndrome.

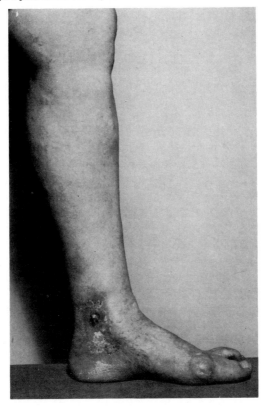

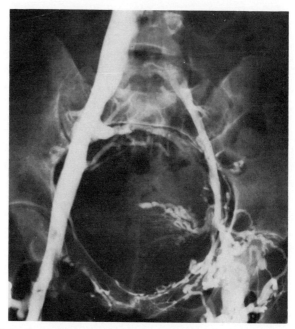

Fig 3. — Obstructed left common iliac vein in type 2 and type 3 post-thrombotic syndrome, due primarily to an iliac compression band at the caval bifurcation.

In post-thrombotic syndromes it is the interplay of perforating vein valve destruction and variable degrees of postcanalization obstruction of the deep veins that causes the ankle venous hypertension, which in turn disrupts the pressure gradient in the capillary loops, leading to cellular necrosis and ulceration. Up until recent years, the postcanalization valve destruction in the deep veins was believed to be the important lesion — it was thought that reflux down the valveless deep veins was a main contributing cause for ankle hypertension. Following this concept, many authors — notably Bauer[3] and, more recently, Linton[4] — have included deep vein ligation in the surgical treatment of post-thrombotic ulceration. However, following the more recent work of May and Thurner[5] and Negus and Cockett,[6] it has been shown that many cases of post-thrombotic syndrome have, in fact, a serious obstruction in the iliac veins at the level of the caval bifurcation (Fig 3). This obstruction is caused by an anatomic developmental anomaly whereby the right common iliac artery crosses the left common iliac vein, compressing it against the convexity of the sacrum behind. In extreme cases the left common iliac vein may be reduced to a wide, flattened, tape-like piece of fibrous tissue behind the artery, sometimes with a few small venous channels still passing through it, but causing almost total obstruction of the left common iliac vein (Fig 4). This "compression band" is the etiologic factor in most cases of iliofemoral thrombosis occurring in relatively young people (age 18–30). After this type of thrombosis, some recanalization occurs up to the iliac compression band, but the patient is left with a serious obstruction to the venous outlet of the limb and numerous venous collaterals develop to overcome this.

Thus, recognition of this condition, which has been named the "iliac compression syndrome,"[7] has now made it possible to accurately sort out the various types of post-thrombotic syndromes. There are three main types or patterns of venous thrombosis in the lower limb as shown in Figure 5.

Fig 4.– A, neoprene cast of the caval bifurcation and the aorta, showing compression and flattening of the left common iliac vein by the overriding right common iliac artery. B, simultaneous arteriogram and venogram, showing a left iliac vein flattened and compressed by overriding right common iliac artery.

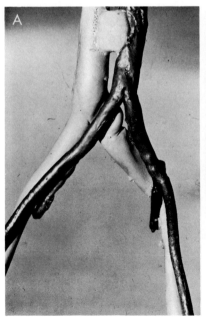
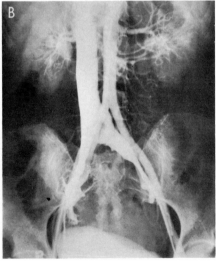

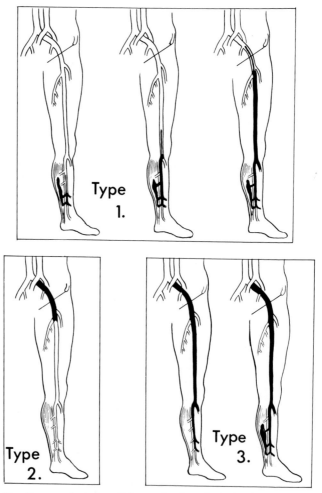

Fig 5.—The three main types of deep vein thrombosis in the lower limb that give rise to the three types of post-thrombotic syndrome.

TYPE 1.—This is the below inguinal ligament type, which starts quietly in the calf and progresses a variable distance up the main deep veins as high as the popliteal or femoral vein. This is the familiar postoperative or stasis thrombosis well known in all hospital patients and most common in older patients.

Patients with type 1 venous thrombosis produce incompetent

ankle perforators as their main post-thrombotic lesion. The popliteal and femoral veins usually recanalize adequately, causing very little deep vein obstruction, and the post-thrombotic ulceration in these patients is due almost entirely to the incompetent perforators. For this reason, if exploration and radical ligation are done before intractable ulceration has been established, a good and permanent cure may be achieved (see Fig 2).

TYPE 2. — This is segmental iliofemoral thrombosis, usually occurring in the left leg and caused by an iliac compression lesion. Typically, this presents as an acute painful swelling of the whole leg — particularly of the thigh — in a young adult. The onset is rapid and dramatic, in sharp contrast to type 1. It usually subsides within a week or two, leaving the patient with a slightly swollen leg that becomes uncomfortable and tense on exercise. These symptoms may subside somewhat with time as the patient gradually develops venous collaterals. As the thrombosis never penetrates down to the calf, the perforating veins and calf pump mechanism remain intact; thus these patients do not develop "explosive" localized perforating vein ulcers. Their ankle skin may remain intact for 10–20 years, after which time some may show mild signs of generalized venous hypertension around the ankle (venules, pigmentation, etc.). Their main post-thrombotic complaint is an uncomfortable aching limb on prolonged standing, with a "bursting feeling" in the calf on exercise (often referred to as venous claudication).

TYPE 3. — This is extended iliofemoral thrombosis, in which the original thrombosis extends right from the iliac vein down to the calf veins and perforating veins. They present in much the same way as type 2 venous thrombosis ulcers but with a more severe clinical picture. A major iliofemoral thrombosis (or "white leg") involves severe swelling of the whole limb, pain, fever and sometimes a cold, blue periphery (the so-called phlegmasia cerulea dolens). As the thrombosis gradually resolves, patients are left with both incompetent perforating veins and an obstructed iliac vein, i.e., both generalized and localized causes of ankle hypertension. They therefore develop the severest form of post-thrombotic syndrome with all the worst characteristics of the previous two groups (gravitational aching, bursting pain *and* severe intractable ankle ulceration).

Such patients need all the resources of treatment to prevent their conditions from deteriorating into the all-too-familiar large ulcers. Early perforator ligation and eradication of any large incompetent superficial veins in the lower part of the limb, continuous strong elastic stocking support and regular periods of rest with elevation of the limb, may all be required at different times throughout life in the management of this condition.

It is also in cases of type 2 and type 3 venous thrombosis ulcers that surgical attempts at dealing with the iliac obstruction by various forms of bypass operation, such as Palma's operation, now are being made.[8]

CLINICAL DIAGNOSIS OF THE VENOUS ULCER

Venous ulcers always have the following characteristics:

SITE. — The ulcer is always somewhere within the so-called gaiter area (the area covered by the gaiter worn by bishops in the present day, and by many famous regiments of foot soldiers during the past century). This area consists of the whole of the lower half of the leg and dorsum of the foot. Venous ulceration may occur anywhere in this area but is, of course, most common on the inner side just above and behind the internal malleolus. This is the area of skin drained directly by the internal ankle perforating veins (in the erect exercising limb). This area also has a relatively slight arterial supply, compared with the profuse supply of the sole of the foot.[9]

THE ANKLE FLARE (Fig 6). — This is always present with a venous ulcer and is a sure sign of pathologic venous hypertension of long standing. It is a flare of dilated venules, particularly on the inner side of the ankle, below the internal malleolus, disappearing into the heel pad.

PIGMENTATION. — There is always some brown pigmentation in the vicinity of a venous ulcer (hemosiderin deposition).

REACTION TO REST WITH ELEVATION. — If the patient is put to bed flat, with the foot of the bed raised just enough to bring the feet at or just above the level of the patient's heart, then the ulcer will rapidly start to heal. Usually there is a marked difference within as few as 48 hours. This position, of course, if maintained rigidly and uninterruptedly, brings the venous pressure in the ankle area down to nearly zero. This early healing reaction, together with respite from pain, etc., can be used as a diag-

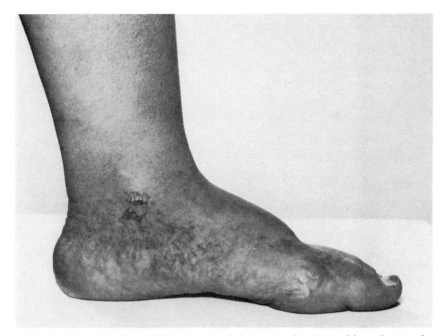

Fig 6.—The ankle flare of dilated venules below an incompetent ankle perforator, the sure sign of a venous ulcer.

nostic test for venous ulceration in doubtful or difficult ulcer cases. However, any ulcer that is due to arterial disease gets more painful and does not heal in this position.

TREATMENT OF VENOUS ULCERATION

The main aim of treatment is to prevent occurrence of an ulcer rather than to treat one after it has occurred. This means that the ulcer precursor signs must be recognized. These are: (1) ankle flare; (2) pigmentation; (3) a patch of fat necrosis or sclerosis in fat legs; and (4) scaling and irritation of the skin in the ankle area.

The occurrence of these signs indicates that ulceration is imminent and that efficient control of the venous hypertension is needed urgently. This may be through surgery (radical control of varicose veins with full perforator surgery in suitable cases) or by external elastic compression; or both may be needed in certain cases (group 3 post-thrombotic syndrome). It cannot be emphasized too strongly that the real place of surgery is in the *prevention* rather than the treatment of established ulceration.

OTHER FACTORS RESPONSIBLE FOR PERSISTENT CHRONIC ULCERATION

Once a breach of the skin of the ankle in a patient with venous hypertension has occurred, then the stage is set for the two complications that are responsible for the persistence of ulcers. These are: infection and skin sensitivity to almost all external applications (ointments, medicated bandages, etc.). Once these complications have been allowed to occur, treatment is urgently needed because the persistence of these two factors in addition to venous hypertension over the years, will produce an almost uncontrollable chronic ulcer.

The treatment of infection is by an oral antibiotic used in adequate dosage over a good two-week course. A red rim around the ulcer and some pain nearly always are indicative of staphylococcal infection. Culture may be difficult because the area may be overgrown by commensals. But regardless of what is grown from the bacteriologic swab (and a great many irrelevant organisms often are grown), an oral antibiotic active against the staphylococcus must be used. The author has always found erythromycin to be by far the best in this context, since sensitivity reactions are almost unknown. This antibiotic also covers less common streptococcal infections. Rarely, where an erythromycin-resistant staphylococcus is present, flucloxacillin may be used. Locally the ulcer should be cleansed with normal saline solution only. On no account should local infection be treated by strong local applications or by local antibiotic treatment.

The treatment of the second complication (skin sensitivity) is to stop applying any medicated dressing, bandage, lotion or ointment to the ulcer. It still is not widely enough known that in an area of venous hypertension — around or near an ulcer — the skin is extremely likely to develop sensitivity to almost any application after even a short period of time (Fig 7). First the skin becomes red and then a mild exfoliative dermatitis with increased serous oozing occurs. This is the ideal medium for bacterial growth; most of the chronic large ulcers that used to be seen in

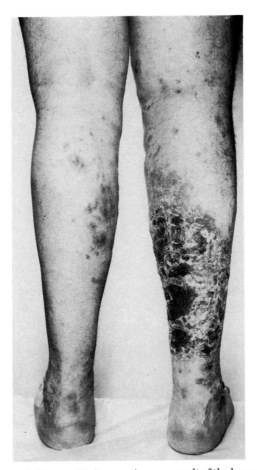

Fig 7. — Widespread skin sensitivity reaction as a result of the long-continued use of a medicated sticky bandage on the skin. Note generalization of skin sensitivity and bilateral eczema.

profusion were due to this combination of skin sensitivity plus infection. All the time-honored ulcer applications have this effect. All medicated creams and ointments (including zinc ointment) usually have lanolin (wool fat) as their base, which is notorious for causing skin sensitivity. All sticky bandages, "tulle gras," and all local antibiotics or antiseptics are bad in this respect. There is no safer application for an ulcer than ordinary plain absorbent gauze.

MANAGEMENT OF THE VENOUS ULCER

The management of an infected eczematous venous ulcer is as follows:

1. Place the patient in bed, recumbent, with the feet higher than the heart (this cures the venous hypertension).
2. Remove all local applications and dressings from the ulcer. Clean away any accumulated discharge or debris daily with a swab soaked in normal saline. No dressings whatsoever should be used. Expose the ulcer to the air by day and simply wrap the leg in a sterile towel by night.
3. Start a two-week course of oral erythromycin.

After four or five days of this regimen the whole condition usually will have settled down and the patient can be allowed up for ambulatory treatment. This is simply a dressing pad made of three or four layers of ordinary gauze and a firm webbing elastic bandage carefully molded around the foot, ankle and calf. The elastic bandage must be stout enough to maintain pressure of at least 70 mm Hg in the ulcer area; otherwise it will not control the ambulatory venous hypertension. If the dressing sticks to the ulcer and is painless it need not be changed, as healing is going on beneath.

The patient is now ready for a full, definitive diagnosis as to the exact venous cause of the condition and for appropriate surgery. On the whole, ankle perforator surgery should not be undertaken until an ulcer has either healed or nearly healed.

Nonvenous Ulcers

Approximately 30% of ulcers of the leg seen in average vascular practice and usually diagnosed as varicose ulcers have little or nothing to do with venous disease. In many patients an ulcer that basically is of venous origin suddenly gets worse and more painful because the patient develops an additional disease that contributes in a major way to the venous problem. In such a patient the ulcer may break down as a complication of gross anemia, polycythemia, leukemia, systemic sclerosis, rheumatoid arthritis or ulcerative colitis, to mention a few of the general conditions.

However, probably the most common cause of sudden breakdown of an ulcer that has been healed for years in an older person (aged 60–70 years) is the appearance of arterial obstruction in the lower limb. Even a straightforward femoral artery block with good collateral, causing only moderate claudication, may cause a healed venous ulcer to start giving pain and to start breaking down. This constitutes a definite indication for direct arterial reconstruction (rather than sympathectomy, which always seems to aggravate venous ulcers).

There is a host of ulcers of the leg that have nothing to do with venous disease. Some of the more common ones are described below.

Ulcers Due to Peripheral Arterial Disease

Ulcers due to peripheral arterial disease and poor peripheral circulation, are seen most often in older people. These really are episodes of trauma or infection that destroy the skin over a more or less limited area of the leg or foot, become infected and then fail to heal because of poor arterial supply. Such ulcers tend to occur on the anterior and outer aspects of the leg (the parts most exposed to trauma); there is no tell-tale "ankle flare," and pain usually is the patient's chief complaint. The ulcers tend to be "punched out" and destroy the whole skin down to deep fascia, unlike venous ulcers. When these ulcers occur on the inner side of the ankle the diagnosis frequently is overlooked.

Martorell's Ulcers

Martorell's ulcers (hypertensive ulcers), first described by Martorell in 1945,[10] are a definite clinical entity and are being seen with great frequency in our aging population. They occur in patients of the upper age group (50–80+ years of age) who usually are hypertensive or arteriosclerotic. They break out quite suddenly, without warning, as a local patch of skin on the back or outer side of the calf necroses and sloughs away (Fig 8). This leaves a punched-out ulcer extending down to the deep fascia. Pain, which may be quite severe and prevent the patient from sleeping, is the presenting and predominant symptom. Martorell's ulcers may be bilateral. The pathology of these ul-

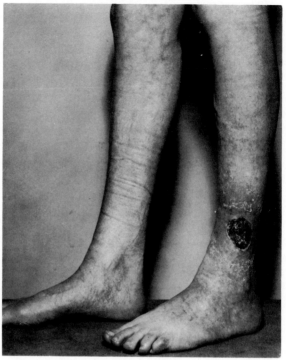

Fig 8.— Martorell's ulcer. Note typical punched-out appearance of the localized area of gangrene. It appeared quite suddenly, causing great pain.

cers lies in a sudden obliteration of the end arterioles of the skin of this region,[9] which has a very sparse arterial supply, either by hypertensive vasculitis or microemboli. It is noteworthy that all peripheral foot pulses usually are present in patients, a few of whom are mildly diabetic.

Since the Martorell's ulcer is an ischemic lesion it has a long, painful course and may take months to heal. If infection takes place, a widespread undermining and gangrene of the skin leading to loss of leg is a risk. In the author's experience, the quickest and best way of curing these ulcers is to excise them with a wide margin of skin until healthy bleeding skin is encountered, and to cover the area with a very thin split-skin graft. In most cases this is combined with a sympathectomy to increase local blood supply, and a course of erythromycin.

BANDAGE PRESSURE ULCERS

These are small, painful, circular ulcers, always occurring right on the prominence of the lateral or medial malleolus. They usually are seen in very elderly patients (70–80 years of age) and are more common on the tip of the lateral malleolus. As their name implies, they are actually a small area of pressure necrosis of skin under an elastic bandage. Even a light elastic bandage on the ankle of an elderly person with perhaps some peripheral arterial occlusion is enough to cause one of these ulcers.

Bandage pressure ulcers are extremely difficult to treat, as they really are a form of peripheral gangrene. Removal of all pressure bandages is essential. Sometimes, when peripheral pulses are present, excision of the area with split-skin grafts will be successful.

INFECTIVE ULCERS

Ulceration due to tuberculosis and syphilis is rare now, but typical multiple serpiginous ulcers of tertiary syphilis occasionally are seen. Other rare organisms occasionally may be the cause of leg ulceration, such as in the epidemic of diphtheritic ulcers that occurred in the Western Desert during the 1939–45 war. However, the most common cause of pure infective ulceration is *Staphylococcus aureus* (occasionally with a streptococcus as well). Chronic staphylococcal ulceration (called impetigo in children) may occur at any age. It usually takes the form of multiple small, red, scabbed sores on the leg and ankle. This type is almost always due to constant reinfection as a result of unclean habits, poor hygiene and inadequate dressings, and rapidly clears up in response to an antistaphylococcal antibiotic taken orally and good dressing technique. These ulcers often are seen in patients with anemia, or in a poor nutritional state. (Fig 9).

Occasionally, particularly in older people, the staphylococcal ulcer can be single and confined to the lower leg and is due to chronic staphylococcal infection of a minor area of trauma, or an insect bite. "Footballers' ulcer" of the shin is due to staphylococcal infection in an area of repetitive trauma.

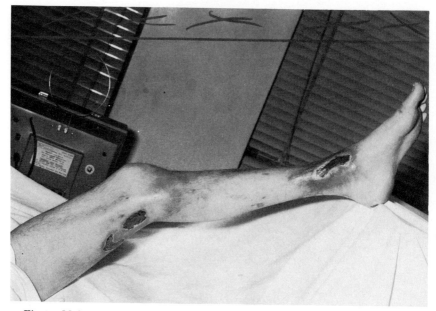

Fig 9.—Multiple staphylococcal ulcers in a drug addict who was dirty, anemic and in a poor nutritional state.

Erythrocyanoid Ulcers

"Erythrocyanosis frigida" or "the erythrocyanoid limb" is a condition frequently seen in the ankles of young women. These patients have thick ankles with an abnormal amount of subcutaneous fat, combined with an abnormally poor arterial supply to the ankle skin. The blood supply of the lower third of the leg and ankle normally is rather poor, consisting of a number of fine perforating arteries arising from the posterior tibial and peroneal arteries. In many erythrocyanoid cases one of these arteries may be abnormally small or even absent altogether, causing chronic low-grade ischemia of the whole ankle region. The patient finds that the ankle skin is abnormally sensitive to temperature changes. When the weather is cold, the ankle is blue and cold and the skin is irritable and often tender. In hot weather a sort of chronic reactive hyperemia is present; the ankle is hot and becomes edematous, swollen and painful. The importance of erythrocyanosis in relation to ulcers is twofold.

1. Anything liable to cause an ulcer (varicose vein, perforating

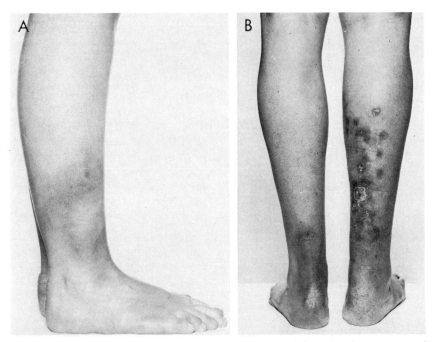

Fig 10.—**A,** a mild case of the erythrocyanoid limb, with blue discoloration around the ankle. **B,** a more advanced case with multiple ulcerating chilblains and areas of fat necrosis.

vein incompetence, trauma, infection, etc.) produces its effect much more quickly and in a more severe degree in the relatively ischemic fat ankle. It therefore is necessary to recognize this condition and to treat conditions such as varicose veins earlier and more vigorously in the erythrocyanoid limb. Once they have occurred in an erythrocyanoid ankle, trauma, ulceration and infection are much slower to heal.

2. Acute fat necrosis sometimes may occur on the back and outer side of the ankle, particularly with chronic exposure to cold external conditions. This may ulcerate through the skin, causing a very chronic painful ulcer, sometimes requiring sympathectomy to manage it.

Ulcerating surface chilblains also may occur in response to cold (Fig 10). These chilblains are due to "rouleaux clumping" of red cells in the static blood in surface capillaries of a relatively ischemic area. This again may be an indication for sympathectomy, particularly if the patient lives in a cold climate.

Chronic ulcers of the ankle that occur in the severe paralyzed postpoliomyelitic leg are of this variety (i.e., localized fat necrosis due to ischemia); this also is an indication for sympathectomy.[7]

CORTISONE ULCERS

During the last decade, ointments containing various cortisone derivatives have become available freely to the medical profession. These often are applied to quite minor abrasions, eczemas and other lesions of the ankle because they tend to damp down local inflammatory reaction, therefore controlling pain. If these local cortisone creams are applied continuously over a period of months or even years, as is often the case, the result may be a large, callous, sluggish ulcer with absolutely no tissue inflammatory response. These ulcers are a great problem and may end up requiring widespread excision and grafting.

Summary

The catalog of possible causes of ulceration of the leg is unending. It has been the purpose of this article to cover in some detail those ulcers seen most commonly in Western Europe and America. Neoplastic ulcers, tropical ulcers, ulcers due to underlying bone disease, ulcers associated with blood dyscrasias, ulcers due to foreign bodies and self-inflicted injury, and injection ulcers all occur but are rare and are covered in detail elsewhere.[7]

In summary, it must be emphasized that an ulcer of the leg needs a correct diagnosis before appropriate treatment can be administered. Diagnosis often is difficult and far from obvious, requiring considerable care and clinical experience.

REFERENCES

1. Gay, J.: On varicose diseases of the lower extremities, in *The Lettsomian Lectures of 1867* (London: Churchill, 1868).
2. Højensgaard, I. C., and Sturup, H.: Static and dynamic pressures in superficial and deep veins of the lower extremity in man, Acta. Physiol. Scand. 27:49, 1952.
3. Bauer, G.: Division of popliteal vein in treatment of so-called varicose ulceration, Br. Med. J. 2:318, 1950.
4. Linton, R. R., and Hardy, I. B., Jr.: Postthrombotic syndrome of lower extremity; treatment by interruption of superficial femoral vein and ligation and stripping of long and short saphenous veins, Surgery 24:452, 1948.

5. May, R., and Thurner, J.: The cause of the predominantly sinistral occurrence of thrombosis of the pelvic veins, Angiology 8:419, 1957.
6. Negus, D., and Cockett, F. B.: Femoral vein pressures in post-phlebitic iliac vein obstruction, Br. J. Surg. 54:522, 1967.
7. Cockett, F. B.: *Pathology and Surgery of the Veins of the Lower Limb* (London: Churchill Livingstone, 1976).
8. Palma, E. C., Passano de Moizo, M., and Guevara, A., et al.: Arteriosclerosis hemodinamica experimental de la arteria coronria, Rev. Cir. Urug. 35: 11, 1965.
9. Arterial supply of the ulcer-bearing area, in *Pathology and Surgery of the Veins of the Lower Limb* (London: Churchill Livingstone, 1976).
10. Martorell, F.: Les ulcères supra-maleolares por arteriolitis de los grandes hipertensos, Actas Polyclin., 1945.

Coronary Artery Surgery

JOSEPH N. CUNNINGHAM, JR., M.D.,
O. WAYNE ISOM, M.D., AND FRANK C.
SPENCER, M.D.

*Department of Surgery, New York University Medical Center,
New York, New York*

Coronary artery disease is a major cause of death in adults over the age of 40 in the western world.[1] In 1973 coronary artery disease was the leading cause of death in men over the age of 35 and in all persons over age 45 in the United States. It accounted for more than 600,000 deaths in this country.[2] About 4 million people in the United States, or about 2% of the total population, have been estimated to have coronary artery disease. These 4 million people have a history of either myocardial infarction or angina pectoris. It is staggering to realize that the incidence of subclinical or unapparent anatomical coronary artery disease may be 5 or even 10 times that of clinical disease.

Surgery for coronary artery disease has evolved over the past 50 years. For almost 30 years, between 1930 and 1960, techniques of denervation such as excision of the upper thoracic ganglia were performed to alleviate angina. Attempts to increase blood supply to the myocardium through development of an inflammatory response between the pericardium and the epicardium were pioneered by Beck between 1935 and 1955.[3] In the late 1940s modification of this procedure was extended by arterialization of the coronary sinus and ligation or decreasing the size of the coronary sinus.[4] In 1950 Vineberg and Walker reported clinical results with implantation of the internal mammary artery in areas of the left ventricular wall.[5] This was performed with varying frequency over the next 20 years.

0065-3411/78/0012-0347 $03.75

Finally, in 1967 and 1968, coronary bypass surgery evolved at the Cleveland Clinic, at the University of Wisconsin in Milwaukee and at New York University in New York City. By 1970 the number of coronary bypass procedures across the country was starting to increase, and it is estimated that about 70,000 to 80,000 of these procedures were performed in 1977.[6] The total number over the past 10 years has been estimated at 400,000. The goals for surgery in coronary artery disease over the past 50 years have been (1) to eliminate symptoms, (2) to prevent or decrease the incidence of myocardial infarction and (3) to increase longevity. All of these goals were to be obtained with a low morbidity.

Prior to direct coronary bypass surgery, many of the previously mentioned procedures were initially accepted with enthusiasm, relief or improvement of symptoms being seen in 70–90% of patients. This relief was short-lived, however, as there was no influence on the incidence of myocardial infarction or longevity. In contrast, direct coronary bypass surgery showed a dramatic relief of symptoms, with marked improvement in 85–90% of patients.[7] Nevertheless, the debate persists, even after 10 years' experience, regarding the ability of the procedure to decrease the incidence of myocardial infarction or to prolong survival.[8] As pointed out in the thoughtful and thorough review by McIntosh and Garcia in 1978, only a few more than 1,000 patients have been studied in a carefully controlled, randomized manner.[6]

It is not the purpose of this discussion to enter the debate on "medical vs surgical therapy." Taking into consideration the advances in surgical techniques in coronary bypass surgery over the past 10 years, we propose to convey our approach to ischemic heart disease in its various manifestations as we see them clinically in our day-to-day practice at the New York University Medical Center. Undoubtedly the various surgeons across the country will consider different modes of therapy according to different clinical manifestations. Our philosophy is that, with the current state of the art in 1978, coronary bypass surgery should be considered part of the armamentarium of both cardiologist and surgeon in treatment of various clinical syndromes. Whether the patient is treated surgically or not, certainly intense medical therapy such as cessation of smoking, control of hyperlipidemia, control of hypertension and drug therapy should be considered of utmost importance.

At NYU Medical Center we classify the manifestations of ischemic heart disease as follows:

I. Incapacitating angina
II. Poor left ventricular function with or without angina
III. Mild stable angina
IV. Asymptomatic patient following myocardial infarction
V. Asymptomatic patient with significant angiographic disease
VI. Crescendo or preinfarction angina
VII. Significant stenosis of left mainstem coronary artery

This discussion will define each of these syndromes and will discuss the indications for surgery, operative mortality, relief of symptoms, influence on myocardial infarction and long-term survival.

Finally, the operative techniques currently used at NYU will be presented with the experimental and clinical results.

Incapacitating Angina

Incapacitating angina is defined as disabling angina that has been unresponsive to medical therapy and limits the patient's life style, either preventing him from working or limiting most recreational activities. Table 1 shows the overall experience with coronary bypass surgery at NYU between 1968 and 1975. A total of 1,172 patients had elective coronary bypass for incapacitating angina during this period. Patients included 967 men between ages 27 and 79, mean age 53 years, and 205 women between ages 26 and 73, mean age 57 years. Patients having emergency operations for crescendo angina (to be discussed later) and those with associated valvular replacement were excluded from this group. Included in this analysis were the 50% of patients who had ventricular impairment, except for those with diffuse hypokinesis (bad left ventricle). These also will be discussed later.

INDICATIONS FOR SURGERY

The only contraindication to surgery was the presence of chronic congestive heart failure (bad left ventricle) without angina. Nonvisualization of vessels beyond arterial obstruction,

TABLE 1.—OVERALL EXPERIENCE IN 1,712 PATIENTS UNDERGOING CORONARY BYPASS SURGERY

YEAR	TOTAL NO. OF PATIENTS	TYPE OF SURGERY*	NO. OF PATIENTS	NO. OF OPERATIVE DEATHS	OPERATIVE MORTALITY (%)
1968	13	SCB	10	3	38.5
		DCB	3	2	
1969	31	SCB	6	0	6.5
		DCB	22	2	
		TCB	3	0	
1970	74	SCB	11	0	12.2
		DCB	59	9	
		TCB	4	0	
1971	156	SCB	24	1	6.4
		DCB	57	4	
		TCB	67	5	
		QCB or more	8	0	
1972	166	SCB	19	0	3.6
		DCB	56	3	
		TCB	91	3	
1973	213	SCB	16	0	4.2
		DCB	61	3	
		TCB	123	6	
		QCB or more	13	0	
1974	244	SCB	31	0	2.7
		DCB	66	1	
		TCB	116	3	
		QCB or more	31	3	
1975	275	SCB	19	0	4.7
		DCB	62	3	
		TCB	108	4	
		QCB or more	86	6	
Totals	1172			61	5.2

*SCB = single coronary bypass; DCB = double coronary bypass; TCB = triple coronary bypass; QCB = quadruple coronary bypass.
From Isom, O. W., et al.: Does coronary bypass increase longevity?, J. Thor. Cardiovasc. Surg. 75:29, 1978. Used by permission.

age, diabetes or hypertension, although clearly complicating the operative procedure, were not major contraindications. Table 1 shows the number of patients operated on annually between 1968 and 1975, the types of bypass grafts performed and the operative mortality. Fewer than 100 patients were operated on annually before 1970, after which the number has gradually increased to well over 200 per year. Because of the limited institutional resources and multiple responsibilities for teaching and research at the Medical Center, the number of bypass operations has been limited to between 200 and 300 a year. This policy has similarly influenced our data, as we have selected more seriously disabled patients for operation.

OPERATIVE MORTALITY

As shown in Table 1, the number of triple bypass grafts increased after 1970 and single bypass grafts decreased. Operative mortality was initially high but has ranged between 2.7% and 4.7% since 1971, with an overall 8-year average of 5.2%. A total of 61 operative deaths (patients who died within the first 30 days or never left the hospital) occurred among the 1,172 patients (Table 2). Of these 61 deaths, 39 clearly resulted from cardiac injury: 14 cases from myocardial infarction, 17 from low-output syndrome and 8 from arrhythmia. Renal failure, sepsis, respiratory problems and neurologic injury were rarely a cause of death, a somewhat surprising finding in these patients with diffuse atherosclerosis. The operative mortality ranged from 1% to 2% in 1976–1977.

TABLE 2.–CAUSES OF OPERATIVE
DEATHS IN 1,172 PATIENTS UNDER-
GOING ELECTIVE CORONARY BYPASS
GRAFTING

CAUSE OF DEATH	NO. OF DEATHS
Myocardial infarction	14
Low output	17
Arrhythmias	8
Renal failure	3
Sepsis	4
Respiratory	5
Neurologic	4
Hemorrhage from peptic ulcer	1
Complications of reoperation	2
Miscellaneous*	3
Total	61 (5.2%)

*Graft occlusion, 1; ruptured aorta, 1; thrombosis of superior mesenteric artery, 1.
From Isom, O. W., et al.: Does coronary bypass increase longevity?, J. Thor. Cardiovasc. Surg. 75:30, 1978. Used by permission.

TABLE 3. – STATUS OF ANGINA IN
1,017 CURRENTLY
SURVIVING PATIENTS

	PATIENTS	
STATUS OF ANGINA	NO.	%
None or less	935	91.9
Equal	56	5.5
Worse	26	2.6

From Isom, O. W., et al.: Does coronary bypass increase longevity?, J. Thor. Cardiovasc. Surg. 75:31, 1978. Used by permission.

RELIEF OF SYMPTOMS

Among 1,017 late survivors, 91.9% were either free of angina or much improved (Table 3). Angina remained the same as before operation in about 5.5% of patients, and was worse than before in only 2.6%. In more than two thirds of the patients, activity levels increased over those before operation, whereas activity levels were decreased in only 12% of patients because of cardiac symptoms. Of the 1,017 survivors, 44% (452) were employed full time and 6% part time; 30% had retired before the operation because of age and had not planned on returning to full-time work even with improvement of symptoms. Thus, the degree of rehabilitation following operation is impressive, especially since many patients were threatened with either retirement or total change in vocation because of disabling angina before the operation.

INFLUENCE ON MYOCARDIAL INFARCTION

PERIOPERATIVE INFARCTIONS. — Perioperative myocardial infarction has been reported to occur in 1 – 2% of patients, based on ECG and enzyme analysis.[9] If rapid sequence isoenzyme CPK-MB analysis is performed (every 15 minutes) during operation and each hour for 8 hours following surgery, myocardial injury will be more apparent.[10] If more sophisticated radioisotope studies are performed, myocardial injury at the time of operation may be more accurately defined. Codd et al. recently compared a group of 50 patients who sustained myocardial infarction, as diagnosed by ECG or enzyme criteria, during surgery

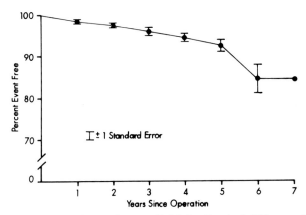

Fig 1.—Cumulative incidence of myocardial infarction in 1,017 currently surviving patients. Deaths, both early and late, have been excluded. (From Isom, O. W., et al.: Does coronary bypass increase longevity?, J. Thor. Cardiovasc. Surg. 75:32, 1978. Used by permission.)

with a similar group of patients undergoing coronary bypass surgery who did not sustain a perioperative myocardial infarction. No difference in long-term survival, relief of angina, congestive heart failure or graft patency could be ascertained.[11]

LATE MYOCARDIAL INFARCTIONS.—Among 1,111 patients surviving operation, there were 16 fatal myocardial infarctions and 41 nonfatal myocardial infarctions in 33 patients (Table 4). Of the 41 nonfatal infarctions, 26 patients had 1, 6 patients had 2 and 1 patient had 3. Therefore, if the frequency of infarction in currently surviving patients is calculated by the actuarial method, 94% of surviving patients remained free of myocardial infarction for 5 years and 91% for 7 years (Fig 1).

TABLE 4.—NUMBER OF LATE
DOCUMENTED MYOCARDIAL
INFARCTIONS IN 1,111 PATIENTS
SURVIVING OPERATION

INFARCTION	NO. OF INFARCTIONS
Fatal	16
Nonfatal	41
Total	57

From Isom, O. W., et al.: Does coronary bypass increase longevity?, J. Thor. Cardiovasc. Surg. 75:31, 1978. Used by permission.

LONG-TERM SURVIVAL

Forty-eight late cardiac-related deaths, a surprisingly small number, occurred among the 1,111 patients discharged from the hospital (Table 5). Of the 48 deaths, 33 apparently were caused by an acute ischemic episode with 16 myocardial infarctions, and 11 sudden unexplained deaths. In 2 of the sudden deaths the patient was found to have the graft occluded at autopsy and, in 4, death was apparently due to an arrhythmia. It seems significant that only 5 patients died of congestive heart failure. Five patients died at reoperation because of occluded previous grafts. Hepatitis (1 patient), pulmonary embolism (1) and renal failure (2) were rare a causes of death.

The long-term survival, calculated by the actuarial method and including operative deaths, was 88% at 5 years and 80% at 7 years (Fig 2). To further emphasize the surprisingly low late mortality, of each 100 patients operated on, 95 were discharged from the hospital and only 7 of these died from cardiac causes in the ensuing 5 years. Hence, once the patient was discharged from the hospital, his chances of dying from heart disease in the next 5 years was 7.4%, or 1.5% annually. This overall survival rate of 88% at 5 years is similar to the frequently quoted Veterans Administration study performed between 1972 and 1974.[12] The additional factor that makes the 88% 5-year survival rate surprising is that the data include our total experience, and, in

TABLE 5.—CAUSES OF LATE CARDIAC-RELATED DEATHS

		YEARS					
CAUSE	TOTAL	1ST	2D	3D	4TH	5TH	6TH
Documented myocardial infarction	16	4	3	5	2	2	0
Congestive heart failure	5	0	0	2	2	0	1
Sudden and unexplained	11	4	2	2	0	0	3
Sudden (grafts occluded at autopsy)	2	1	0	0	0	0	1
Arrhythmia	4	1	1	0	0	1	1
Reoperation for cardiac disease	5	2	1	0	1	1	0
Pneumonia	1	1	0	0	0	0	0
Pulmonary embolus	1	1	0	0	0	0	0
Hepatitis	1	1	0	0	0	0	0
Renal failure	2	1	0	0	1	0	0
Total	48	16	7	9	5	4	6

From Isom, O. W., et al.: Does coronary bypass increase longevity?, J. Thor. Cardiovasc. Surg. 75:31, 1978. Used by permission.

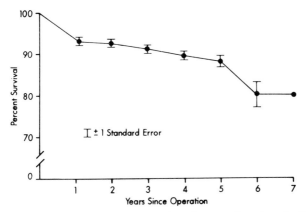

Fig 2. — Actuarial survival curve for 1,172 patients undergoing elective coronary bypass grafting from 1968 to 1972. All cardiac-related deaths, both early and late, are included. Noncardiac-related deaths and patients who were lost to follow up are excluded as withdrawn alive. (From Isom, O. W., et al.: Does coronary bypass increase longevity: J. Thor. Cardiovasc. Surg., 75:32, 1978. Used by permission.)

retrospect, the techniques used between 1968 and 1971 were considerably inferior to those used subsequently. Such improvement in operative mortality and long-term survival, has also been reflected in other reports.[13-15] This improvement is almost surely due not only to more complete revascularization but also to less injury to the myocardium at operation.

The magnitude of injury to the myocardium at operation remains one of the most elusive aspects of coronary bypass surgery and is undoubtedly one of the principal reasons for the conflicting data in many reports. Chemical measurements of myocardial injury have shown clearly that not only may a patient survive operation despite extensive myocardial injury but the injury may not even be clinically recognizable. As pointed out earlier and supported by the recent report by Codd et al., the degree of injury cannot be ascertained by current ECG or enzyme analysis.[11] However, the relative proportion between the degree of injury and the degree of benefit from revascularization most assuredly determines the eventual results.

The 2 most significant factors in medical therapy appear to be cessation of smoking and control of hypertension. After the patient has undergone surgery, these 2 factors are vigorously encouraged. The value of decreased lipid intake is strongly supported on theoretical grounds but unfortunately has not been proved with long-term data. Nevertheless, this therapeutic approach certainly is recommended. Exercise programs, weight reduction and other measures to increase collateral circulation, although theoretically sound, also have not yet been demonstrated to have a major impact on the course of the disease. Fortunately, atherosclerosis developing in vein grafts, which can readily be demonstrated in the experimental laboratory, has not been a significant factor in causing late occlusion of vein grafts.

Poor Left Ventricle With or Without Angina

This manifestation of coronary disease is defined as diffuse hypokinesia of the left ventricle involving 3 or more planes with an end diastolic pressure of 20 or above or an ejection fraction of less than 25%. Most of these patients have sustained myocardial infarctions in the past. In the early years of coronary bypass surgery, significant impairment of left ventricular function was considered a contraindication to this therapeutic approach because of the high operative mortality.[16] There has been a drastic reversal in therapeutic philosophy concerning this group of "previously inoperable" patients: this group is now more than ever considered to be in more urgent need of coronary revascularization, as further infarction may result in such severe ventricular impairment that cardiac failure will supervene.

Even though the long-term effect of bypass surgery on increasing longevity and decreasing late infarction is important, the operative technique in this group of patients with borderline myocardial tissue assumes even greater significance. Many perioperative infarctions occurred in the early years of bypass surgery, making these patients a high-risk surgical group. Over the past 5 years, however, methods of myocardial preservation during coronary revascularization have been refined, lowering significantly perioperative infarction rate and thereby the operative mortality.

INDICATIONS FOR SURGERY

Any patient with incapacitating angina should be considered for bypass surgery, regardless of the degree of left ventricular dysfunction or the severity of congestive heart failure symptoms. Patent distal vessels for bypass grafting should be visualized beyond stenotic lesions or by retrograde filling of completely obstructed vessels through collateral circulation. The only contraindication to bypass surgery is chronic congestive heart failure without angina or diffusely diseased distal vessels unacceptable for grafting. This anatomical state probably represents a more severe form or further advanced stage of coronary arteriosclerosis. The presence of hypertension, diabetes or congestive heart failure with angina is not considered a contraindication to surgery.

OPERATIVE MORTALITY

Table 6 shows the number of operative and late deaths in 87 patients operated on by three surgeons at NYU Medical Center from 1971 through 1975. These patients had diffuse hypokinesia and left ventricular end diastolic (LVED) pressures of 20 or above (mean 27, range 20–45). The number operated on each year rose from 12 in 1971 to 28 in 1975. Among the 87 patients there were 9 operative deaths, an operative mortality of 10.3%. There were only 5 late deaths during a follow up of 4–64 months. The causes of the operative deaths were low output, and causes of late deaths either congestive heart failure or recurrent myocardial infarction.

RELIEF OF SYMPTOMS

The relief of angina was gratifying in this group. Although all patients had angina in varying degrees preoperatively (most

TABLE 6.—OPERATIVE EXPERIENCE IN 87
PATIENTS WITH IMPAIRED LEFT
VENTRICULAR FUNCTION

	NO. OF PATIENTS	OPERATIVE DEATHS	LATE DEATHS
1971	12	3	0
1972	10	1	3
1973	18	1	1
1974	19	0	1
1975	28	4	0
Total	87	9	5

From Isom, O. W., et al.: Coronary revascularization with significant impairment of left ventricular contractility, Cardiovasc. Clin. 8:269, 1977. Used by permission.

TABLE 7.—STATUS OF ANGINA IN
87 PATIENTS FOLLOWING SURGERY

None	60.6%
Less	32.4%
Unchanged	7.0%

From Isom, O. W., et al.: Coronary revascularization with significant impairment of left ventricular contractility, Cardiovasc. Clin. 8:269, 1977. Used by permission.

TABLE 8.—STATUS OF CONGESTIVE HEART
FAILURE IN 87 PATIENTS FOLLOWING SURGERY

	FREE OF SYMPTOMS OR SIGNS %
Dyspnea on exertion	60
Paroxysmal nocturnal dyspnea	80
Orthopnea	76
Pulmonary or pedal edema	77

From Isom, O. W., et al.: Coronary revascularization with significant impairment of left ventricular contractility, Cardiovasc. Clin. 8:270, 1977. Used by permission.

had incapacitating angina), 93% were either free of angina or significantly improved after operation (Table 7). Only 7% of patients were not improved postoperatively. Of the patients, 60% were free of symptoms of dyspnea on exertion, and nearly 80% were free of more severe symptoms of paroxysmal nocturnal dyspnea, orthopnea or pulmonary edema (Table 8). The lack of dramatic improvement in the symptoms of congestive heart failure is not surprising, since the most likely benefit of operation is to *preserve* myocardium rather than improve contractility. Although improvement in contractility is desirable, realistically this probably occurs in only a small percentage of patients undergoing operation. Therefore, the goal of the operation should be to preserve the myocardium during the surgical procedure and, with improvement in blood supply, decrease the incidence of myocardial injury in the late postoperative period.

INFLUENCE ON MYOCARDIAL INFARCTION

As mentioned earlier, the 9 operative deaths were due to low-output syndrome, probably as a result of perioperative infarc-

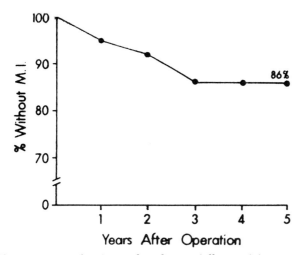

Fig 3.—The percentage of patients, plotted actuarially, surviving operation 5 years without a myocardial infarction *(M.I.)* (From Isom, O. W., et al.: Coronary revascularization with significant impairment of left ventricular contractility, Cardiovasc. Clin. 8: 271, 1977. Used by permission.)

tion. Figure 3 shows the percentage of patients, plotted actuarily, surviving operation 5 years without a myocardial infarction. A remarkable level of 86% is noted. Thus, only 14% of the surviving patients suffered a myocardial infarction, an incidence of less than 3% a year.

Long-Term Survival

Figure 4 shows the 5-year survival to be 83% including operative deaths, plotted actuarily, in the 87 patients operated on at NYU. Although no recent studies have been presented with 5-year survivals in unoperated on groups, this is certainly a marked improvement in survival over that in similar patients who were treated medically in the 1960s.[17]

Mild Stable Angina

Mild stable angina is defined as nondisabling angina that occurs once or twice a week or less. Patients are usually well controlled with medical therapy (usually beta-blockers) and vasodilators. The key point in the status of this syndrome is that

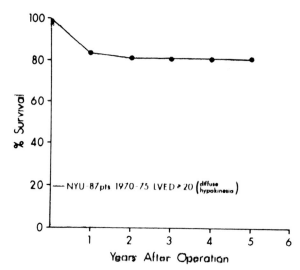

Fig 4.—Five-year survival of 87 patients operated on with left ventricular end dia-stolic pressures of 20 mm Hg or above and diffuse hypokinesia. (From Isom, O. W., et al.: Coronary revascularization with significant impairment of left ventricular contractility, Cardiovasc. Clin. 8:271, 1977. Used by permission.)

the patient is not significantly limited in work or recreational activity.

The indications for surgery in this group remain debatable in most institutions across the country. Some medical groups will catheterize these patients and, if the lesions are operable, will recommend surgery.

The NYU Medical Center is presently participating in a na-tional, collaborative, prospective, randomized study involving a number of major centers in the United States. This study has been in progress for the past 3 years, but to date no significant data are available. At present, at NYU, unless the patient with mild stable angina accepts randomization, we do not recommend surgery. The only exclusion in this group would be the patient with significant left main-stem disease or the patient with ste-nosis of 90% or more in the left anterior descending artery proxi-mal to the first septal perforator.

The Asymptomatic Patient After Myocardial Infarction

These patients usually are seen initially with minimal or ab-sent symptoms following a myocardial infarction. Upon resuming previous activities, no angina and no limitation in function are noted.

The indications for angiography and possible surgery in this group are also debatable, and are being evaluated in the previously mentioned study under the auspices of the National Institutes of Health. Unless such patients accept randomization, we do not recommend them for bypass surgery. As in the mild, stable angina patients, the only exceptions are those with left main-stem stenoses and high-grade stenosis of the left anterior descending artery proximal to the first perforator.

The Asymptomatic Patient With Significant Angiographic Disease

This group of patients is defined as having no symptoms and are usually identified by an abnormal stress ECG. Following cardiac catheterization, they are found to have significant coronary disease. As in the previous 2 groups, debate exists in major centers across the country as to whether this group of patients should undergo coronary bypass. At present, we are not considering these patients for surgery unless there is significant left main-stem disease or high-grade stenosis of the proximal left anterior descending artery. As additional data are accumulated over the next several years, perhaps the indications for surgery in this group of patients will change.

Preinfarction or Crescendo Angina

Preinfarction angina, or intermediate coronary syndrome, has been described as being between intermittent angina pectoris and myocardial infarction. It is characterized by continued angina at rest, associated with reversible ECG changes, but the natural history of patients with this clinical syndrome is not homogeneous. About 85% of patients treated with adequate doses of beta-blockers experience complete relief of chest pain and regression of ECG abnormalities.[18] The 1-year mortality from this disease in medically treated groups is reported to be 18–20%.[19, 20] In patients who fail to respond to medical therapy and continue to experience pain and ECG changes, the outlook appears grim. This high-risk group described by Gazes et al. had a 12-month mortality of 43% and a cumulative 24-month mortality of 53%.[19]

The risk of acute myocardial infarction appears to be very

significant in preinfarction angina patients. Krauss, Hutter and DeSantis[20] observed 6 myocardial infarctions in 36 patients before discharge (18%), and Gazes et al.[19] reported 19 myocardial infarctions in 54 patients within 3 months (60%).

INDICATIONS FOR SURGERY AND OPERATIVE MORTALITY

In light of the high incidence of myocardial infarction and death, emergency coronary bypass surgery has been proposed as an alternative in most patients with preinfarction angina who fail to respond to appropriate medical therapy. The results of coronary artery bypass in preinfarction angina are varied. The mortality has been reported as low as 2.5% and as high as 22%.[21, 22] Most groups, however, report an operative mortality of 8–10%, which is about 3 times as high as the mortality for elective bypass procedures.[23, 24] Impaired ventricular function, unrecognized acute myocardial infarction, and pre-bypass hemodynamic instability all have been cited as factors that contribute to this higher operative mortality.[22, 24, 25]

The relatively high operative mortality and incidence of perioperative infarction (about 10% in most series) has prompted investigators to examine various modalities of myocardial preservation in attempts to reduce the risk of emergency coronary artery bypass.[21, 23, 24] Some have advocated the use of balloon counterpulsation prior to operation to alleviate continued ischemia and to prevent hemodynamic instability associated with induction of anesthesia.[26, 27] Gold et al. have demonstrated morbidity and mortality with this modality that approach those of stable angina patients undergoing elective revascularization.[26] Adams et al. reported emergency surgery in 25 consecutive patients with preinfarction angina (uncontrolled by medical therapy) in whom counterpulsation was not used.[28] They reported an overall incidence of perioperative infarction and mortality of 4% in this group of patients (1 death occurring in a patient with left main-stem occlusion). In this particular series of patients, these impressive results were attributed to three factors: (1) avoidance or early treatment of hemodynamic instability at the time of induction of anesthesia, (2) utilization of profound hypothermia with potassium cardioplegic arrest and (3) limitation of cross-clamp times to less than 50 minutes' total ischemia.

In summary, therapeutic goals in patients with preinfarction angina remain relief of recurrent ischemic chest pain and prevention of myocardial infarction and death. Medical modalities of strict bed rest and beta-adrenergic blockade are often successful for patients with this syndrome, and control of the patient with unstable or preinfarction angina should always be attempted initially from a medical standpoint.[18] However, if adequate control is not readily obtained from medical maneuvers, the immediate mortality is significant, and emergency coronary bypass surgery should be performed.[19, 20, 29]

MYOCARDIAL PROTECTION AND PREOPERATIVE ASSESSMENT

The key factor in successfully performing such emergency surgery relates to protective measures during the period of induction pre-bypass, as well as adequate measures of myocardial protection during the operation itself. All attempts should be made to rule out a preexisting myocardial injury by use of such measures as specific CPK-MB isoenzyme data, myocardial scanning techniques and ECGs in order to avoid performing revascularization in a setting of a preexisting myocardial infarction. Such revascularization generally is associated with an unacceptable mortality because of further injury resulting from myocardial hemorrhage and extension of the preexisting infarct.[30] Utilization of careful preoperative patient assessment as well as strict intraoperative measures for myocardial preservation should result in an acceptably low morbidity and mortality (under 5%) and longevity approaching those of patients undergoing surgery for incapacitating angina of the non-preinfarction variety.[7]

Left Main-Stem Coronary Occlusion

Left main-stem coronary occlusion represents a difficult management problem from both surgical and medical standpoints. Surgical intervention in this particular group of patients, because of uncontrollable angina, is usually associated with a higher than normal morbidity and mortality than in the patient operated on electively for stable angina with more distal occlusion only. Obstruction of the left main-stem coronary artery occurs in about 8–12% of patients with angina pectoris, and more often than not is associated with concomitant distal coronary occlusive disease.[31] Isolated stenosis of the left main coronary is unusual and occurs in less than 1% of patients.[32]

INDICATIONS FOR SURGERY

Although there is still considerable controversy concerning surgical intervention in patients with asymptomatic left main-stem coronary stenosis, there appears to be almost no disagreement that the symptomatic individual with left main-stem coronary stenosis should undergo aortocoronary bypass grafting at the earliest possible interval to avoid progression of unstable angina to overt myocardial infarction. No data exist in the literature, however, to support the premise that surgery prevents myocardial infarction in asymptomatic patients with left main-stem coronary occlusion. Some investigators report that the occurrence of myocardial infarction with such occlusion is uncommon despite a large amount of jeopardized myocardium.[31] Nevertheless, most surgeons have concluded that *urgent coronary bypass grafting* in the patient with left main-stem coronary occlusion will improve the clinical course. In many institutions the discovery of a left main-stem occlusion (asymptomatic or symptomatic) is considered a situation of surgical urgency.[31, 33-35]

OPERATIVE MORTALITY, TECHNIQUE AND PERIOPERATIVE INFARCTION

A retrospective review of about 400 consecutive patients undergoing cardiac catheterization and subsequent coronary bypass surgery at NYU Medical Center during the period from April 1976 through October 1977 revealed an approximate 12% incidence of left main-stem coronary occlusions. All of these stenotic patients (55) underwent aortocoronary bypass grafting at the earliest possible time following stabilization of symptoms. Absence of symptoms was not considered a contraindication for revascularization. The critical nature of this particular type of stenosis is evidenced by the fact that patients undergoing revascularization have a mortality of about 10% (2 – 3 times that of elective patients) and a perioperative infarction rate ranging from 12 – 22% depending on the method of myocardial preservation chosen.[36]

Before surgical intervention, all attempts at stabilization of symptoms, including maximum medical therapy, should be used. Often when patients continue to have symptoms despite adequate medical management, it is necessary to apply balloon counterpulsation judiciously prior to the period of induction and bypass. This latter approach may ultimately prove to be a method of myocardial preservation that should be used in all patients with significant left main-stem coronary stenoses. The reasons for this statement are based on evidence that more than 50% of patients undergoing bypass grafting for left main-stem coronary occlusion experience some significant degree of instability in the period during induction before bypass.[36] It is during this period that the majority of myocardial injuries occur as a result of alterations in the supply-demand ratio due to the critical nature of the left main-stem coronary occlusion. Minor changes in blood pressure, heart rate or oxygen demands may cause occult subendocardial necrosis, with resultant pump failure in the post-bypass period. All measures to monitor the patient via arterial catheters and Swan-Ganz wedge pressures should be carried out to detect and quickly treat pre-bypass instability. With careful planning, adequate monitoring, pre-bypass balloon counterpulsation (if indicated), and rapid treatment of hemodynamic instability, the surgeon should be able to achieve acceptable rates of perioperative infarction and mortality following revascularization in this tenuous group of patients.

Specific Operative Techniques and Considerations

Two methods of myocardial protection have been used and therefore both techniques will be mentioned. One technique is *intermittent* cross-clamping with hypothermic ischemic arrest and the other is *pharmacologic* hypothermic arrest.

INTERMITTENT HYPOTHERMIC ARREST

Table 9 shows the operative guidelines for intermittent hypothermic ischemic arrest. Patients should be premedicated 30 – 45 minutes before arrival in the operating room so that they are well sedated and experience minimum anxiety. Coronary vasodilators should be available as the patient is delivered to the operating room or upon induction, since anginal attacks are frequent during this period. Induction should be gradual, with avoidance of both hypertension and hypotension. If hypertension develops, nitroprusside in low doses should be administered

TABLE 9. – OPERATIVE GUIDELINES
FOR INTERMITTENT HYPOTHERMIC
ARREST

Adequate premedication
Smooth induction
Proximal anastomosis first (limit bypass time)
Systemic cooling – 25 C, supplemented by
   topical cooling to 4 C
Ischemic intervals limited to 15 minutes or less
Ischemic intervals followed by 10 – 15 minutes
   perfusion

From Isom, O. W., et al.: Coronary revascularization with significant impairment of left ventricular contractility, Cardiovasc. Clin. 8: 267, 1977. Used by permission.

---

and, if hypotension occurs, low doses of inotropic drugs may be given while pulmonary wedge pressure is monitored.

TECHNIQUE. – The vein is removed from the thigh and leg while the chest is being opened. Veins are stored in cold (25 C) heparinized blood while preparation is made to initiate bypass. Ordinarily, the internal mammary artery is not used in this group of patients because of the increased length of time required to mobilize this vessel.

As soon as the pericardium is opened, left atrial pressure is monitored and cannulation of the ascending aorta and venae cavae is accomplished. With continual monitoring of left atrial pressure and systemic blood pressure, a partial occlusion clamp is placed on the aorta. Vein grafts for the left anterior descending and circumflex coronary arteries are anastomosed to an area of aorta after a pledget about 10 mm long in the shape of an isosceles triangle has been removed. The graft for the right coronary artery is anastomosed through a longitudinal slit in the aorta. If the blood pressure falls or left atrial pressure rises, cardiopulmonary bypass is instituted; otherwise, bypass is started as the last proximal anastomosis is completed. A standard cardiopulmonary bypass is used with a Temptrol bubble oxygenator and DeBakey roller pumps. A non-blood balanced electrolyte solution is used as a pump prime with 25 gm/L of albumin. Perfusion is usually carried out at a flow rate of 3 L/m²/minute. During perfusion, the mean blood pressure is kept at the level existing before induction of anesthesia. The systemic blood temperature is lowered to 25 C and iced saline at 4 C is introduced into the pericardial space. In most instances, a left ventricular vent is inserted, but occasionally a left atrial vent is used. Ordinarily the heart spontaneously fibrillates as a result of the hypothermia. Myocardial temperatures at this point are usually 20–22 C. Usually the aorta is cross-clamped while the distal anastomosis is completed, and the completely obstructed vessels are bypassed first. A 10-mm arteriotomy is made at the site of anastomosis, and the size of the vessel is calibrated with a probe passed distally and proximally. Distal anastomosis is usually accomplished with 6–0 or 7–0 Prolene in a running or interrupted fashion. If a running suture is used, care is taken not to stenose the proximal or distal portion of the arteriotomy.

Even if cross-clamping of the aorta is not required during performance of the circumflex anastomosis, retraction of the heart to the right with fibrillation during this anastomosis is considered to be an ischemic interval, just as if the aorta were cross-clamped. Aortic cross-clamping is limited to 15 minutes or less. After the aorta is cross-clamped and the anastomosis begun, the blood is warmed. As the anastomosis is finished, the cross-clamp is removed, air is vented from the left ventricle and aorta, and the heart is defibrillated and allowed to beat for 10–15 minutes. During this period of beating, the blood is again cooled to 25 C, and iced saline is introduced into the pericardial space. This entire sequence is repeated for each distal anastomosis.

After completing the last anastomosis, the heart is defibrillated and allowed to beat for 10–15 minutes while warming takes place. The left ventricular vent is clamped, and a determination is made regarding myocardial function as bypass is slowed.

Pharmacologic Hypothermic Arrest

Pharmacologic arrest has recently been repopularized in the United States after a period of several years during which such agents were avoided because of fear of left ventricular damage following cardioplegia. Most of the fears of reported left ventricular damage resulted from use of hypertonic potassium citrate in the early days of cardiac surgery.[37] It is now apparent that pharmacologic and hypothermic arrest are advantageous in terms of immediate alteration of the supply-demand ratio of energy for myocardial tissue. As a consequence, an alternative method of myocardial preservation during coronary bypass surgery is comprised of techniques utilizing *immediate* pharmacologic arrest with solutions containing small amounts of potassium (30 mEq/L) in either crystalloid or blood-containing solutions. Augmentation of myocardial preservation after initial arrest can be obtained by maintaining myocardial temperatures at less than 20 C by direct thermister measurement.

The widespread popularity of potassium cardioplegia is based on excellent studies demonstrating its safety for 60 – 90 minutes of ischemia in several laboratories including those of Buckberg and Maloney at UCLA as well as our own.[38-41] Reports from our Medical Center have confirmed a superior degree of myocardial protection when hypothermic potassium arrest is used clinically during cardiac surgical procedures. We have shown that this method of myocardial protection offers a high degree of preservation during prolonged periods of ischemia in patients undergoing surgery for valve replacement and coronary bypass, either elective or in unstable anginal syndromes.[28, 42] Use of these techniques of cardioplegia has resulted in a significant diminution in the perioperative infarction rate and postoperative low-output syndrome. It should be recognized, however, that despite its wide popularity, very little is known about potassium cardioplegia, except that it is associated with a low operative mortality and an apparently low perioperative infarction rate. Almost no data are available regarding long-term influences on ventricular function or the duration of the safe limits of tolerable ischemia (60, 90, 120 minutes or longer?).

TECHNIQUE. – When pharmacologic hypothermic arrest is performed during coronary artery bypass grafting at NYU Medical Center, we currently use an arrest solution containing 30 mEq/L of potassium in cold blood obtained from the heart-lung machine at 10 C. Proximal anastomoses are performed on or off bypass utilizing partial aortic occlusion. Bypass is then begun and systemic cooling at 20 C is carried out. After aortic cross-clamping is performed, the blood-cardioplegia solution is injected directly into the aortic root at sufficient pressure to obtain arrest (with the realization that critical coronary stenoses exist and greater pressure than normal will probably be required). Myocardial temperature is measured with a constantly indwelling thermister probe and kept at less than 20 C by topical iced Ringer's lavage. Reinjection of the arrest solution is carried out every 20 minutes, and the cross-clamp is not released until the final distal anastomosis is performed. When uncross-clamping is carried out, perfusion pressure is dropped for 2–5 minutes to prevent occurrence of myocardial edema resulting from exposure of the dilated coronary bed to high perfusion pressures. Preliminary data utilizing this current technique appear to be promising in that the perioperative infarction rate is low (less than 3%), and mortality remains in the 2–3% range for elective bypass procedures.

CLINICAL AND EXPERIMENTAL RESULTS OF PHARMACOLOGIC HYPOTHERMIC ARREST.—From April 1976 to January 1977, 231 consecutive patients undergoing elective coronary bypass grafting at NYU were studied to determine the incidence of perioperative infarction in relation to 4 different methods of myocardial preservation. Ventricular function and severity of disease were comparable in each of the groups, and the operative mortality for all 231 patients was 2.2%. Assessment of the 4 approaches to myocardial preservation appears to illustrate some of the advantages of single cross-clamp potassium arrest for coronary bypass surgery.

NEW YORK UNIVERSITY MEDICAL CENTER

Surgical status	Elective coronary bypass grafting
Period	April 1976 – January 1977
No. of patients	231
Average no. of bypasses	2.7 per patient
Overall mortality	2.2%

Group I had proximal anastomoses performed on bypass at normothermia with distal anastomoses constructed during intermittent periods of cross-clamping and ventricular fibrillation at 30 C. After performance of each distal anastomosis, the aorta was uncross-clamped and the heart allowed to beat for 10–12 minutes.

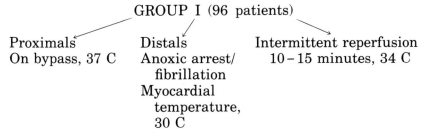

GROUP I (96 patients)

Proximals	Distals	Intermittent reperfusion
On bypass, 37 C	Anoxic arrest/ fibrillation Myocardial temperature, 30 C	10–15 minutes, 34 C

Group II also had distal anastomoses performed during intermittent aortic cross-clamping at 30 C. This group differed from group I in 2 respects: (1) proximal anastomoses were performed prior to institution of bypass, and (2) topical iced saline lavage was used intermittently to augment myocardial cooling.

GROUP II (58 patients)

Proximals	Distals	Intermittent reperfusion
Pre-bypass, 37 C	Anoxic arrest/	10 – 15 minutes, 34 C
	fibrillation	
	topical cold	
	lavage	
	myocardial	
	temperature 30 C	

Group III had proximal anastomoses performed on bypass at normothermia. After aortic cross-clamping, 500 – 600 cc of the arrest solution at 8 – 10 C was instilled into the aortic root and reinjection of the solution carried out every 20 – 30 minutes, as described earlier. Myocardial temperature was monitored with an indwelling thermister probe and maintained at less than 20 C by continuous cold lavage. All distal anastomoses were performed during a *single* uninterrupted ischemic period.

GROUP III (58 patients)

Proximals	Distals
On bypass, 37 C	single cross-clamp
	K+ arrest
	myocardial temperature, 18 C

In group IV, hypothermia and potassium arrest were also utilized; however, after performance of each distal anastomosis, the aorta was again unclamped and the heart allowed to beat at normothermia for 10 – 15 minutes before reclamping.

GROUP IV (19 patients)

Proximals	Distals	Intermittent reperfusion
On bypass, 37 C	K+ arrest	10 – 15 minutes, 34 C
	myocardial	
	temperature 18 C	

A comparison of myocardial protection during bypass grafting offered by each of the 4 approaches is shown in Table 10. The data indicate that a combination of uninterrupted aortic cross-clamping, potassium arrest, and profound myocardial hypothermia for performance of all distal anastomoses was advantageous in this group. ECG evidence of infarction was significantly lower in this group (only 3%), despite the fact that the average single longest cross-clamp time was 49 minutes (about twice as long as in any other group). Total or cumulative cross-clamp time did not differ significantly in the 4 groups.

Of particular interest is the rate of perioperative infarction and need for inotropic support in group IV (*intermittent* potassium arrest with *reperfusion*). The data suggest that this method is not a viable substitute for more conventional approaches. The infarction rate was quite unacceptable (ranging from 11–20%, depending on the criteria used), and the need for inotropic support postoperatively was at least twice as frequent in this group as in the groups using topical hypothermia or single cross-clamp potassium arrest.

Of equal importance clinically, with respect to the duration of safe ischemia tolerated during single cross-clamp potassium arrest, is onset time of injury compared to length of the single longest cross-clamp time (Fig 5). A significant difference is noted among the 4 groups of elective coronary patients previously mentioned. It becomes readily apparent from the graph that poor protection against intraoperative infarction exists after 15–20 minutes of ischemia, except when potassium arrest is combined with profound hypothermia and uninterrupted cross-clamping. This group not only has the lowest rate of infarction but appears to be adequately protected for periods of 60–70 minutes. This differs markedly from the degree of protection observed in the other 3 groups in which about 50% of the expected infarcts had occurred when cross-clamp times approached 20–24 minutes. Need for inotropic support postoperatively in relation to duration of single longest cross-clamp time has virtually the same pattern as does this rate of perioperative infarction. In essence the use of uninterrupted potassium arrest and profound hypothermia almost tripled the length of tolerable ischemia time before vasopressors were needed postoperatively.

These clinical data support previous observations from our experimental studies on normal dog hearts from which we con-

TABLE 10.–CORONARY BYPASS SURGERY: MYOCARDIAL PROTECTION VS PERIOPERATIVE INJURY

	GROUP I INTERMITTENT CROSS-CLAMP	GROUP II INTERMITTENT CROSS-CLAMP– TOPICAL HYPOTHERMIA	GROUP III SINGLE CROSS-CLAMP– K+ ARREST < 20 C	GROUP IV INTERMITTENT CROSS-CLAMP– K+ ARREST < 20 C
Single longest cross-clamp (minutes ± SD)	21 ± 4	22 ± 7	49 ± 18	27 ± 10
Cumulative cross-clamp	56 ± 20	40 ± 16	49 ± 18	56 ± 17
Infarction (ECG)	12%	31%	3% (p < 0.05)	11%
Infarction (total)	19%	33%	3% (p < 0.05)	21%
Inotropic support	37%	21%	23%	42%
Mortality	2%	2%	3%	0

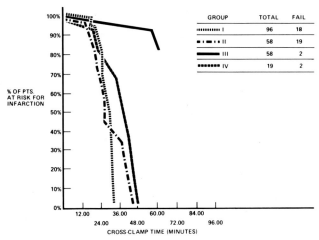

GROUP	TOTAL	FAIL
I	96	18
II	58	19
III	58	2
IV	19	2

Fig 5. — Rate of infarction vs single longest cross-clamp time.

cluded that use of hypothermic pharmacologic arrest during a single period of aortic cross-clamping (60 minutes) was safer than use of the same arrest technique during several shorter cross-clamp intervals.[43] When *intermittent* potassium arrest and cross-clamping are used for short repetitive intervals, depression of left ventricular performance, compliance and metabolism occurred following even 2–3 short intervals of ischemia of only 10–12 minutes. Mechanisms for the injury occurring when intermittent potassium arrest is used are unclear but may be related to (1) changes in vascular permeability, causing myocardial edema, (2) resultant reperfusion injury following repeated unclamping into a maximally dilated and previously ischemic coronary bed and (3) microembolization of air or particulate matter associated with repeated unclamping.

Table 11 compares the changes in left ventricular function and metabolism occurring when uninterrupted vs intermittent cross-clamping with potassium arrest is used in normal animal hearts. These data correlate well with our clinical findings, i.e., that potassium arrest when used as a means of myocardial preservation during coronary bypass surgery should be performed under a *single uninterrupted* cross-clamp period.

In summary, myocardial (and subendocardial) necrosis continues to be the most common cause of low-output syndrome and mortality following coronary bypass operations. The best meth-

TABLE 11.—MYOCARDIAL METABOLISM, LV COMPLIANCE, PERFORMANCE AND CORONARY FLOW*

GROUP	LV† FUNCTION	LV† COMPLIANCE	O_2 CONSUMPTION (ML/100 GM/BEAT)	LACTATE EXTRACTION	LV FLOW (ML/100 GM/MINUTE)	ENDO/EPI FLOW
Control (No. = 10)	...	...	0.05 ± 0.010	0.14 ± 0.04	60 ± 3	1.23 ± .06
Group 1 (No. = 5) cardioplegia, single cross-clamp (60 minutes)	↓ 5%	↓ 19%	0.04 ± 0.004	0.18 ± 0.03	97 ± 8‡	1.08 ± .06
Group 2 (No. = 5) cardioplegia, intermittent cross-clamp (3 20-minute periods)	↓ 50%‡	↓ 250%‡	0.03 ± 0.004‡	−0.06 ± 0.02‡	91 ± 18‡	0.74 ± .12‡

*Values are mean ± SE; LV = left ventricle; ENDO = left ventricular subendocardial muscle; EPI = left ventricular epicardial muscle.
†Measured as % change from control in area under isovolumetric ventricular function and compliance curves; intraventricular balloon volumes from 0 to 40 ml.
‡P < 0.05 (from control).
From Pappis, M. L., et al.: Comparison of the myocardial protection offered by intermittent vs. continuous potassium hypothermia cardioplegia during cardiopulmonary bypass, Surg. Forum 28:285, 1977. Used by permission.

od of myocardial preservation during revascularization surgery for the patient with ischemic heart disease has not yet been determined. Early indications are that diligent attempts at reducing the supply-demand ratio of the myocardium during the period of aortic cross-clamping by whatever means possible is the most efficacious approach toward preventing the recurrent and still prevalent problem of late cardiac failure or death secondary to intraoperative myocardial injury.

Anesthetic Management and Monitoring during Coronary Bypass Surgery

An initial study by Isom et al. at New York University revealed that the isoenzyme CPK-MB was detected before cardiopulmonary bypass in about 36% of patients in whom it appeared perioperatively.[10] A similar study by Oldham and colleagues revealed a 16% incidence prior to bypass in a similar population.[44] These results strongly suggest the importance of the pre-bypass interval and specifically the peri-induction period in the evolution of early myocardial injury in patients undergoing coronary artery bypass surgery. Since Isom's original study, the anesthetic and pharmacologic management of coronary artery bypass patients has changed markedly at New York University. Emphasis is currently placed on attaining a deep level of anesthesia to prevent or attenuate the sympathetic responses of hypertension and tachycardia, both known to increase myocardial oxygen consumption. Should such hemodynamic changes occur or electrocardiographic evidence of myocardial ischemia appear, treatment is promptly instituted.

The new management technique is as follows:

Premedication:	Morphine, 0.1 mg/kg
	Scopolamine, 0.3–0.4 mg
	± Diazepam, 0.1 mg/kg by mouth
Monitoring:	After additional sedation with diazepam:
	14- or 16-gauge peripheral intravenous
	Central venous pressure
	20-gauge radial or 18-gauge femoral
	arterial line
	7 Fr thermodilution Swan-Ganz catheter
	ECG (6 standard leads, 1 precordial)

Induction:	Diazepam, 0.3 mg/kg (including sedation)
	Fentanyl, 0.005 mg/kg
	Halothane, 0.2 – 1.5%, as needed
	Nitrous oxide, 50%
	Pancuronium, 0.1 mg/kg or succinylcholine
	by infusion
Maintenance:	Nitrous oxide, 50%
	Halothane
	Incremental diazepam
	Fentanyl

A major feature of the newer management technique is hemodynamic measurements, which include radial artery and pulmonary artery pressures, pulmonary capillary wedge or left atrial pressures, central venous pressure, heart rate and repetitive cardiac output determinations. The following derived measurements are also obtained: SVR, PVR, RVSWI, LVSWI, CI, and HR-systolic pressure product.* Intraoperatively, ECG leads II and V_5 or any other that has shown ischemic changes while on the ward or during exercise testing are closely monitored. Complete 12-lead ECG tracings are obtained preoperatively, immediately postoperatively, on the third postoperative day and before discharge. These are routinely analyzed with respect to the patient's course. Serial isoenzyme CPK-MB measurements are obtained preoperatively and at frequent intervals throughout the pre-bypass, bypass and post-bypass periods for determination of isoenzyme liberation.

Our previous studies of coronary artery bypass grafting in collaboration with several other institutions have shown that the CK-MB isoenzyme was observed perioperatively in 70–80% of patients. It was recognized that in over 90% of patients in whom CK-MB is detected, the isoenzyme was first observed in the operating room and that it persists for a variable period, often implicating injury during the pre-bypass and peri-induction interval.[45] Since we have recently directed our effort toward improved anesthetic management as described above, it has been possible to reevaluate operative myocardial protection as related to anesthetic management in several populations. Recent review of data accumulated over the past 12 months has re-

---

*SVR, systemic vascular resistance; PVR, pulmonary vascular resistance; RVSWI, right ventricular stroke work index; LVSWI, left ventricular stroke work index; CI, cardiac index; HR, heart rate.

vealed a significant reduction in evidence of peri-induction injury, resulting in diminution of pre-bypass liberation of CK-MB from 35.7% 3 years ago to 0 since August 1977.[45] Although the studies are preliminary at this stage, the data suggest that strict attention to anesthetic management in the pre-bypass period, as well as aggressive monitoring techniques, will play an increasingly important role in prevention of perioperative myocardial infarction in the coronary bypass patient.[46, 47]

THERMODILUTION AND CARDIAC OUTPUT MEASUREMENTS

Cardiac output is not routinely measured in most medical centers following open heart surgery despite the inherent value of this determination to the clinician during the critical phase of the patient's recovery. Thermodilution techniques are easily adaptable for use in a variety of clinical situations and appear to correlate well with conventional methods of cardiac output determinations.[48-51] These techniques allow multiple measurements of cardiac output, which can be obtained on a minute-by-

Fig 6.—Insertion and placement of thermistor in pulmonary artery *(PA)* prior to pericardial closure. *SVC* = superior venae cava. (From Kohanna, F. H., and Cunningham, J. N., Jr.: Monitoring of cardiac output by thermodilution after open heart surgery, J. Thorac. Cardiovasc. Surg. 73:452, 1977. Used by permission.)

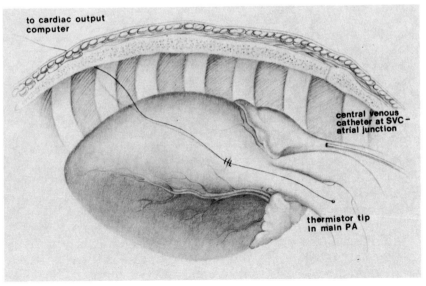

minute basis. Such determinations have depended on accurate placement of a Swan-Ganz type of catheter with a thermister tip in the main pulmonary artery (Fig 6).

We advocate routine introduction of Swan-Ganz catheters into the pulmonary artery prior to induction of anesthesia in every patient undergoing coronary bypass surgery. Such catheter placement not only allows constant monitoring of wedge pressure, with treatment of sudden rises in wedge pressure as a result of ventricular dysfunction with nitroprusside or nitroglycerin, but also makes available constant monitoring of cardiac output by thermodilution measurements.[52]

Cardiac output measurements generally are obtained prior to induction of anesthesia, pre-bypass, immediately post-bypass and at serial intervals during recovery. The importance of monitoring cardiac output levels in the immediate period following cardiopulmonary bypass has been emphasized since the early years of cardiac surgery. A close correlation between cardiac output and the clinical course of the patient has been established. Boyd and associates, reported a mortality of 67% in a group of patients whose cardiac indices were less than 2 $L/m^2/minute$ in the immediate period following cardiac surgery.[53] Evaluation of cardiac output (especially when cardiac index falls below 2 L/minute) can be used as a method of assessment of the need for institution of artificial left ventricular assist devices, left atrial femoral bypass or intra-aortic balloon counterpulsation. For these reasons, it is recommended that routine cardiac output measurements be utilized not only in all coronary bypass patients but in any functional class III-IV cardiac surgical patient.[54]

Importance of Pericardial Closure after Coronary Bypass Surgery

Pericardial closure following coronary bypass surgery should be considered an extremely important aspect of the operation. The pericardium has long been recognized as a protective sac that not only allows the heart to move in a frictionless chamber but also provides support and limits displacement.[55, 56] Great care should be taken to cover coronary bypass grafts with pericardium or pleural flaps following operation. This should be coupled with adequate intrapericardial and substernal drainage to prevent tamponade and accumulation of blood in the peri-

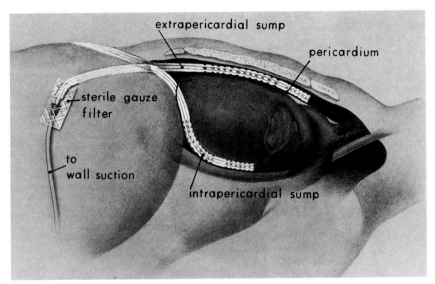

Fig 7.—Lateral view of differential sump drainage, pericardium closed. (From Cunningham, J. N., Jr., et al.: Influence of primary closure of the pericardium after open heart surgery on the frequency of tamponade, post cardiotomy syndrome, pulmonary complications, J. Thorac. Cardiovasc. Surg. 70:121, 1975. Used by permission.)

cardial sac postoperatively (Fig 7). Stretching of the pericardium, utilizing weights attached to its lateral edges, or procedures to tack the pericardium up to the anterior sternal table will allow pericardial closure over bypass grafts in most cases following surgery (Fig 8). Paradoxically, closure of the pericardium combined with differential drainage from intrapericardial and extrapericardial sump tubes discloses that most postoperative bleeding originates from extrapericardial rather than intrapericardial sources. As a result, tamponade apparently results when blood from extrapericardial sources drains into the pericardial cavity and clots. This observation yields further credence to the importance of pericardial closure following operation for coronary bypass surgery.

Further reasons for pericardial closure and use of mediastinal sumps alone for drainage are related to notions that the incidence of postcardiotomy syndrome (usually occurring in 10 and 40% of patients postoperatively) is much less (about 3%) when this method of closure and drainage is used. Table 12 clearly indicates these factors and summarizes the morbidity of differ-

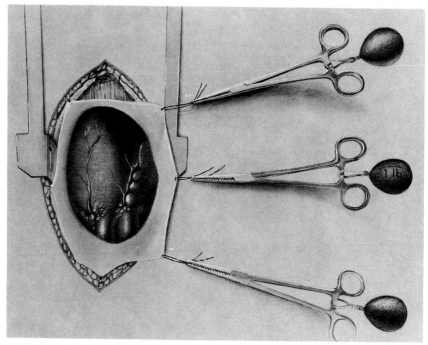

Fig 8.—A, pericardium tacked up to anterior sternal table and heart suspended anteriorly. B, pericardium stretched by lead weights. (From Cunningham, J. N., Jr., et al.: Influence of primary closure of the pericardium after open heart surgery on the frequency of tamponade, post cardiotomy syndrome, pulmonary complications, J. Thorac. Cardiovasc. Surg. 70:121, 1975. Used by permission.)

ent drainage techniques in 100 consecutive bypass patients studied at NYU recently.[57] The long-term implications of this in terms of graft patency are obvious. With a lowered frequency of postcardiotomy syndrome, we should expect less scar tissue formation and improved graft patency on this basis alone.

Finally, an advantage of primary closure of the pericardium is evident when a repeat operation is necessary months or years after the original procedure. The hazards of reopening a previous sternotomy incision when the pericardium has been left open are well known: the right ventricle may be adherent to the undersurface of the sternum, so that laceration or even fatal hemorrhage may occur if the heart is injured when the sternum is reopened. By contrast, in patients in whom the pericardium has been closed at the previous operation, the degree of adhe-

TABLE 12.—EFFECT OF MODE OF CHEST
DRAINAGE ON POSTOPERATIVE MORBIDITY IN
OPEN-HEART SURGERY PATIENTS

MORBIDITY	CHEST TUBES PLUS MEDIASTINAL SUMPS	MEDIASTINAL SUMPS ONLY
No. of patients	28	72
Incidence of tamponade	0	0
Reoperation for bleeding	1	4
Postoperative bleeding (cc)		
12 hr	639	428
24 hr	761	553
Pleural effusion (%)	34	22
Atelectasis (%)	61	41
Postoperative fever > 100 F.		
(days)	6	4.7
Mediastinal infection	0	0
Postcardiotomy syndrome		
(%)	10.7	2.8
Postoperative hospital stay		
(days)	14	13

From Cunningham, J. N., Jr., et al.: Influence of primary
closure of the pericardium after open heart surgery on the frequency of tamponade post cardiotomy syndrome and pulmonary
complications. J. Thor. Cardiovasc. Surg. 70:121, 1975. Used
by permission.

sions in the pericardial cavity is strikingly less. The difference
in degree of adhesion formation provides further indirect support of the hypothesis that the inflammatory reaction around
the heart following coronary bypass surgery is much less if the
pericardium is closed. When primary pericardial closure cannot
be achieved, use of substitutes such as autologous fascia lata or
porcine pericardium have been suggested and offer viable substitutes (Fig 9).[58]

Summary

Coronary bypass surgery has become an extremely popular
operative procedure in this country, about 100,000 procedures
having been performed in 1977. The popularity of the operation
stems to a great degree from the marked improvement in symptoms gained by the patient with severe or incapacitating angina. Certain other areas in which this surgical procedure de-

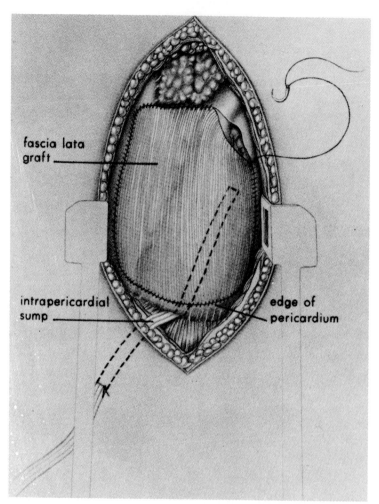

Fig 9.—Closure of pericardium with free fascia lata graft. (From Kohanna, F. H., et al.: Use of autologous fascia lata as a pericardial substitute following open heart surgery, J. Thorac. Cardiovasc. Surg. 74:15, 1977. Used by permission.)

serves special attention include patients with left main-stem coronary disease or severe proximal lesions of left anterior descending arteries (before the first septal perforator arises), minimally symptomatic patients and asymptomatic patients with severe triple coronary vessel disease and a history of numerous infarctions. Although there is general agreement that the left main-stem coronary lesion is a condition of surgical urgency and that bypass relieves the pain of incapacitating angina, only time will tell whether bypass surgery is indicated in the many other borderline areas along the wide spectrum of coronary artery disease. As previously stated, the purpose of this chapter was not to argue the benefits of surgical vs medical therapy, but to indicate our current views and philosophies of management of coronary artery disease. Many questions remain unanswered.

Since it is quite clear that symptomatic relief occurs in about 90% of patients who are operated on for incapacitating angina, the principal question concerning coronary bypass surgery is its influence on longevity. Nonrandomized studies in coronary bypass grafting at our Medical Center and other institutions indicate an improvement not only in survival but also in prevention of future myocardial infarctions and in the ability of the patient to return to worth-while socioeconomic endeavors. No study currently exists, nor are there data available to support either medical or surgical therapy as a treatment of choice for patients in many categories other than incapacitating angina.

Whether the asymptomatic patient with severe angiographic disease should be operated on is a typical unresolved question. Should a patient who has had 3 previous infarctions but is currently asymptomatic be catheterized and considered for surgery? Is it appropriate to perform coronary artery bypass on a patient with mild stable angina? These and similar questions will of course be answered over the next 5–10 years. But such answers can only arise from careful scrutiny of collaborative and cooperative studies among numerous institutions such as the prospective study for coronary artery disease supported by the National Institutes of Health. This particular study will require about 7 years and several 100 or more patients before statistically significant and meaningful data can be derived through a randomized process. Nevertheless, it can be expected that many of the questions that have been left unanswered in these pages will some day be resolved. As a result, it can be anticipated that an intelligent approach combining surgical and medical therapy can be applied in a rational manner for the best interests of the patient with coronary artery disease.

REFERENCES

1. Vital Statistics and Causes of Death, *World Health Statistics Annual, 1967,* Vol. 1. (Geneva: World Health Organization, 1970).

2. *Heart Facts* (New York: American Heart Association, 1975).
3. Beck, C. S.: The development of a new blood supply to the heart by operation, Ann. Surg. 102:801, 1935.
4. Beck, C. S., and Brofman, B. L.: The surgical management of coronary artery disease: Background, rationale, clinical experiences, Ann. Intern. Med. 45:975, 1956.
5. Vineberg, A., and Walker, J.: Six months' to six years' experience with coronary insufficiency treated by internal mammary artery implantation, Am. Heart J. 54:851, 1957.
6. McIntosh, H. D., and Garcia, J. A.: The first decade of aortocoronary bypass grafting: 1967–1977. A review, Circulation 57:405, 1978.
7. Isom, O. W., Spencer, F. C., Glassman, E., Cunningham, J. N., Jr., Teiko, P., Reed, G. E., and Boyd, A. D.: Does coronary bypass increase longevity?, J. Thorac. Cardiovasc. Surg. 75:28, 1978.
8. Braunwald, E.: Coronary artery surgery at the crossroads, N. Engl. J. Med. 297:661, 1977.
9. Rose, M. R., Glassman, E., Isom, O. W., and Spencer, F. C.: Electrocardiographic and serum enzyme changes of myocardial infarction after coronary artery bypass surgery, Am. J. Cardiol. 33:215, 1974.
10. Isom, O. W., Spencer, F. C., Feigenbaum, H., Cunningham, J. N., Jr., and Roe, C.: Prebypass myocardial damage in patients undergoing coronary revascularization; an unrecognized vulnerable period, Circulation 52 (Suppl. 2):119, 1975.
11. Codd, J. E., Wiens, R. D., Kaiser, G. C., Barner, H. B., Tyras, D. H., Mudd, J. G., and Willman, V. L.: Late sequelae of perioperative myocardial infarction. Presented at Society of Thoracic Surgeons, Orlando, Fla., January 1978.
12. Murphy, M. L., Hultgren, H. N., Detre, K., Thomsen, J., Takaro, T., and participants of VA Cooperative Study: Treatment of chronic stable angina – a preliminary report of survival data of the randomized VA Cooperative Study, New Engl. J. Med. 297:621, 1977.
13. Stiles, Q. R., Lindesmith, G. G., Tucker, B. L., Hughes, R. K., and Meyer, B. W.: Long-term follow-up of patients with coronary artery bypass grafts, Circulation 54 (Suppl. 3):32, 1976.
14. Sheldon, W. C., and Loop, F. D.: Direct myocardial revascularization – 1976, Cleve. Clin. Q. 43:97, 1976.
15. Tecklenberg, P. L., Alderman, E. L., Miller, D. C., Shumway, N. E., and Harrison, D. C.: Changes in survival and symptom relief in a longitudinal study of patients after bypass surgery, Circulation 51–52 (Suppl. I):98, 1975.
16. Spencer, F. C., Green, G. E., Tice, D. A., Wallsh, E., Mills, N. L., and Glassman, E. G.: Coronary artery bypass grafts for congestive heart failure, J. Thorac. Cardiovasc. Surg. 63:353, 1971.
17. Bruschke, A., Proudfit, W. L., and Sones, F. M.: Progress study of 590 consecutive nonsurgical cases of coronary disease followed 5–9 years. II. Ventriculographic and other correlations, Circulation 47:1154, 1973.
18. Fischl, S. J., Herman, M. V., and Gorlin, R.: The intermediate coronary syndrome: Clinical, Angiographic, and Therapeutic Aspects, N. Engl. J. Med. 288:755, 1973.

19. Gazes, P. C., Mobley, N., Jr., and Faris, H. M., Jr.: Pre-infarctional (unstable) angina: A prospective study: 10-year follow-up: Prognostic significance of electrocardiographic changes, Circulation 48:331, 1973.
20. Krauss, K. R., Hutter, A. M., Jr., and DeSantis, R. W.: Acute coronary insufficiency: Cause and follow-up, Circulation 45 (Suppl. 1):66, 1972.
21. Bonchek, L. I., Rahimtoola, S. H., Anderson, R. P., et al.: Late results following an emergency saphenous vein bypass grafting for unstable angina, Circulation 50:972, 1974.
22. Conti, C. R., Brawley, R. K., Triffth, L. S. C., et al.: Unstable angina pectoris: Morbidity and mortality in 57 consecutive patients evaluated angiographically, Am. J. Cardiol. 32:745, 1973.
23. Scanon, P. J., Nemickus, R., Moran, J. F., et al.: Accelerated angina pectoris: Clinical, hemodynamic, arteriographic, and therapeutic experience in 85 patients, Circulation 47:19, 1973.
24. Seybold-Epting, W., Oglietti, J., Wukasch, D. C., et al.: Early and late results after surgical treatment of pre-infarction angina, Ann. Thorac. Surg. 21:97, 1976.
25. Klein, N. S., Ludbrook, P. A., Mimbs, J. W., et al.: Perioperative mortality rate in patients with unstable angina selected by exclusion of myocardial infarction, J. Thorac. Cardiovasc. Surg. 73:253, 1977.
26. Gold, H. K., Lunbach, P. C., Buckley, M. J., et al.: Refractory angina pectoris: Follow-up after intra-aortic balloon pumping and surgery, Circulation 54 (Suppl. 3):41, 1976.
27. Weintraub, R. M., Voukydis, P. C., Aroestz, J. M., et al.: Treatment of pre-infarction angina with intra-aortic balloon counterpulsation and surgery, Am. J. Cardiol. 34:809, 1974.
28. Adams, P. X., Cunningham, J. N., Jr., et al.: Technique and experience using potassium cardioplegia during myocardial re-vascularization for pre-infarction angina, Surgery 83:12, 1978.
29. Vakil, R. J.: Pre-infarction syndrome: Management and follow-up, Am. J. Cardiol. 14:55, 1972.
30. Roberts, R., and Sobel, B. E.: Coronary revascularization during evolving myocardial infarction – the need for caution, Circulation 50:67, 1974.
31. Cohen, M. V., and Gorlin, R.: Main left coronary occlusive disease. Clinical experience from 1964–1974, Circulation 52:275, 1975.
32. Takaro, T., Hultgren, H. N., Lipton, M. J., and Detrek, M.: The VA cooperative randomized study of surgery for coronary occlusive disease. II. Sub group with significant left main lesions, Circulation 54(Suppl. 3):107, 1976.
33. Oberman, A., Harrell, R. R., Russell, R. O. Jr., Kouchoukos, N. T., Holt, J. H. Jr., and Rackley, C. E.: Surgical vs. medical treatment of the left main coronary artery, Lancet 2:591, 1976.
34. Zeft, H. J., Manley, J. C., Huston, J. H., Tector, A. J., Auer, J. E., and Johnson, W. D.: Left main coronary artery stenosis. Results of coronary bypass surgery, Circulation 49:68, 1974.
35. DeMots, H., Bonchek, L. I., Rosch, J., Anderson, R. P., Starr, A., and Rahimtoola, S. H.: Left main coronary artery disease. Risks of angiography, importance of co-existing disease of other coronary arteries and effects of revascularization, Am. J. Cardiol. 36:136, 1975.

36. Cunningham, J. N. Jr., Adams, P. X., Isom, O. W., and Spencer, F. C.: Unpublished data from New York University, 1978.
37. Waldhausen, J. A., Braunwald, N. S., Bloodwell, R. D., et al.: Left ventricular function following elective cardiac arrest, J. Thorac. Cardiovasc. Surg. 39:813, 1960.
38. Buckberg, J.: Left ventricular subendocardial necrosis, Ann. Thorac. Surg. 24:379, 1977.
39. Trehan, N., Adams, P. X., Cunningham, J. N. Jr., et al.: Clinical experience using potassium induced cardioplegia with hypothermia in aortic valve replacements, Circulation 54(Suppl. 3):181, 1976.
40. Hearse, D. J., Garlick, P. D., and Humphrey, F. M.: Ischemic contracture of the myocardium: Mechanisms and prevention, Amer. J. Cardiol. 39:986, 1977.
41. Hearse, D. J., Stewart, D. A., and Brainbridge, M. V.: Cellular protection during myocardial ischemia: The development and characterization of a procedure for induction of reversible ischemic arrest, Circulation 54:193, 1976.
42. Cunningham, J. N. Jr., Adams, P. X., et al.: Potassium arrest, profound hypothermia, and uninterrupted aortic cross-clamping — a superior technique for myocardial protection in coronary bypass surgery, Abstracts of the XIII World Congress of the International Cardiovascular Society, B-6-14, 1977.
43. Pappis, M. L., DeRossi, J. F., Basuk, R., Puma, F., Adams, P. X., and Cunningham, J. N. Jr.: Comparison of the myocardial protection offered by intermittent continuous potassium hypothermic cardioplegia during cardiopulmonary bypass, Surg. Forum 28:285, 1977.
44. Oldham, H. N., Roe, C. R., Young, W. H., and Dixon, S. H.: Intraoperative detection of myocardial damage during coronary artery surgery by plasma creatine phosphokinase isoenzyme analysis, Surgery 74:917, 1973.
45. Roe, C. R.: Personal communication.
46. Roe, C. R.: Diagnosis of myocardial infarction by serum isoenzyme analysis, Ann. Clin. Lab. Sci. 7:201, 1977.
47. Warren, S. G., Wagner, G. S., Bethea, C. F., Roe, C. R., Oldham, H. N., and Kong, Y.: Diagnostic and prognostic significance of electrocardiographic and CPK isoenzyme changes following coronary bypass surgery: Correlation with findings at one year, Am. Heart J. 93:189, 1977.
48. Ganz, W., Donoso, R., Marcs, H., Forrester, J. S., and Swan, H. J. C.: A new technique for measurement of cardiac output by thermodilution in man, Am. J. Cardiol. 27:392, 1971.
49. Forrester, J. S., Ganz, W., Diamond, G., McHugh, T., Chonette, D. W., and Swan, H. J. C.: Thermodilution cardiac output determination with a single flow-directed catheter, Am. Heart. J. 83:306, 1972.
50. Baranthwaite, M. A., and Bradley, R. D.: Measurement of cardiac output by thermal dilution in man, J. Appl. Physiol. 24:434, 1968.
51. Sorensen, M. B., Bille Brahe, N. E., and Engell, H. C.: Cardiac output measurement by thermal dilution: Reproducibility and comparison with dye dilution technique, Ann. Surg. 183:67, 1975.
52. Lappas, D. G., Lowenstein, E., et al.: Hemodynamic effect of nitroprusside infusion during coronary artery operation in man, Circulation 54(Suppl. 3): 1; 4–10, 1976.

53. Boyd, A. D., Tremblay, R. E., Spencer, F. C., and Bahnson, H. T.: Estimation of cardiac output soon after intra-cardiac surgery with cardiopulmonary bypass, Ann. Surg. 150:613, 1959.
54. Kohanna, F. H., and Cunningham, J. N. Jr.: Monitoring of cardiac output by thermodilution after open heart surgery, J. Thorac. Cardiovasc. Surg. 73:415, 1977.
55. Boyd, L. J., and Elias, H.: Contributions to diseases of the heart and pericardium. I. Historical introduction, Bull. N.Y. Acad. Med. 18:1, 1955.
56. Spodick, D. H.: Medical history of the pericardium: The hairy hearts of hoary heroes, Am. J. Cardiol. 26:447, 1970.
57. Cunningham, J. N. Jr., Spencer, F. C., Zeff, R., Williams, C. D., Cukinghan, R., Mullin, M.: Influence of primary closure of the pericardium after open heart surgery on the frequency of tamponade, post cardiotomy syndrome, pulmonary complications, J. Thorac. Cardiovasc. Surg. 70:119, 1975.
58. Kohanna, F. H., Adams, P. X., and Cunningham, J. N., Jr.: Use of autologous fascia lata as a pericardial substitute following open heart surgery, J. Thorac. Cardiovasc. Surg. 74:14, 1977.

Author Index

Subject Index